T0192369

Innovative Strategies, Statistical Solutions and Simulations for Modern Clinical Trials

Chapman & Hall/CRC Biostatistics Series

Shein-Chung Chow, Duke University School of Medicine
Byron Jones, Novartis Pharma AG
Jen-pei Liu, National Taiwan University
Karl E. Peace, Georgia Southern University
Bruce W. Turnbull, Cornell University

Recently Published Titles

Repeated Measures Design with Generalized Linear Mixed Models for Randomized Controlled Trials
Toshiro Tango

Clinical Trial Data Analysis Using R and SAS, Second Edition
Ding-Geng (Din) Chen, Karl E. Peace, Pinggao Zhang

Clinical Trial Optimization Using R
Alex Dmitrienko, Erik Pulkstenis

Cluster Randomised Trials, Second Edition
Richard J. Hayes, Lawrence H. Moulton

Quantitative Methods for HIV/AIDS Research
Cliburn Chan, Michael G. Hudgens, Shein-Chung Chow

Sample Size Calculations in Clinical Research, Third Edition
Shein-Chung Chow, Jun Shao, Hansheng Wang, Yuliya Lokhnygina

Randomization, Masking, and Allocation Concealment
Vance Berger

Statistical Topics in Health Economics and Outcomes Research
Demissie Alemayehu, Joseph C. Cappelleri, Birol Emir, Kelly H. Zou

Applied Surrogate Endpoint Evaluation Methods with SAS and R
Ariel Alonso, Theophile Bigirumurame, Tomasz Burzykowski, Marc Buyse, Geert Molenberghs, Leacky Muchene, Nolen Joy Perualila, Ziv Shkedy, Wim Van der Elst

Medical Biostatistics, Fourth Edition
Abhaya Indrayan, Rajeev Kumar Malhotra

Self-Controlled Case Series Studies: A Modelling Guide with R
Paddy Farrington, Heather Whitaker, Yonas Ghebremichael Weldeselassie

Bayesian Methods for Repeated Measures
Lyle D. Broemeling

Modern Adaptive Randomized Clinical Trials: Statistical and Practical Aspects
Oleksandr Sverdlov

Medical Product Safety Evaluation: Biological Models and Statistical Methods
Jie Chen, Joseph Heyse, Tze Leung Lai

Statistical Methods for Survival Trial Design
With Applications to Cancer Clinical Trials Using R
Jianrong Wu

Bayesian Applications in Pharmaceutical Development
Satrajit Roychoudhury, Soumi Lahiri

Platform Trials in Drug Development: Umbrella Trials and Basket Trials
Zoran Antonjevic and Robert Beckman

Innovative Strategies, Statistical Solutions and Simulations for Modern Clinical Trials
Mark Chang, John Balser, Jim Roach and Robin Bliss

For more information about this series, please visit: https://www.crcpress.com/go/biostats

Innovative Strategies, Statistical Solutions and Simulations for Modern Clinical Trials

Mark Chang
John Balser
Jim Roach
Robin Bliss

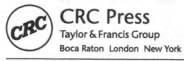

CRC Press
Taylor & Francis Group
Boca Raton London New York

CRC Press is an imprint of the
Taylor & Francis Group, an Informa business

A CHAPMAN & HALL BOOK

CRC Press
Taylor & Francis Group
6000 Broken Sound Parkway NW, Suite 300
Boca Raton, FL 33487-2742

First issued in paperback 2021

© 2019 by Taylor & Francis Group, LLC
CRC Press is an imprint of Taylor & Francis Group, an Informa business

No claim to original U.S. Government works

Version Date: 20190201

ISBN-13: 978-1-03-209350-5 (pbk)
ISBN-13: 978-0-8153-7944-7 (hbk)

This book contains information obtained from authentic and highly regarded sources. Reasonable efforts have been made to publish reliable data and information, but the author and publisher cannot assume responsibility for the validity of all materials or the consequences of their use. The authors and publishers have attempted to trace the copyright holders of all material reproduced in this publication and apologize to copyright holders if permission to publish in this form has not been obtained. If any copyright material has not been acknowledged please write and let us know so we may rectify in any future reprint.

Except as permitted under U.S. Copyright Law, no part of this book may be reprinted, reproduced, transmitted, or utilized in any form by any electronic, mechanical, or other means, now known or hereafter invented, including photocopying, microfilming, and recording, or in any information storage or retrieval system, without written permission from the publishers.

For permission to photocopy or use material electronically from this work, please access www.copyright.com (http://www.copyright.com/) or contact the Copyright Clearance Center, Inc. (CCC), 222 Rosewood Drive, Danvers, MA 01923, 978-750-8400. CCC is a not-for-profit organization that provides licenses and registration for a variety of users. For organizations that have been granted a photocopy license by the CCC, a separate system of payment has been arranged.

Trademark Notice: Product or corporate names may be trademarks or registered trademarks, and are used only for identification and explanation without intent to infringe.

Publisher's Note
The publisher has gone to great lengths to ensure the quality of this reprint but points out that some imperfections in the original copies may be apparent.

Library of Congress Cataloging-in-Publication Data

Names: Chang, Mark, author. | Balser, John, author. | Bliss, Robin, author. | Roach, Jim (James Michael), 1959- author.
Title: Innovative strategies, statistical solutions and simulations for modern clinical trials / Mark Chang, John Balser, Jim Roach and Robin Bliss.
Description: Boca Raton : Taylor & Francis, 2019. | Includes bibliographical references and index.
Identifiers: LCCN 2018044542| ISBN 9780815379447 (hardback : alk. paper) | ISBN 9781351214544 (ebook)
Subjects: | MESH: Clinical Trials as Topic | Statistics as Topic | Research Design | Drug Approval
Classification: LCC RM301.27 | NLM QV 771.4 | DDC 615.1072/4--dc23
LC record available at https://lccn.loc.gov/2018044542

Visit the Taylor & Francis Web site at
http://www.taylorandfrancis.com

and the CRC Press Web site at
http://www.crcpress.com

Contents

Preface

The pharmaceutical industry's approach to drug discovery and development has rapidly transformed in the last decade from the more traditional Research and Development (R & D) approach (e.g., "sequential" progression from phase 1 to phase 2 to phase 3) to a more innovative approach in which strategies are employed to compress and optimize the clinical development plan and associated timelines. To date, this paradigm shift, although real, has been mostly limited within a small scope of the development spectrum. For example, adaptive trial designs are increasingly being used to achieve higher power and mitigate the risk at interim analyses. However, these strategies are generally being considered on an individual trial basis and not as part of a fully integrated overall development program. Such optimization at the trial level is somewhat near-sighted and does not ensure cost, time, or development efficiency of the overall program. For this reason, the purposes of this book are set to establish a statistical framework for overall/global clinical development optimization and provide tactics or techniques to support such optimization, including clinical trial simulations. Under such a framework, depending on the unique circumstances of each development program, a mix of "classical" and "adaptive" trial designs can be implemented to achieve such an overall optimization.

It has been reported that among the reasons for failure of a clinical development program between 2013 to 2015, efficacy issues account for 52% of all failures, whereas the figures for safety, strategy, commercial and operational failures are 24%, 15%, 6%, and 3%, respectively (Harrison, 2016). Innovative statistical methodologies, employed wisely, can mitigate these risks and have the potential to significantly reduce the risk of a development program failing. Optimization tools, such as adaptive designs and other innovative approaches require strong collaborations among and between different stakeholders.

Statisticians are key members of the team tasked with assembling the clinical development strategy and plan and need to work very closely with these different stakeholders who represent different perspectives, all of which need to be considered in order to meet all program goals. As such, it is important for statisticians to possess a deep knowledge of the drug development process beyond statistical considerations. For these reasons, this book was written to incorporating both statistical and "clinical/medical" input.

The book is structured as follows:

Chapter 1, Overview of Drug Development, introduces the key elements of the "sequence" of the drug development process from inception through approval, including drug discovery, preclinical development, and clinical development. Chapter 2, Formulating Clinical Development Plan and Trial Design, describes the role and the key components of a clinical development program, followed by a review of critical concepts of clinical trial designs. Chapter 3, Clinical Development Program (CDP) Optimization, analyzes the benchmarks in clinical development, including determination of the net present value (NPV), Clinical Program Success Rates and Reasons for Failure, deconstructing costs associated with clinical trials, timelines associated with advancing through each phase of development, regulatory review time after a file is submitted, and competitive landscape as well. In the second part of the chapter, Stochastic Decision Process as a statistical model is introduced as a method to incorporate into CDP optimization. Chapter 4, Global-Optimal Adaptive Trial Designs, provides different examples of how to design an adaptive trial that achieves global optimization. These first four chapters serve as the framework or foundation that is necessary to achieve global optimization in drug development. The rest of chapters describe specific techniques to support such optimization. Specifically, Chapter 5, Designing Trials for Precision Medicine, discusses marker-adaptive designs, basket, and population-adaptive designs. Chapter 6, Clinical Trial with Survival Endpoint, given the complexity and richness of survival endpoint trials, discusses a variety of challenging issues and how best to mitigate or resolve them, including delayed drug effect, treatment switching, and competing risks. Chapter 7, Practical Multiple Testing Methods in Clinical Trials, discusses different multiplicity issues that often arise in clinical trials, including dose-finding, coprimary, multiple-endpoint and mixed-endpoint trials. Many different testing procedures are compared, including some new powerful testing procedures. Chapter 8: Missing Data Handling in Clinical Trials, discusses practical approaches to missing data handling in SAS. Chapter 9: Special Issues and Resolutions is a collection of statistical issues and resolutions in clinical trials, including the drop-loser design with efficacy and safety, Estimation of Treatment Effect with Interim Blinded Data, and the relative advantages and disadvantages associated with choosing either the Fisher or the Barnard exact tests. Chapter 10, Controversies in Statistical Science and Applications, addresses key controversial issues in statistics from the perspectives of both "general science" and "statistical science", and discusses how these various perspectives can be applied to resolving some of these controversies for both statistical considerations as well as a decisions or choices we make in our daily lives.

The book includes a large amount of SAS code. To reduce the burden of retyping, relevant programming code is available at www.statisticians.org

Mark Chang, PhD
John Balser, PhD
Jim Roach, MD
Robin Bliss, PhD

Author Bio

Dr. Mark Chang is Sr. Vice President, Strategic Statistical Consulting at Veristat, an elected fellow of the American Statistical Association, and adjunct professor of Biostatistics at Boston University. He has been an active member in the statistical community, including a co-founder of the International Society for Biopharmaceutical Statistic, Co-Chair of the Biotechnology Innovation Organization Adaptive Design Working Group, and a member of the Multiregional Clinical Trial Expert Group.

Before joining Veristat, Chang served in various strategic roles including as Vice President of Biometrics at AMAG Pharmaceuticals and director and scientific fellow at Millennium /Takeda Pharmaceuticals. Dr. Chang has served as associate editor for *Journal of Pharmaceutical Statistics*, and has published eight books in biostatistics and science, including *Principles of Scientific Methods, Paradoxes in Scientific Inference, Modern Issues and Methods in Biostatistics, Adaptive Design Theory and Implementation Using SAS and R*, and *Monte Carlo Simulation for the Pharmaceutical Industry*.

John Balser, PhD, co-founder and President of Veristat, has developed the company as industry leaders in areas of clinical monitoring, data management, biostatistics and programming, medical writing, and project management. John is actively involved with clinical projects in his role as one of Veristat's principal statistical consultants. In this role, he assists clients with clinical study design and program development based on his many years of experience in the statistical aspects of clinical research. He is often called upon to assist clients on a variety of statistical issues at meetings with regulatory agencies. Prior to founding Veristat in 1994, John served as Vice President, Biostatistics, and Data Management at Medical & Technical Research Associates, Inc. He has held positions of increasing responsibility in the biostatistics departments at various pharmaceutical companies including E.R. Squibb, Biogen, and Miles. John received his MS and PhD in Biometrics from Cornell University, and has been actively engaged in clinical biostatistics for over 25 years. John is an avid runner and has competed in the Boston Marathon.

James M. Roach, MD, FACP, FCCP joined Pulmatrix as their Chief Medical Officer (CMO) in November 2017. Dr. Roach served as the CMO at Veristat, Inc for the year prior to joining Pulmatrix, and prior to Veristat served as the Senior Vice President, Development and CMO at Momenta Pharmaceuticals, Inc. from 2008-2016. From 2002-2008 Dr. Roach was the Senior Vice President, Medical Affairs at Sepracor, Inc. Dr. Roach has also held senior clinical research and/or medical affairs positions at Millennium

Pharmaceuticals, Inc., LeukoSite, Inc., Medical and Technical Research Associates, Inc. and Astra USA. Dr. Roach held an academic appointment at Harvard Medical School for close to 25 years and has been an Associate Physician at Brigham and Women's Hospital (BWH) and member of the BWH Pulmonary and Critical Care Medicine Division since 1993. He received his B.A. in Biology and Philosophy from the College of the Holy Cross and his M.D. from Georgetown University School of Medicine. Dr. Roach completed his residency in Internal Medicine and fellowships in Pulmonary Disease and Critical Care Medicine at Walter Reed Army Medical Center in Washington, D.C., and served in the US Army Medical Corps for ten years. Dr. Roach is board certified in Internal Medicine and Pulmonary Disease, and is a Fellow of the American College of Physicians (ACP) and the American College of Chest Physicians (ACCP).

Robin Bliss, PhD joined Veristat in October, 2011 and has served as Director, Biostatistics since October, 2017. Through her experience at Veristat, Dr. Bliss has implemented complex adaptive designs across clinical trials in Phases I, II, and III as well as seamless Phase I/II and II/III trials. She has also provided strategic advice to sponsor companies, including representation of such companies at regulatory agencies, participation with scientific advisory committees, performance of simulation studies, and other consulting services. Dr. Bliss has taught conference short courses in adaptive design as well as statistical courses as a university adjunct faculty member. Prior to Veristat, Dr. Bliss held a post-doctoral fellowship position at Brigham and Women's Hospital (Boston) in the Orthopedic and Arthritics Center for Outcomes Research. Dr. Bliss earned her PhD in Biostatistics from Boston University where her research focused on spatial and environmental statistics.

1

Overview of Drug Development

1.1 Introduction

Pharmaceutical research and biotechnology companies are "devoted to inventing medicines that allow patients to live longer, healthier, and more productive lives".

— "Who We Are", PhRMA, www.phrma.org.

A pharmaceutical or biopharmaceutical company is a commercial business licensed to research, develop, market and/or distribute drugs, most commonly in the context of healthcare. They are subject to a variety of laws and regulations regarding the patenting, testing and marketing of drugs, particularly prescription drugs. From its beginnings at the start of the 19th Century, the pharmaceutical industry is now one of the most successful and influential, attracting both praise and controversy. Most of today's major pharmaceutical companies were founded in the late 19th and early 20th centuries. The origins of the Food and Drug Administration (FDA) as a federal consumer protection agency can be traced back to the passage of the Pure Food and Drug Act, which was signed into law by President Theodore Roosevelt in 1906. This law was prompted by egregious marketing practices within the industry, and prohibited the introduction of adulterated or misbranded drugs. At this time, however, there was no mandate to require evidence of efficacy or safety of drugs prior to marketing. Key discoveries of the 1920s and 1930s, such as insulin and penicillin, became mass-manufactured and distributed. Switzerland, Germany and Italy had particularly strong industries, with the UK and US following suit.

Over time, attempts were increasingly made to increase regulation and to limit financial links between pharmaceutical companies and prescribing physicians, including by the relatively new US FDA (which became known "formally" as FDA in 1930). In 1938, the Federal Food, Drug and Cosmetic Act (FDCA) was enacted, which required manufacturers to demonstrate evidence of safety prior to obtaining approval by FDA. Such calls increased in the 1960s after the thalidomide tragedy came to light, in which the use of a new tranquilizer in pregnant women caused severe birth defects. The Kefauver-Harris amendments were implemented in 1962, further strengthening the provisions of the FDCA and requiring pharmaceutical manufacturers to also demonstrate evidence of efficacy to FDA prior to approval, and in 1964, the World Medical Association issued its Declaration of Helsinki, which set standards for clinical research and demanded that subjects give their informed consent before enrolling in an experiment.

The industry remained relatively small scale until the 1970s when it began to expand at a greater rate. Legislation allowing for strong patents, to cover both the process of manufacture and the specific composition of matter of the products themselves, came in to force in most first world countries. Different from traditional pharmaceuticals, most of which are "small molecule drugs" that are relatively easy to manufacture, biopharmaceuticals are "large molecule drugs" produced using biotechnology. They are usually proteins (including antibodies) or nucleic acids (DNA, RNA or antisense oligonucleotides) used for therapeutic or in vivo diagnostic purposes, and are produced by means other than direct extraction from a native (non-engineered) biological source. By the mid-1980s, small biotechnology firms started to form, and since that time the growth of biotechnology companies has been explosive. Based on market capitalization, many biotechnology companies are now represented in the list of the top 20 most successful firms. Additionally, the majority of drugs now approved by FDA originated in biotechnology companies. Many biotech companies have also forged mutually beneficial partnerships with large pharmaceutical companies and/or have been acquired. Since the early 1990s, costs of drug development have increased dramatically, and the productivity from internal Research and Development (R&D) efforts has not followed suit. In 2004 FDA released the Drug Modernization Act – Innovation/Stagnation: Challenge and Opportunity on the Critical Path to New Medical Products. Pharmaceutical industries are clearly seeking new and more efficient ways to develop drugs such as genomic & biomarker utilization, adaptive design, targeted molecular design, and computer simulations.

In the new millennium, drug development is increasingly characterized by Globalization. According to ASPE's estimates in 2016, prescription drug spending in the United States was about $457 billion in 2015, or 16.7 percent of overall personal health care services. Of that $457 billion, $328 billion (71.9 percent) was for retail drugs and $128 billion (28.1 percent) was for non-retail drugs

Bringing a drug to market requires extensive and lengthycollaborations among people from dozens of disciplines. The entire development process includes multiple stages or phases: from Discovery, Preclinical, Clinical Trials, through Phase IV commitments and Marketing (Figure 1.1). Interactions with regulatory authorities usually start before starting phase I clinical trials. All clinical trial protocols (see later in this chapter) have to be approved by an Institutional Rreview Board (IRB) as well as the relevant competent regulatory authorities before conducting clinical trials. It is estimated that, on average, a drug takes 10 to 12 years from initial research to reach the commercialization stage. The cost of this process is estimated to be more than US $2.5 billion.

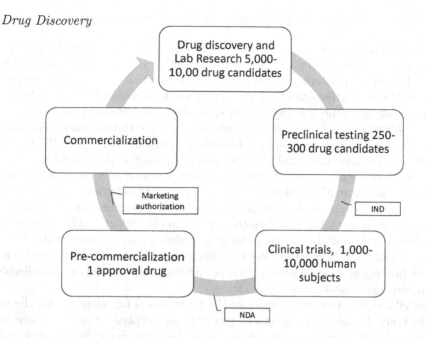

FIGURE 1.1
The Drug Development Life Cycle (Source: Venture Pharma).

1.2 Drug Discovery

Drug discovery involves: (1) identifying and defining medical needs, i.e., an effective prophylactic or therapeutic intervention, (2) researching on disease mechanism, i.e., identifying and validating target(s) (receptors) involved in disease processes, (3) searching for lead compounds that interact with the target, and (4) optimizing the properties of the lead compounds to generate potential drug molecules.

1.2.1 Target Identification and Validation

For a drug to work, it has to interact with a disease target in the human body. In most situations, it is the proteins or receptors that drug molecules are developed to interact with to provide the therapeutic benefit. The exceptions are in cases such as antisense drugs and gene therapy, where the nucleotides and genes are targeted, respectively. When presented to the target, drug molecules can elicit reactions to switch on or switch off certain biochemical reactions. The main drug targets in the human body can be classified into three categories: enzymes, intracellular receptors, and cell surface receptors. Enzymes are biomolecules that catalyze (i.e. increase the rates of) chemical reactions. Drugs can interact with enzymes to modulate their enzymatic activities. Intracellular receptors are in the cytoplasm or nucleus. Drugs or endogenous ligand molecules have to pass through the cell membrane (a lipid bilayer) to interact with these receptors. The molecules must be hydrophobic or coupled to a hydrophobic carrier to cross the cell membrane. Cell surface receptors are on the cell surface and have an affinity for hydrophilic binding molecules. Signals are transduced from external stimuli to the cytoplasm, and affect cellular pathways via these surface receptors. There are three main superfamilies (groups) of cell surface receptors: G-protein coupled receptors (GPCRs), ion channel receptors, and catalytic receptors using enzymatic activities.

When the action of the drug is to activate or switch on a reaction, the drug is called an 'agonist'. On the other hand, if the drug switches off the reaction, or inhibits or blocks the binding of other agonist components onto the receptor, it is called an 'antagonist'. When the interaction is with an enzyme, the terms 'inducer' and 'inhibitor' are used to denote drugs that activate or deactivate the enzyme. The interactions between drug molecules and targets are desired to be binding-specific: binding occurs at particular sites in the target molecule, and binding is most often reversible.

Cells communicate to coordinate the biochemical functions within the human body. If the communication system is interrupted or messages are not conveyed fully, our bodily functions can go haywire. For example, if the p53 protein is mutated, cell growth is unchecked and cancer can form. G-protein coupled receptors (GPCR5) represent possibly the most important class of target proteins for drug discovery. They are always involved in signaling from outside to inside the cell. The number of diseases that are caused by a GPCR malfunction is enormous, and therefore it is not surprising that most commonly prescribed medicines act on a CPCE. It is estimated that more than 30% of drugs target this receptor superfamily.

For most diseases, genetic makeup and variations determine a person's individuality and susceptibility to diseases, trauma, pathogens and drug responses. The current method of drug discovery is to break down the disease process into the cellular and molecular levels such that more specific (fewer side effects) and effective (high therapeutic index) drugs can be discovered and manufactured to intervene or restore the cellular or molecular dysfunction. Among approximately three billion base pairs that make up the DNA module, about $30,000 - 40,000$ genes (DNA segments) encode proteins. Based these genes, many thousands of proteins are produced. Common drug targets are protein or glycoprotein molecules because proteins are the ingredients for enzymes and receptors, with which drugs interact.

After a potential disease-causing target has been identified, validation is necessary to confirm the functions and effects of the target. Validations are carried out in two ways: in vitro laboratory tests, and in vivo disease models using animals. Typically, in vitro tests are cell- or tissue-based experiments. The aim is to study the biochemical functions of the target as a result of binding to potential drug ligands. Parameters such as ionic concentrations, enzyme activities, and expression profiles are studied.

For in vivo studies, animal models are set up and how the target is involved in the disease is analyzed. One such model is the mouse knockout model. It should be borne in mind, however, that there are differences between humans and animals in terms of gene expression functional characteristics and biochemical reactions. Nevertheless, in addition to in vitro tests, animal models can provide the results to further inform the biology and pathophysiology associated with human disease.

1.2.2   Irrational Approach

There are two main approaches to discovering small molecule drugs (molecular weights < 500 Da): the irrational approach, or the rational approach.

The steps in the traditional irrational approach include: (1) target identification, (2) target purification, and (3) modification of lead compound.

To find lead compounds or potential drug molecules that bind with receptors and modulate disease pathways, thousands of compounds (through natural product collection or lab-produced) are screened using high throughput screening (HTS) or ultra-HTS (UHTS?). When an interaction happens, it is referred to as 'a hit'. The so-called lead compounds are those that have shown some desired biological activities when tested against the assays. However, these activities are not optimized. Modifications to the lead compounds are necessary to improve the physicochemical, pharmacokinetic, and toxicological properties for clinical applications.

Following 'hits', the lead compounds are purified using chromatographic techniques and their chemical compositions identified via spectroscopic and chemical means. Structures may be elucidated using X-ray or nuclear magnetic resonance (NMR) methods. Protein purification is a series of processes intended to isolate a single type of protein from a complex mixture. Protein purification is an important step in the characterization of the function, structure and interactions of the protein of interest.

Further tests are carried out to evaluate the potency and specificity of the lead compounds isolated. This is usually followed up with modifications of the compounds to improve properties through synthesis of variations to the compounds via chemical processes in the laboratory and frequently with modifications to the functional groups.

The lead compounds go through processes with many iterations to keep improving and optimizing the drug interaction properties to achieve improved potency and efficacy.

Potency is an important consideration and is a measure of drug activity expressed in terms of the amount required to produce an effect of given intensity. A highly potent drug evokes a larger response at low concentrations. It is proportional to Affinity and Efficacy, as well as on-target toxicity. Affinity is the ability of the drug to bind to a receptor. Efficacy is the relationship between receptor occupancy and the ability to initiate a response at the molecular, cellular, tissue or system level. On-target toxicity, which is also referred to as mechanism-based toxicity, relates to adverse effects that occur because of interactions of the drug with its intended target.

After all these exhaustive tests, a few candidates are selected for preclinical in vivo studies using animal disease models. Many tests based on tissue cultures or cell-based assays, as they are less costly and provide results more readily. At the end of this long process is the identification of selected drug candidates with sufficient efficacy and safety to support the initiation of human clinical trials.

1.2.3 Rational Approach

The rational approach is based on an understanding of the geometric structure of molecules/proteins to predict and define structure-activity relationships (SARs) and the knowledge to identify the genes that are involved in disease pathogenesis, or nanotechnology.

Computer aided molecular design and modeling is the central part of computational chemistry, which use 3-D structures of compounds in virtual chemical compound libraries to determine the SARs of ligand-protein receptor binding. The aim of computational chemistry is to perform virtual screening using computer-generated ligands. Libraries of virtual ligands are generated on computer based on certain building blocks or framework (scaffolds) of chemical compounds. Methods such as genetic algorithm and genetic programming can be used, which simulates the genetic evolutionary process to produce 'generations' of virtual compounds with new structures that have improved ability to bind the receptor protein, similar to the concept of 'survival for the fittest' in the biological process. See Chapter 13 for more discussion.

Combinatorial chemistry is a laboratory chemistry technique to synthesize a diverse range of compounds through methodical combinations of building block components.

The aim of antisense therapy is to identify the genes that are involved in disease pathogenesis. A strategy for antisense therapy is based on the binding of oligodeoxyribonucleotides to the double helix DNA. This stops gene expression either by restricting the unwinding of the DNA or by preventing the binding of transcription factor complexes to the gene promoter. Another strategy centers on the messenger RNA (mRNA). Oligoribonucleotides form a hybrid with the mRNA. Such a duplex formation ties up the mRNA, preventing the encode translation message from being processed to form the protein.

Although all these seem like elegant ways to stop the disease at the source, at the DNA or mRNA level, there are practical problems. First, the antisense drug has to be delivered to the cell interior, and the polar groups of oligonucleotides have problems crossing the cell membrane to enter the cytoplasm and nucleus; secondly, the oligonucleotides have to bind to the intended gene sequence through hydrogen bonding; and, thirdly, the drug should not exert toxicities or side effects as a result of the interaction. For these reasons, there have been difficulties in bringing antisense drugs to the market.

1.2.4 Biologics

Unlike the small molecule drugs (pharmaceuticals), large molecule drugs (bio-pharmaceuticals) are mainly protein-based and similar to natural biological compounds found in the human body or they are fragments that mimic the active part of the natural compounds. Today biopharmaceuticals discovery is largely based on examining the compounds within human body, for example, hormones or other biological response modifiers, and determining how they affect the biological process.

Pharmaceuticals are new chemical entities (NCEs) and they are produced (synthesized) in manufacturing plants using techniques based on chemical reactions of reactants. Biopharmaceuticals are made using totally different methods. These protein-based drugs are 'manufactured' in biological systems such as living cells, producing the desired protein molecules in large reaction vessels or by extraction from animal serum.

Biopharmaceuticals are products which are derived using living organisms to produce or modify the structure and/or functioning of plants or animals with a medical or diagnostic use. Biopharmaceuticals are becoming increasingly important because they are more potent and specific, as they are similar to the proteins within the body, and hence are more effective in treating our diseases. There are three major areas in which biopharmaceuticals are used: as prophylactic (preventive, as in the case of vaccines), therapeutic (antibodies) and replacement (hormones, growth factors) therapy. Another term that is used for protein-based drugs is biologics.

Vaccines

The basis of vaccination is that administering a small quantity of a vaccine (antigen that has been treated) stimulates the immune system and causes antibodies to be secreted to react against the foreign antigen. Later in life, when we are exposed to the same antigen again, the immune system will evoke a 'memory' response and activate the defense mechanisms by generating antibodies to combat the invading antigen.

In cancer, the immune system does not recognize the changes in cancer cells. Cancer vaccines seek to mimic cancer-specific changes by using synthetic peptides to challenge the immune system. When these peptides are taken up by T cells, the immune system is activated. The T cells search for cancer cells with specific markers and proceed to kill them.

Antibodies

The human immune system is a remarkable system for combating against foreign substances that invade the body. It protects us from infections by pathogens such as viruses, bacteria, parasite and fungi. An important aspect of the immune system is the self-non-self recognition function, by means of markers present on a protein called the major histocompatibility complex (MHC). Substances without such markers are discerned and targeted for destruction (Ng, 2005).

When this aspect of the immune system is not regulated properly, this gives rise to autoimmune diseases such as rheumatoid arthritis, diabetes, and multiple sclerosis. However, mistakes can happen occasionally when the immune system responds to the environment, leading to allergies, as in the case of asthma and hay fever.

B cells are produced by the bone marrow. In response to activation of $CD4^+$ T helper cells, B cells proliferate and produce antibodies. The antibodies produced by B cells circulate in the bloodstream and bind to antigens. When this happens, other cells are in turn activated to destroy the antigens.

T-cells are lymphocytes produced by the thymus gland. $CD4^+$ (CD positive, helper cells) and $CD8^+$ (CD positive also called T killer, or suppressor cells) are the two types of T cells involved in immune response. When the antigen-presenting cells (APCs) present the antigens to $CD4^+$ helper T cells, the secretory function is activated and growth factors such as cytokines are secreted to signal the proliferation of $CD8^+$ killer T cells and B cells. When the $CD8^+$ cells are activated by the APCs, the $CD8^+$ killer T cells directly kill those cells expressing the antigens. Activated B cells produce antibodies, as described above (Ng, 2005).

Cytokines and Hormones Therapies

Cytokines are produced mainly by leukocytes (white blood cells). They are potent polypeptide molecules that regulate the immune and inflammation functions, as well as hemopoiesis (production of blood cells) and wound healing.

Hormones are intercellular messengers. Hormones maintain homeostasis — the balance of biological activities in the body; for example, insulin controls blood glucose level, epinephrine and norepinephrine mediate response to external environment, and growth hormone promotes normal healthy growth and development.

Diabetes mellitus occurs when the human body does not produce enough insulin. Production of insulin is triggered when there is a rise in blood sugar, for example after a meal. Most of our body cells have insulin receptors which bind to the insulin secreted. When the insulin binds to the receptor other receptors on the cell are activated to absorb sugar (glucose) from the bloodstream into the cell.

When there is insufficient insulin to bind to receptors the cells are starved because sugar cannot reach the interior to provide energy for vital biological processes Patients with insulin-dependent diabetes mellitus (IDDM) become unwell when this happens. They depend on insulin injection for survival.

Gene Therapies

Gene therapy is the technology involves the transfer of normal functional genes to replace genetically faulty ones so that proper control of protein expression and biochemical processes can take place. However, it is challenging to get the normal genes to the intended location using delivery tools or vehicles, called vectors (gene carriers). Whether using the in vitro or in situ method, genes are first loaded onto the vectors, which usually are viruses. Retroviruses are the preferred candidates, as they are efficient vectors for entering humans and replicating their genes within human cells. The hurdle of gene therapy is to overcome toxicities associated with immune and inflammatory response.

Stem Cell Therapies

Stem cell treatment is a cell therapy that introduce new cells into damaged tissue in order to treat a disease or injury. The ability of stem cells to self-renew and give rise to subsequent generations that can differentiate offers a large potential to culture tissues that can replace diseased and damaged tissues in the body, without the risk of rejection. However, cell rejection due to the host's immune system recognizing the cells as foreign has to be overcome to ensure stem cell therapy as a viable treatment

Bone-marrow is the spongy tissue inside the cavities of bones. Bone marrow stem cells grow and divide into the various types of blood cells: white-blood cells (leukocytes) that fight infection, red blood cells (erythrocytes) that transport oxygen, and platelets that are the agents for clotting.

1.2.5   NanoMedicine

Nanomedicine is an application of nanotechnology in medical science. Nanotechnologies study features of materials on the scale of nanometers or billionths of a meter. In biology the scale of a single human hair is about 80,000 nanometers wide and a red blood cell is about 7,000 nanometers wide. Nanoscale materials often have novel properties related to their high ratio of surface area and quantum effects. The current research and development efforts on Nanomedicine are concentrated in six primary categories (The Royal Society, 2004, Tegart, 2003):

1. Antimicrobial Properties. Investigating nanomaterials with strong antimicrobial properties. Nanocrystalline silver, for example, is already being used for wound treatment.

2. Biopharmaceutics. Applying nanotechnology to drug delivery system, e.g., using nanomaterial coatings to encapsulate drugs and to serve as functional carriers. Nanomaterial encapsulation could improve the diffusion, degradation, and targeting of a drug.

3. Implantable Materials. Using nanomaterials to repair and replace damaged or diseased tissues. Nanomaterial implant coatings could increase the adhesion, durability, and lifespan of implants, and nanostructure scaffolds could provide a framework for improved tissue regeneration. Nanomaterial implants could be engineered for biocompatibility with the host environment to minimize side effects and the risk of rejection.

4. Implantable Devices. Implanting small devices to serve as sensors, fluid injection systems, drug dispensers, pumps and reservoirs, and aids to restore vision and hearing functions. Devices with nanoscale components could monitor environmental conditions, detect specific properties, and deliver appropriate physical, chemical, or pharmaceutical responses.

5. Diagnostic Tools. Utilizing lab-on-a-chip devices to perform DNA analysis and drug discovery research by reducing the required sample sizes and accelerating the chemical reaction process. Moreover, imaging technologies such as nanoparticle probes and miniature imaging devices as well as IV imaging agent could promote early detection and diagnosis of disease.

6. Understanding Basic Life Processes. Using nanoscale devices and materials to learn more about how biological systems self-assemble, self-regulate, and self-destroy at the molecular level. Insights into basic life processes will overlap multiple disciplines and could yield scientific breakthroughs.

1.3   Preclinical Development

1.3.1   Objectives of Preclinical Development

Pre-clinical development is a stage of research that bridges between Discovery and Clinical Trials (trials in human subjects/patients). After a lead compound has been identified, it is subjected to a development process to optimize its properties. The development process includes pharmacological studies of the lead compound to influence and optimize the therapeutic index. Pre-clinical research includes in vitro (in tubes), ex vivo (in cells/tissues but outside an organism), and in vivo (in animals) tests. Preclinical research includes pharmacology and toxicology studies as well as pharmacodynamics and pharmacokinetics studies. Many iterations are carried out and at the end of this process, an optimized compound will hopefully be selected to move forward into clinical studies.

Two different animal species are typically required for toxicology studies. The most commonly used species are murine and canine, although primate and porcine are also used. The choice of species is based on which are anticipated to be most predictive of response in humans. Differences in the gut, enzyme activity, circulatory system, or other considerations make certain models more appropriate in terms of the dosage form, site of activity, or noxious metabolites. For example, rodents cannot act as models for antibiotic drugs because the resulting alteration to their intestinal flora causes significant adverse effects. Studies are sometimes performed in larger species such as dogs, pigs and sheep which allow for testing in a similar sized model as that of a human. Some species are used for similarity in specific organs or organ system physiology. Such examples are: swine for dermatological and coronary stent studies; goats for mammary implant studies; dogs for gastric studies.

Drug development also extends to formulation and delivery. Most drugs that are administered to patients contain more than just the active pharmaceutical ingredients (the drug molecules that interact with the receptors or enzymes). Other chemical components are often added to improve manufacturing processing, or the stability and bioavailability of drugs. Effective delivery of drugs to target sites is an important factor to optimize efficacy and reduce side effects.

An ideal drug is potent, efficacious and specific, that is, it must have strong effects on a specific targeted biological pathway and minimal effects on all other pathways, to reduce side effects. Potency is the dose required to generate an effect. A potent drug elicits an effect at a low dose. An important concept is so-called therapeutic Index *(window)*. The index is defined by the ratio of TD_{50}/ED_{50}, where TD_{50} is the toxic dose for 50% of the population, and ED_{50} is the effective dose for 50% of the population. A high value of the index is preferable. The lower this index, the less likely that the compound could be considered as a viable drug candidate. Another commonly used team is the so-called standard safety margin (SSM) defined as

$$SSM = \frac{LD_1 - ED_{99}}{ED_{99}} 100\%$$

where LD_1 is the lethal dose for 1% of the population, and ED_{99} is the effective dose for 99% of the population. Again, a high SSM is desirable.

As stated in European Pharmaceutical Review (EPR, 2009), the journey from molecular target and early drug lead to the clinic is an arduous one with many hurdles to cross prior to developing a successful clinical candidate. The high rate of attrition of drug molecules has forced drug researchers to pay greater attention to drug metabolism and pharmacokinetics (DMPK) of lead molecules at even the earliest stages of drug discovery. Throughout the development of a successful molecule the researcher must bear in mind three important questions: will enough drug reach the target (pharmacokinetics)? What form will it arrive in (metabolism)? And what will it do when it gets there (pharmacodynamics)? These are the main questions that the DMPK scientist attempts to answer.

1.3.2 Pharmacokinetics

Pharmacokinetics is often studied in conjunction with pharmacodynamics. Pharmacodynamics explores what a drug does to the body, whereas pharmacokinetics explores what the body does to the drug. Specifically, pharmacokinetics is the study of drug Absorption, Distribution, Metabolism, and Excretion (ADME). Absorption is the process of a substance entering the body. Distribution is the dispersion or dissemination of substances throughout the fluids and tissues of the body. Metabolism is the irreversible transformation of parent compounds into daughter metabolites. Excretion is the elimination of the substances from the body. In rare cases, some drugs irreversibly accumulate in a tissue in the body.

Drug administration (Absorption)

Pharmacokinetic properties of drugs may be affected by elements such as the site of administration and the rate of drug administration. There are several ways to administer a drug such as oral and intravenous. With intravenous administration, a drug is injected directly into the bloodstream, oral administration requires the drug to be absorbed through the gastrointestinal tract before it can enter the bloodstream for distribution to target sites and metabolism may precede the distribution to the site of action.

The oral route is the most common way of administering a drug. For a drug to be absorbed into the bloodstream, it has to be soluble in the fluids of our gastrointestinal tract. Drugs are often formulated with excipients (components other than the active drug) to improve manufacturing and dissolution processes. The gastrointestinal tract is lined with epithelial cells, and drugs have to cross the cell membrane. In the stomach with low pH, drugs that are weak acids are absorbed faster. In the intestine, where pH is high, weak basic drugs are absorbed preferentially.

When a drug is injected (intravenous administration), the entire dose can be considered as being available in the bloodstream to be distributed to the target site. Hence, the dosage can be controlled, unlike with other routes of administration where the bioavailability of the drug is difficult to predict because of complex diffusion processes. Intravenous injection is the normal route for administration of protein-based drugs, as they are likely to be destroyed when taken orally because of the pH conditions in the gastrointestinal tract and/or too large to be effectively absorbed. The onset of drug action with intravenous injection is quick, therefore it is especially useful for emergency cases, but also potentially the most dangerous. Once a drug is injected, it is almost impossible to remove it.

Distribution

The distribution patterns of a drug from the bloodstream to various tissues depends on a number of factors such as (1) vascularity of the tissue, (2) binding of the drug to protein molecules in blood plasma, and (3) drug substance transportation types: perfusion or diffusion of the drug.

Drugs absorbed through the gastrointestinal tract pass into the hepatic portal vein, which drains into the liver. The liver metabolizes the drug, thus potentially reducing the availability of the drug for interaction with receptors. At a certain time after administration when the rate of drug absorption equals the rate of clearance, it reaches an equilibrium condition called 'steady state'. The area under the concentration curve represents the total amount of drug in the blood, which measures the bioavailability of the drug. Comparison of drug concentrations in the bloodstream administered via intravenous injection and oral route provides information for the bioavailability of the oral drug.

Drug molecules in the blood are transported to the tissue until equilibrium is reached. The transporting speed depends the transportation types: perfusion (fast) and diffusion (slow). Acid drugs usually bind to albumins and basic drugs to glycoproteins. When the drug bind to albumin and proteins in the blood, it becomes less available for distribution to tissues. Lastly, lipid-soluble drugs can cross the cell membrane more readily than polar drugs and move into the tissues to interact with receptors.

Metabolism

Most drugs are metabolized in the body, though different in extent. Metabolism changes the chemical structures and generally reduces pharmacological activity of a new molecular entity (NME) (although sometimes metabolites are active as well). The liver is the major organ for metabolizing drugs, followed by the kidneys. Some drugs also are metabolized in tissue systems.

Two types of biochemical metabolism reactions take place in the liver: (1) Phase I reactions include oxidation, reduction and hydrolysis, which transform the drugs into metabolites by means of the family enzymes, cytochrome P-450. They convert lipid-soluble drugs to more water-soluble metabolites. (2) Phase II reactions involve the addition or conjugation of subgroups, such as -OH, -NH and -SH to the drug molecules. Enzymes other than P-450 are responsible for these reactions. These reactions give rise to less lipid-soluble or more polar molecules and are excreted from the body (Ng, 2005).

Excretion

Drug excretion is the process of discharging medical waste matter from the blood, tissues, or organs. The common routes for drugs to excrete from the body are: kidneys, lungs, intestine and colon, and skin. The kidneys are the primary organs for clearing drugs from the body. Water-soluble drugs are usually cleared more quickly than lipid-soluble drugs. Some drugs may be re-absorbed into the intestine and colon and later passed out as solid waste.

Clearance is a measure of drug elimination from the body without identifying the mechanism or process. Clearance considers the entire body as a drug-eliminating system from which many elimination processes may occur. The clearance of a drug is given by the following expression:

$$CL = \frac{\text{Rate of drug elimination}}{\text{Drug concentration in blood}}$$

In general, drugs that are highly bound to plasma protein have reduced overall drug clearance. Drug elimination is governed mainly by renal and other metabolic processes in the body. When a drug is tightly bound to a protein, only the unbound drug is assumed to be metabolized — restrictively eliminated. In contrast, some drugs may be eliminated even when they are protein bound — nonrestrictively eliminated.

Albumin is a protein (molecular weight about 70k Da) synthesized in the liver and is the major component of plasma proteins responsible for reversible drug binding. In the body, albumin is distributed in the plasma and in the extracellular fluids of skin, muscle, and various other tissues. The elimination half-life of albumin is about 18 days. Albumin is responsible for maintaining the osmotic pressure of the blood and for the transport of endogenous and exogenous substances (Shargel, et al., 2005).

PK Analysis Method

Pharmacokinetic analysis is traditionally performed by noncompartmental or compartmental methods. Noncompartmental methods estimate the exposure to a drug by estimating the area under the curve of a concentration-time curve, whereas compartmental methods estimate the concentration-time curve using kinetic models.

Noncompartmental PK analysis is highly dependent on estimation of total drug exposure. Total drug exposure is most often estimated by Area Under the Curve (AUC) methods using the trapezoidal rule. In this method, the area estimation is highly dependent on the blood/plasma sampling schedule and the closer the time points are, the closer the trapezoids are to the actual shape of the concentration-time curve. Other important PK parameters include $C_{\max}$ (maximum concentration), $T_{\max}$ (the time to $C_{\max}$), and the half-time $T_{1/2}$ (time to $C_{\max}/2$).

Compartmental PK analysis uses kinetic models to describe and predict the concentration-time curve. The advantage of compartmental to noncompartmental analysis is the ability to predict the concentration at any time. The disadvantage is that the results are model-dependent and it is often difficult to validate these models. The simplest PK compartmental model is the one-compartmental PK model with oral dose administration and first-order elimination (Figure 1.2). The most complex PK models are based on physiological information, which hopefully can more precisely model each organ PK compartment. Some typical PK parameters of interest are presented in Table 1.1.

TABLE 1.1
Example of Preclinical PK Parameters.

	Dose (mg/kg)		
	20	100	200
$C_{\max}(\mu g/ml)$	99.2 ± 22.3	502 ± 142.2	1261 ± 83
$T_{1/2}$ (hr)	0.86	0.72	0.67
AUC ($\mu g/hr/ml$)	14.2	83.3	248.1
Clearance ($l\ h/kg$)	1.42	1.18	0.82

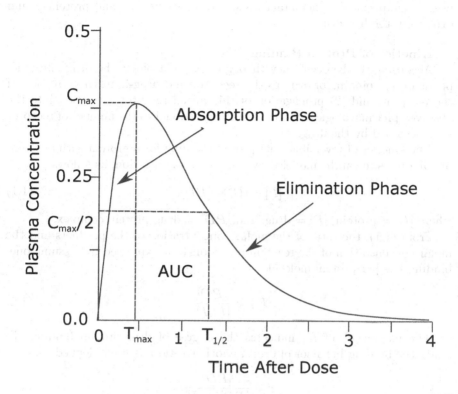

FIGURE 1.2
Concentration Curve of Oral Administration.

1.3.3 Pharmacodynamics

Pharmacodynamics is the study of the biochemical and physiological effects of drugs on the body. Mechanisms of most drugs either mimic or inhibit normal physiological processes or inhibit pathological processes in animals. The drug actions can be classified into five main categories: depressing, stimulating, destroying cells (cytotoxic), irritation, and replacing substances.

Many drugs interact with proteins or other macromolecules (e.g., melanin and DNA) to form a so-called drug-protein complex. Most drug-protein binding is reversible. Unlike free or unbound drug, the protein-bound drug can't easily transverse cell or possibly even capillary membranes. The drug in the form of "drug-complex" is usually pharmacologically inactive. Studies that critically evaluate drug-protein binding are usually performed in vitro using a purified protein such as albumin. The commonly used methods to determine the protein-binding are equilibrium dialysis and ultrafiltration, each of which uses a semipermeable membrane to separate the protein and protein-bound drug from the free drug.

Kinetics of Protein Binding

According to the occupancy theory in pharmacology, the drug effect depends on (1) binding of drug to the receptor and drug-induced activation of the receptor, and (2) propagation of this initial receptor activation into the observed pharmacological effect that is proportional to the number of receptor sites occupied by the drug.

The kinetics of reversible drug-protein binding for a protein with one simple binding site can be modeled by the law of mass action, as follows:

$$[P] + [D] = [PD], \tag{1.1}$$

where $[P]$ = protein, $[D]$ = drug, and $[PD]$ = drug-protein-complex.

From (1.1), the ratio of the molar concentration of the products and the molar concentration of the reactants is a constant expressed by (assume one-binding site per protein molecule).

$$K_a = \frac{[PD]}{[P][D]} \tag{1.2}$$

The magnitude of K_a indicates the degree of drug-protein binding. To study the binding behavior of drugs, another ratio r is used, defined as:

$$r = \frac{[PD]}{[PD] + [P]} \tag{1.3}$$

where $[PD] + [P]$ is the total moles of protein and $[PD]$ is the moles of drug bound.

$$r = \frac{K_a[D]}{1 + K_a[D]} \tag{1.4}$$

Pharmacodynamic Drug Interactions

Pharmacodynamic interactions can occur when two or more drugs have mechanisms of action that result in the same physiological outcome. Most drugs are metabolized to inactive or less active metabolites by enzymes in the liver and intestine. Inhibition of this metabolism can increase the effect of the object drug and increase the chance of drug toxicity.

Pharmacodynamic interactions can be characterized into: (1) synergistic when the effect of two drugs is greater than the sum of their individual effects, (2) antagonistic when the effect of two drugs is less than the sum of their individual effects, (3) additive when the effect of two drugs is merely the sum of the effects of each, and (4) sequence-dependent when the order in which two drugs are given governs their effects.

1.3.4   Toxicology

Study of the toxicology of a potential drug is critical to determine the anticipated safety profile of a drug before it is given to humans in clinical trials.

Toxicological studies show the functional and morphological effects of the drug, including the mode, site and degree of action, dose relationship, sex differences, latency and progression, and reversibility of these effects.

To study the toxicity of a drug, the maximum tolerable dose and area under curve are generally established in-rodents and non-rodents. There are two types of toxicity studies: single dose and repeated dose. Single dose acute toxicity testing is conducted for several purposes, including the determination of the doses selected for repeated dose studies, identification of target organs subjected to toxicity, and provision of data to be incorporated into the selection of a starting dose in human clinical trials.

The experiments are carried out on animals, usually on two mammalian species: a rodent (mouse or rat) and a non-rodent (rabbit). Two different routes of administration are generally studied; one is the intended route for human clinical trials, and the other is intravenous injection. Various characteristics of the animals are monitored, including weights, clinical signs, organ functions, biochemical parameters, and mortality. At the completion of the study, autopsies are performed to analyze the organs histopathologically, especially the targeted organ for the drug.

Repeated dose chronic toxicity studies are also generally performed on two species of animals, a rodent and non-rodent. The aim is to evaluate the longer-term effects of the drug in animals. Plasma drug concentrations are measured and pharmacokinetics analyses are performed. Vital functions studied include cardiovascular, respiratory and nervous systems. Animals are retained at the end of the study to check toxicity recovery.

Carcinogenicity studies are performed to identify the tumor-causing potential of a drug. Drugs are administered to rates or rodent continuously for months. Data for hormone levels, growth factors and tissue enzymatic activities are analyzed after the experiments.

Genotoxicity studies are to determine if the drug compound can induce mutations to genes, including: assessment of genotoxicity in a bacterial reverse mutation test, detection of chromosomal damage using in vitro method, and detection of chromosomal damage using rodent hematopoietic cells.

The aim of **reproductive toxicology** studies is to assess the effect of the potential drug on mammalian reproduction. All the stages, from pre-mating through conception, pregnancy and birth, to growth of the offspring, are studied on rats and/or rabbit.

The outcomes of all of the toxicity studies provide the basis for the selection of the starting dose for clinical trials in humans. The FDA Guidance — Estimating the Safe Starting Dose in Clinical Trials for Therapeutics in Adult Healthy Volunteers outlines the derivation of the maximum recommended starting dose (MRSD) for a drug to be used in humans for the first time. This MRSD is based on (1) no observed adverse effect level (NOAEL) in animals-the highest dose level that does not produce a significant increase in adverse effects, and (2) conversion of the NOAEL to human equivalent dose (HED) using the following formula:

$$HED = (\text{animal dose in mg/kg}) \times (\text{animal weight/human weight})^{0.33}$$

1.3.5 Intraspecies and Interspecies Scaling

DMPK study concerns the animal subjects, while clinical PKPD study concerns human sibjects. However, the principles are the same for the two studies. Interspecies scaling is a method used in toxicokinetics and the extrapolation of therapeutic drug doses in humans from nonclinical animal drug studies. Toxicokinetics is the application of pharmacokinetics to toxicology and pharmacokinetics for interpolation and extrapolation based on anatomic, physiologic, and biochemical similarities (Shargel, et al., 2005; Mordenti and Chappell, 1989; Bonate and Howard 2000; Mahmood, 2000).

The basic assumption in interspecies scaling is that physiologic variables, such as drug concentration, clearance, heart rate, organ weight, and biochemical processes, are related to the weight or body surface area of the animal species. It is commonly assumed that all mammals use the same energy source (oxygen) and energy transport systems are similar across animal species (Hu and Hayton, 2001). The general allometric equation obtained can be written as (Shargel, et al., 2005)

$$\theta = \beta \omega^a, \tag{1.5}$$

where θ is the pharmacokinetic or physiologic property of interest, β is an allometric coefficient, ω is the weight or surface area of the animal species, and constant a is the allometric exponent.

The allometric equation (1.5) can also be derived based on assumption about fractal structures of animals. As we discussed earlier the fractal structure leads to a power-law for a geometric or physiologic property. A list of allometric relationships for interspecies parameters is presented in Table 1.2.

1.4 Clinical Development

1.4.1 Overview of Clinical Development

After a lead compound has successfully progressed through the preclinical testing phase, the next step is clinical trials. Clinical trials are trials conducted on human subjects in accordance with Good Clinical Practice (GCP) regulations (in the US, these regulations are governed by the FDA). Clinical development is a joined effort by different stakeholders including but not limited to clinical research scientists, study coordinators, clinical and medical monitors, clinical investigators, physicians, medical liaisons, statisticians, data management professionals, CMC professionals, regulatory affairs professionals, project managers, financial managers, sales managers, and strategic

TABLE 1.2

Allometric Relationship for Interspecies Parameters.

Physiologic or Pharmacokinetic Property	Allometric Exponent a	Allometric Coefficient b
Basal O_2 consumption (mL/hr)	0.734	3.8
Endogenous N output (g/hr)	0.72	0.000042
O_2 consumption by liver slices (mL/hr)	0.77	3.3
Creatinine Clearance (mL/hr)	0.69	8.72
Methotrexate apparent volume (L/kg)	0.92	0.859
Kidney weight (g)	0.85	0.0212
Uver weight (g)	0.87	0.082
Heart weight (g)	0.98	0.0066
Stomach and intestines weight (g)	0.94	0.112
Blood weight (g)	0.99	0.055
Total volume (mL)	1.0 1	0.0062
Methotrexate half-life (min)	0.23	54.6

Source: adapted from Ritschel and Banerjee, 1986

planners. The traditional approach is to divide the development process into stages, from phase I to phase IV trials (Figure 1.3).

However, before we design clinical trials, we have some important up-front work to do, including the clinical development plan (CDP), which is a integrated document to describe the master plan outlining the development of a compound from phase I to phase IV. It is a bird eye's view of the plan for all the sequential trials regarding this compound, starting with verification of medical needs, which is usually done through literature review, and consulting with KOLs (key opinion leaders) in the field. The key issues to consider while developing a CDP may include the size of the target population, the feasibility of running such trials, the key inclusion/exclusion criteria to identify the target population, and major competitors/challenges. Meanwhile, the commercial and marketing groups of the company also will gather information regarding the size of the target population to inform different CDP options and return on investment (ROI) through a net present value (NPV) analysis. The company has to evaluate their core competence against their goals and will also develop risk mitigation plans. After several iterations of this process, the team has to make the decision on market position and deliver a sound CDP.

1.4.2 Classical Clinical Trial Paradigm

As mentioned early, clinical trials are divided into phases chronologically. The size of the trial generally increases gradually from phase I to phase III to maximize patients safety and to advance development in a cost-effective manner.

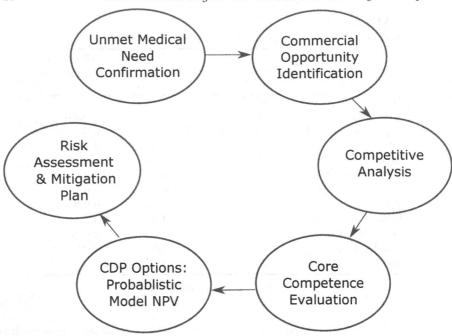

FIGURE 1.3
Clinical Development Process.

Phase I Trial

Traditionally, Phase I trials are the first stage of testing in human subjects. Normally, a small (6-60) group of healthy volunteers will be selected with the exception of some special diseases such as oncology and HIV in which these studies may be conducted in patients with the disease under evaluation. The objectives of the phase trials are to assess/explore the safety, tolerability, pharmacokinetics, and pharmacodynamics of a drug. These trials are often conducted in an inpatient clinic, where the subject can be closely monitored. The subject who receives the drug is usually observed until a minimum of five half-lives of the drug have passed. A Phase I trial is often a dose escalation study to determine the appropriate dose for therapeutic use. If the drug is intended to be used for multiple dose, then phase I trials will usually include a single ascending dose (SAD) study followed by a multiple ascending dose (MAD) trial.

SAD studies are those in which small groups of subjects are given a single dose of the study drug while they are observed for a period of time. If there are no sufficient adverse side effects observed, and the pharmacokinetic data is in line with predicted safe values, the dose is escalated to treat a new group of subjects. This is continued until pre-calculated pharmacokinetic safety levels are reached, and/or intolerable side effects start showing up. MAD are conducted to better understand the pharmacokinetics & pharmacodynamics associated with multiple doses of the drug. In these studies, a group of patients receives multiple low doses of the drug, whilst samples (of blood, and other fluids) are collected at various time points and analyzed to understand how the drug is processed within the body. In addition to SAD and MAD, a study for food effect may also be conducted, which is designed to investigate any differences in absorption of the drug by the body, caused by eating before the drug is given. These studies are usually run as a crossover study, with volunteers being given two identical doses of the drug on different occasions following a washout period; one while fasted, and one after being fed.

Phase II Trial

Once the initial safety of the study drug has been confirmed in Phase I trials, Phase II trials are performed on larger groups (20-300) and are designed to assess how well the drug works, as well as to continue to assess safety in a larger group of patients. In phase I, the dose range that will produce some biological effects with tolerable side-effects has been estimated. In phase II, the dose range will be further explored to identify/confirm the dose(s) that can be expected to be clinically effective with an acceptable safety profile. Therefore, Phase 2 endpoints are usually clinical endpoints instead of biomarker or PD markers.

Phase II studies are sometimes divided into Phase IIA and Phase IIB. Phase IIA is specifically designed to assess dosing requirements (how much drug should be given), whereas Phase IIB is specifically designed to study efficacy (how well the drug works at the prescribed dose(s)).

Many drug programs are discontinued in phase II if the data generated is not compelling because the next phase (phase III) is the most expensive phase of drug development in terms of both cost and time. Unless Phase II has clearly demonstrated that the drug is likely to prove to be both safe and effective in the confirmatory Phase III studies, sponsors will often choose not to make further investment in the program.

Phase III

A Phase III study is usually a randomized controlled multicenter trial including a large number of patients (300–10,000) and are aimed at being the definitive assessment of how effective and safe the drug is, in comparison with current 'gold standard' treatment. Because of their size and comparatively long duration, Phase III trials are the most expensive, time-consuming and difficult trials to design and run (the cost for a typical oncology trial is over $50,000 per patient). The results from Phase III trials (noting that usually two "adequate and well-controlled trials" are required) are the basis for drug approval for marketing.

Upon the completion of Phase III trials, the efficacy and safety results are presented in a so-called integrated efficacy summary (IES or ISE), which includes the analysis of all the efficacy data from all of the relevant trials conducted, and also integrated safety summary (ISS), which includes all the relevant safety data regarding the NME. These integrated results as well as other documents are organized according to ICH guidance and submitted to the regulatory agency for approval. In the United States, generally after a 10-month review process, the sponsor will receive a response from FDA regarding their NDA. The FDA response letter can be three possible types: (1) Approval for marketing the drug, (2) Application denied, and (3) Complete response - request for more information.

Phase IV Trial

After drug approval, a Phase IV trial may sometimes be required by regulatory agencies. A Phase IV trial is sometimes called a Post Marketing Surveillance Trial. Phase IV trials often mandate additional safety surveillance (pharmacovigilance) and ongoing technical support of a drug after it receives permission to be sold. Phase IV studies may be required by regulatory authorities because of potential long-term safety concerns or for label expansion (e.g., extend the use for pediatric population). The safety surveillance is designed to detect any rare or long-term adverse effects over a much larger patient population and longer period than was possible during the Phase I-III clinical trials. Harmful effects discovered by Phase IV trials may result in a drug being no longer sold, or restricted to certain uses.

1.4.3   Adaptive Trial Design Paradigm

In recent years, the cost for drug development has increased dramatically, but the success rate of new drug applications (NDAs) remains low. The Pharmaceutical industry has devoted a significant amount of effort in innovative approaches to clinical development, including adaptive design. An adaptive design is a clinical trial design that allows adaptations or modifications to aspects of the trial after its initiation without undermining the validity and integrity of the trial (Chang 2007). The adaptation can be based internal or external information to the trial.

The purposes of adaptive design trials are to increase the probability of success, reduce the cost and the time to market, and deliver the right drug to the right patient.

1.4.4   New Drug Application

According to the FDA, the regulation and control of new drugs in the United States has been based on the New Drug Application (NDA). Since 1938, every new drug has been the subject of an approved NDA before U.S. commercialization. The NDA application is the vehicle through which drug sponsors formally propose that the FDA approve a new pharmaceutical for sale and marketing in the U.S. The data gathered during the animal studies and human clinical trials of an Investigational New Drug (IND) become part of the NDA.

The goals of the NDA are to provide enough information to permit the FDA review team to reach the following key decisions:

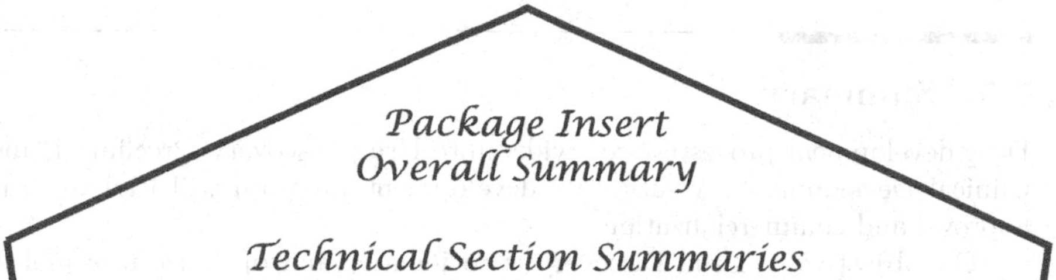

Package Insert
Overall Summary

Technical Section Summaries
Integrated Efficacy Summary
Integrated Safety Summary

Technical Section
Chemistry, Manufacture, and Control (CMC)
Preclinical Pharmacology Toxicology
Microbiology (if appripriate)
Human Pharmacokinetics and Bioavaribility

Row Data
Case Report Form
Case Report Form Tabulation

FIGURE 1.4
A Simplified View of the NDA.

- Whether the drug is safe and effective in its proposed use(s), and whether the benefits of the drug outweigh the risks.

- Whether the drug's proposed labeling (package insert) is appropriate, and what it should contain.

- Whether the methods used in manufacturing the drug and the controls used to maintain the drug's quality are adequate to preserve the drug's identity, strength, quality, and purity.

The documentation required in an NDA is supposed to tell the drug's whole story, including what happened during the clinical tests, what the ingredients of the drug are, the results of the animal studies, how the drug behaves in the body, and how it is manufactured, processed and packaged. The following resources (Figure 1.4) provide summaries on NDA content, format, and classification, plus the NDA review process:

1.5   Summary

Drug development processes are divided into Drug Discovery, Preclinical, and Clinical Development. A successful development program will lead to drug approval and commercialization.

The objective of Drug Discovery is to identify and optimize new molecular entities. There are the traditional irrational approaches or the rational approaches. Pharmaceutical and biotech companies increasingly are transitioning away from irrational approaches into rational approaches thanks to the advancement in genomics, molecular and system biology, computational chemistry, and bioinformatics in general.

When a leading compound is identified and confirmed, further in vitro, ex-vivo, and in vivo tests of the NCE will be conducted in the Preclinical phase to optimize the properties. Preclinical research includes pharmacology, toxicology, pharmacokinetics, and pharmacodynamics studies. Pharmacokinetics is the study of drug absorption, distribution, metabolism, and excretion (AMDE). Pharmacodynamics is the study of the biochemical and physiological effects of drugs on the body. In layman's terms, pharmacokinetics is the study of what the body does to the drug, whereas pharmacodynamics is the study of what a drug does to the body. Toxicological studies explore the adverse functional and morphological effects of the drug, including the mode, site and degree of action, dose relationship, sex differences, latency and progression, and reversibility of these effects.

Clinical Development traditionally includes phase I to Phase IV clinical trials. Clinical trials are experiments of the test drug conducted on human subjects in accordance with Good Clinical Practice (GCP) guidances and regulations. Phase I trials are usually conducted on a small group healthy volunteers. The objectives of a phase I trial are typically to assess the safety, tolerability, pharmacokinetics, and pharmacodynamics of a drug in humans. Successful Phase I trials will lead to a further test of the NCE in a Phase II trial with an increased sample-size to further define the safety profile, preliminary efficacy, and optimal dose range, and to mitigate risks of investing an ineffective NCE in a large scale. If the Phase II results show the test drug is safe and efficacious enough to warrant for further study. Phase III trials are launched with the objective of providing definitive trial data regarding the safety and efficacy for the target indication. The size of the populations in the trials or sample-size should be sufficiently large so that there are adequate probabilities (power) to demonstrate statistical significance if the test drug in fact is effective. Successful Phase III trials lead ultimately to approval and commercialization of the drug. However, a Phase IV trial may sometimes be be conducted as a requirement for the conditional regulatory approval.

Bibliography

Bonate, P.L. and Howard, D. Prospective allometic scaling: Does the emperor have clothes? Journal of Clinical Pharmacology. 40:665-670, 2000.

Chang, M. (2014). Adaptive Design Theory and Implementation Using SAS and R. 2nd Edition. Chapman & Hall/CRC, Taylor & Francis. Boca Raton, FL.

DHHS (2016). ASPE ISSUE BRIEF: Observations on Trends in Prescription Drug Spending, Office of the Assistant Secretary for Planning and Evaluation (ASPE), Department of Health and Human Services, USA, March 8, 2016. https://aspe.hhs.gov/system/files/pdf/187586/Drugspending.pdf

EPR. (2009). Drug Metabolism and Pharmacokinetics – an overview. European Pharmaceutical Review, Issue 6, 2009.

Hu, T.M. and Hayton, W.L. (2001). Allometric scaling of xenobiotic clearance: Uncertainty versus universality. AAPS PharmSci 3(4) , article 29, 2001

Mahmood, I. (2000). Critique of prospective allometric scaling: Does the emperor have clothes? Journal of Clinical Pharmacology. 40:671-674, 2000.

Mordenti, J. and Chappell, W (1989): The use of interspecies scaling in toxicology. In Yacobi A, Skelly jP, Batra VK (eds), Toxicokinetic and Drug Development. New York, Pergamon.

Ng, R. (2005). Drugs, from discovery to marketing. John-Wiley.

Ritschel, W.A., Banerjee PS (1986): Physiological pharmacokinetic models: Principles, applications, limitations and outlook. Methods & Findings in Experimental & Clinical Pharmacology. 8:603-614, 1986.

Shargel, L., Wu-Pong, S., and Yu, A,B.C. (2005). Applied biopharmaceutics & pharmacokinetics. 5th Ed. The McGraw-Hill Companies. USA.

Tegart, G. (2003). Nanotechnology: The Technology for the 21st Century. The APEC Center for Technology Foresight. Bangkok, Thailand. Presented at the Second International Conference on Technology Foresight, Tokyo, Feb. 27-28, 2003.

2

Clinical Development Plan and Clinical Trial Design

2.1 Clinical Development Program

2.1.1 Unmet Medical Needs & Competitive Landscape

Introducing new or revised pharmaceutical drugs to the market requires a team effort to understand the competitive landscape and the best positioning for the new product. Pharmaceutical competitor analysis is essential, to establish key contenders, pricing and forecasted success in delivery. Assessing patients' needs and demands gives the ability to predict sales and return on clinical trials and licences, but success will only be realized if you can be a competitive market player. It is imperative to understand competition and to identify the strengths, weaknesses, opportunities, and threats (SWOT) related to your product Determining the target product profile, optimum formulation for drug, and competitive marketing and commercialization strategy are key elements of the transition from development to market. Pricing research, patient research, physician and patient segmentation, clinical trials, testing demands and assessments are all critical pieces of information to bring a new product to market (Cello Health, 2017).

Drug Profiling is undertaken to predict the efficacy, safety and toxicity at the Preclinical stage of drug development and also to explore the targeted competitive products to enhance market prospects and market penetration estimation before launching a product. A therapeutic Clinical Intelligence study can also be conducted which provides detailed information and analysis of competitive products in the development pipeline, competitive landscape of the drug and identifying the potential collaborators.

It is also critical to understand the Unmet Medical Need in the indication/therapeutic area that the product is being evaluated in. Typically, considerations in this determination include information about the disease incidence, prevalence, the impact on patients' quality of life and work productivity, the associated cost, current treatment available, and why new treatment is needed. An example of addressing Unmet Medical needs is provided by (Mittermayer, et al., 2015)

The increasing global burden of type 2 diabetes (T2D) makes this a disease of considerable concern at the individual patient level and also at the public health level given the direct health costs and indirect costs of loss of work productivity. As a country-specific example, the 2014 National Diabetes Statistics Report, released on June 10th 2014, revealed that from 2010 to 2012 the number of Americans with diabetes increased from 25.8 million to 29.1 million, and that the prevalence rate for adults aged 20 years and older increased from 11.3% to 12.3%. With regard to the pediatric population in the United States, Dabelea et al. reported that the prevalence of T2D increased from 0.34 to 0.46 per 1,000 from 2001 to 2009: when adjusted for completeness of ascertainment these figures represent a 30.5% increase. Total estimated costs of diagnosed diabetes increased 41% from 2007's figure of $174 billion to $245 billion for 2012, with $176 billion associated with direct medical costs and $69 billion with reduced productivity.

The nature of the unmet medical need for T2D is captured by the European Medicines Agency's (EMA's) 2012 guideline addressing the clinical investigation of medicinal products in the treatment or prevention of diabetes......

2.1.2 Therapeutic Areas

Knowledge of the landscape of drug development across many different therapeutic areas is important for key stakeholders and statisticians who would be involved in strategic decisions in drug development.

There are nearly 50 therapeutic areas, some cover very broad scope like oncology, whereas others may be restricted to disease areas (such as rare metabolic diseases). Information regarding approved medications in different areas, including but not limited to General Information, Clinical Results, Side Effects, Mechanism of Action, Additional Information can be found at CenterWatch (2017) and general information about medicines under evaluation in clinical trials can be found at www.clinicalTrials.gov.

FDA Approved Drugs are divided by Therapeutic Area (CenterWatch, May 3, 2017) and include as of this date Cardiology/Vascular Diseases (118 drugs), Dental and Oral Health (7 drugs), Dermatology (89), Devices (1), Endocrinology (221), Family Medicine (619), Gastroenterology (95), Genetic Disease (50), Healthy Volunteers (2), Hematology (100), Hepatology (Liver, Pancreatic, Gall Bladder) (46), Immunology (199), Infections and Infectious Diseases (179), Internal Medicine (1), Musculoskeletal (91), Nephrology (86), Neurology (168), Nutrition and Weight Loss (12), Obstetrics/Gynecology (Women's Health) (103), Oncology (206), Ophthalmology (47), Orthopedics/Orthopedic Surgery (5), Otolaryngology (Ear, Nose, Throat) (23), Pediatrics/Neonatology (112), Pharmacology/Toxicology (28), Podiatry (8), Psychiatry/Psychology (71), Pulmonary/Respiratory Diseases (123), Rheumatology (43), Sleep (3), Trauma (Emergency, Injury, Surgery) (8), Urology (46), and Vaccines (30).

One can further find the information about each drug at CenterWatch. Using Avastin as an example, the information is organized as follows:

Avastin (bevacizumab)

The following drug information is obtained from various newswires, published medical journal articles, and medical conference presentations.

Company: Genentech

Approval Status: Approved February 2004

Specific Treatments: Colorectal Cancer

Therapeutic Areas: Gastroenterology, Oncology, Family Medicine

General Information

Avastin is an anti-VEGF monoclonal antibody for the treatment of solid tumors.

Avastin, used in combination with intravenous 5-fluorouracil-based chemotherapy, is indicated for first-line treatment of patients with metastatic carcinoma of the colon or rectum.

The recommended dose of Avastin is 5 mg/kg given once every 14 days as an IV infusion until disease progression is detected.

Clinical Results

FDA approval of Avastin for colorectal cancer was based on two (STUDY 1 / STUDY 2) randomized, controlled trials in combination with intravenous 5-fluorouracil-based chemotherapy.

Study 1 was a double-blind trial enrolling 813 subjects with metastatic carcinoma of the colon or rectum. Subjects were randomized to bolus-IFL (irinotecan 125 mg/m2 IV, 5-fluorouracil 500 mg/m2 IV, and leucovorin 20 mg/m2 IV given once weekly for 4 weeks every 6 weeks) plus placebo (Arm 1), bolus-IFL plus Avastin (5 mg/kg every 2 weeks) (Arm 2) or 5-FU/LV plus Avastin (5 mg/kg every 2 weeks) (Arm 3). Among the subjects, 57% had an ECOG performance status of 0. The primary endpoint of this trial was overall survival. Results showed that the overall survival in Arms 1 & 2 was 20.3 months with Avastin compared with 15.6 months with placebo. The median progression-free survival was 10.6 months with Avastin compared with 6.4 months with placebo. Data showed that the median overall survival in Arm 3 was 18.3 months, median progression-free survival was 8.8 months, overall response rate was 39%, and median duration of response was 8.5 months.

Study 2 tested Avastin in combination with 5-FU/LV and enrolled as first-line treatment of metastatic colorectal cancer. Subjects were randomized to receive 5-FU/LV (5-fluorouracil 500 mg/m2, leucovorin 500 mg/m2 weekly for 6 weeks every 8 weeks) or 5-FU/LV plus Avastin (5 mg/kg every 2 weeks) or 5-FU/LV plus Avastin (10 mg/kg every 2 weeks). The primary endpoints of the trial were objective response rate and progression-free survival. Results showed that progression-free survival was significantly better in subjects receiving 5-FU/LV plus Avastin at 5 mg/kg when compared to those not receiving Avastin. However, overall survival and overall response rate were not significantly different. Results for subjects receiving 5-FU/LV plus Avastin at 10 mg/kg were not significantly different than without Avastin.

Side Effects

Adverse events associated with the use of Avastin may include (but are not limited to) the following: Asthenia, Abdominal Pain, Pain, Deep Vein Thrombosis, Hypertension, Intra-Abdominal Thrombosis, Syncope, Diarrhea, Constipation, Leukopenia, and Neutropenia

Mechanism of Action

Bevacizumab binds VEGF and prevents the interaction of VEGF to its receptors (Flt-1 and KDR) on the surface of endothelial cells. The interaction of VEGF with its receptors leads to endothelial cell proliferation and new blood vessel formation in in vitro models of angiogenesis.

In preclinical studies, administration of bevacizumab to xenotransplant models of colon cancer in nude mice caused reduction of microvascular growth and inhibition of metastatic disease progression. In January 2000, preclinical results showed that bevacizumab was more effective at preventing growth of tumor cell lines in animal models when it was combined with sub-threshold doses of cisplatin or trastuzumab.

The websites for obtaining further information about the drug are provided. You can also find information regarding competitive intelligence and current on-going trial information and search information from the large collection of trial information included in this database. Another source of information you can use is BiomedTracker, Informa.

2.1.3   Value proposition

Determining the value proposition is not the same as the providing the evidence to support/prove the efficacy or safety of the drug or the proposed scientific hypothesis about the mechanism of action. The following four questions are often considered in the European healthcare system when determining the value proposition of a drug (noting these questions are also applicable irrespective of region) . First, does it work? This is a holistic assessment of the benefits/risk ratio of a drug at launch with continued assessment over time. Second, does it add value to society? That is, the efficiency of the healthcare system improved by addressing a given unmet medical need. Third, is it a reasonable cost to the public? Finally, is it the best way of delivering the service? All those need to be addressed in a value proposition (social.eyeforpharma.com, 2017).

Historically, value in healthcare and determination of pricing was focused on individual patient outcome related to performance of a particular drug. Recently, people have voiced that value proposition needs to be addressed

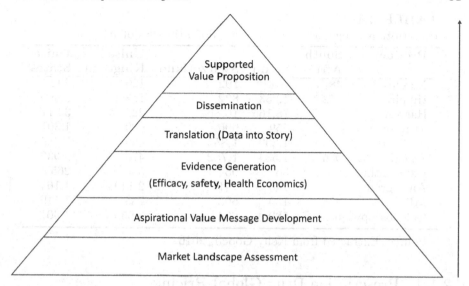

FIGURE 2.1
Supported Value Proposition.

on a community level, with evidence showing how a product will impact the overall health care system and impact on society as a whole. It is also the case that payer demand for post-approval evidence is on the rise. What's needed is the development of formal relationships with regulators, payers, and Health Technology Assessments to establish common evidence requirements, with an increasingly broad and sensitive post-market detection of adverse events. HTA is a systematic process which evaluates on a broad scale the economic, organizational, social and ethical issues associated with the use of a health intervention or health technology.

Opportunities for new indications for drugs need to be continuously reevaluated throughout the discovery, development, and life-cycle management of a compound. Optimizing the value proposition involves several components: drug branding, distribution channels of prescription drugs, source of payment for pharmaceuticals, global pricing policy, etc. Even if one is not seated in the commercial group, basic knowledge about sources for value proposition is informative in the optimization of the drug development program. It is equally important to generate data that payers will want to see in order to reimburse the drug as it is to meet requirements for approval. The pharmaceutical industry is moving from the traditional value proposition to a so-called supported value proposition (Figure 2.1).

TABLE 2.1

Prescription Drug Costs Around the Globe (in US dollar).

Product	South Africa	Spain	Switzerland	United Kingdom	United States
Xarelto	48	101	102	126	292
Humira	552	1,253	822	1,362	2,669
Harvoni		18,165	16,861	22,554	32,114
Truvada		559	906	689	1,301
Tecfidera		1,399	1,855	663	5,089
Avastin	956	1,534	1,752	470	3,930
OxyContin	84	36	95	590	265
Angiogram		240	191	2,149	1,164
MRI	455	130	503	788	1,119
Colonoscopy	632	589	604	3,059	1,301

Source: Extracted from Kelly Gooch, 2016

2.1.4 Prescription Drug Global Pricing

Knowing prescription drug global pricing policy and dynamics is important to drug developers in their decision-making whether to develop the drug for local marketing or global marketing. The challenge to policymakers in the United States and abroad is to ensure that residents have appropriate access to drugs and that drug manufacturers have adequate incentive to continue developing important products (AARP, 2006). The International Federation of Health Plans has released its 2015 Comparative Price Report, highlighting the variation in healthcare prices around the world. The report examines the price of medical procedures, tests, scans and treatments in different countries (Table 2.1).

The data for the report was gathered from participating iFHP member organizations in each country. Prices for the United States came from more than 370 million medical claims and more than 170 million pharmacy claims that reflect prices negotiated and paid to healthcare providers.

WHO reported in 2016: Medicines account for 20–60% of health spending in low- and middle-income countries, compared with 18% in countries of the Organization for Economic Cooperation and Development. Up to 90% of the population in developing countries purchase medicines through out-of-pocket payments, making medicines the largest family expenditure item after food. As a result, medicines, particularly those with higher costs, may be unaffordable for large sections of the global population and are a major burden on government budgets. The Millennium Development Goals include the target: "[I]n cooperation with pharmaceutical companies, provide access to affordable, essential drugs in developing countries."

To study how the price policy affects drug development in a nation and different drug policies affect drug development in the world under economic globalization, it is relevant to review the analysis from the document "Prescription Drug Prices in Canada, Europe, and Japan - Prepared by Minority Staff Special Investigations Division Committee on Government Reform U.S. House of Representatives" (oversight.house.gov, 2017):

The United States is unique among industrialized countries because it is the only country that fails to protect its citizens from discriminatory pricing of prescription drugs. Canada, France, Italy, Germany, Japan, and the United Kingdom all negotiate on behalf of their citizens to obtain lower prices for brand name drugs. As a result, purchasers in these countries pay significantly less for prescription drugs than uninsured senior citizens in the United States.

Drug Pricing in Canada

In Canada, the Patent Medicine Prices Review Board establishes and enforces guidelines that determine the maximum prices at which manufacturers can sell brand name drugs. Under these guidelines, the introductory prices of "breakthrough" drugs must not exceed the median of the prices of the drugs in other industrialized countries. Prices of patented drugs that do not provide a significant breakthrough in treating diseases must not exceed the maximum price of other drugs that treat the same disease. Once the introductory price is established, subsequent price increases are limited to changes in the Consumer Price Index. The Canadian pricing system results in brand name drug prices that are an average of 38% lower than prices in the United States.

Drug Pricing in Germany

Germany has a decentralized national health care system, with coverage provided by over 700 insurance funds. With the exception of innovative drugs that have been patented since 1996, pricing is determined by a reference system, with prices for new drugs based upon the prices of existing drugs that provide the same therapeutic benefit. Prices for innovative drugs that were patented after 1995 are not restricted by the government. However, each individual insurance fund can negotiate with pharmaceutical manufacturers on behalf of their covered patients. The German pricing system results in brand name drug prices that are an average of 35% lower than prices in the United States.

Drug Pricing in the United Kingdom

The National Health Service in the United Kingdom differs from national healthcare providers in other countries because it does not negotiate the prices of individual drugs with manufacturers. Instead, drug companies in the United Kingdom are free to establish their own prices for individual drugs. However, under the country's pharmaceutical laws, the maximum profit that drug manufacturers can earn on sales in the United Kingdom is limited. Companies that set their prices so high that they exceed maximum allowable profit rates must reimburse the government. Allowable profits are based on several factors, including the company's investments in the United Kingdom and the level of long-term risk. Generally, companies are allowed to earn returns of 17% - 21% on capital investments. The pricing system in the United Kingdom results in brand name drug prices that are an average of 31% lower than prices in the United States.

Drug Pricing in Japan

Japan, like other industrialized countries, has a national health care system. The prices paid by this health care system are generally determined via a reference system. Prices for new drugs are determined by comparing them with similar drugs that are already on the market. Prices are based upon the safety and effectiveness of the drug; drugs that are shown to be more effective or innovative than existing drugs are priced higher. If there is no comparable drug on the market, the price of the drug is determined by factors such as manufacturing cost and the price of the drug in other countries.

Price structure of branded drugs is the key determinant of profitability for pharmaceutical companies. How to maximize the profit within the time period of patent protection (e.g., 12 years — typically an innovative drug has 20 years of patent protection in the US, however it generally takes on average approximately 8 years after the patent is filed to advance the drug to market by determining an appropriate international price structure for a brand drug is of great interest to pharmaceutical manufacturers. An unreasonably high drug price beyond consumer's affordability is not desired, and there is a tremendous (and increasing) amount of pressure being placed on pharmaceutical companies to ensure fair pricing. On the other hand, disproportionately low pricing in an ex-US country relative to the price in US may lead to drug importation into to the US at these lower prices, i.e., the so-called reimportation or parallel trade.

Exclusivity was designed to promote a balance between new drug innovation and greater public access to drugs that result from generic drug competition (FDA, 2017a). Patents and exclusivity work in a similar fashion but are distinct from one another and governed by different statutes. Exclusivity refers to certain delays and prohibitions on approval of competitor drugs available under the statute that attach upon approval of a drug or of certain supplements. A new drug application (NDA) or abbreviated new drug application (ANDA) holder is eligible for exclusivity if statutory requirements are met (see 21 C.F.R. 314.108). The exclusivity period depends on what type of exclusivity is at issue: 7 years for Orphan Drug Exclusivity (ODE), 5 years for New Chemical Entity Exclusivity (NCE) and Generating Antibiotic Incentives Now (GAIN) Exclusivity, and 3 years for New Clinical Investigation Exclusivity.

There are also legal complications of drug marketing. Compulsory licenses are licensees that are granted by a government to use patents, copyrighted works or other types of intellectual property. Compulsory licenses are an essential government instrument to intervene in the market and limit patent and other intellectual property rights (IPRs) in order to correct market failures. As concerns public health and compulsory licensing, the restrictions imposed by the IPRs system on access to (patented) drugs must be reasonable, not creating situations where entire populations are denied access to known therapies. Therefore, the 1994 WTO TRIPs Agreement contains provisions on safeguards, exceptions and mechanisms to protect essential public health interests. The TRIPS provides for compulsory licenses of patents, but also provides a number of restrictions on the use of compulsory licenses.

The propriety of parallel trade is a matter of intense policy debate in a number of countries and in the World Trade Organization (WTO). At present, WTO provisions allow member countries to establish their own rules for the "exhaustion" of intellectual property rights (IPR). If a country opts for national exhaustion of IPR, a rights holder there may exclude parallel imports, because intellectual property rights continue until such a time as a protected product is first sold in that market. If a country instead chooses international exhaustion of IPR, parallel imports cannot be blocked, because the rights of the patent, copyright, or trademark holder expire when a protected product is sold anywhere in the world. The United States practices national exhaustion for patents and copyrights, but permits parallel imports of trademarked goods unless the trademark owner can show that the imports are of different quality from goods sold locally or otherwise might cause confusion for consumers. The European Union provides for regional exhaustion of IPR whereby goods circulate freely within the trading bloc but parallel imports are banned from nonmember countries. Japanese commercial law permits parallel imports except when such trade is explicitly excluded by contract provisions or when the original sale is made subject to foreign price controls (Grossman and Lai, 2009).

2.1.5 Clinical Development Plan

Before individual clinical trials are designed, it is important to consider the goals of the overall development program and pull together a comprehensive clinical development plan (CDP). The CDP is a critical document in the clinical development of a drug candidate.

A CDP is a bridge between the purely strategic asset management planning process on the one hand, and, on the other, the highly tactical scientific and operational realms of the clinical trial process. Its creation is generally spearheaded by the clinical research department, which then becomes accountable for its execution. Clinical research professionals are responsible for ensuring that every protocol contributes to the body of knowledge specified by the CDP, and that the resulting data are expressed and communicated in a way

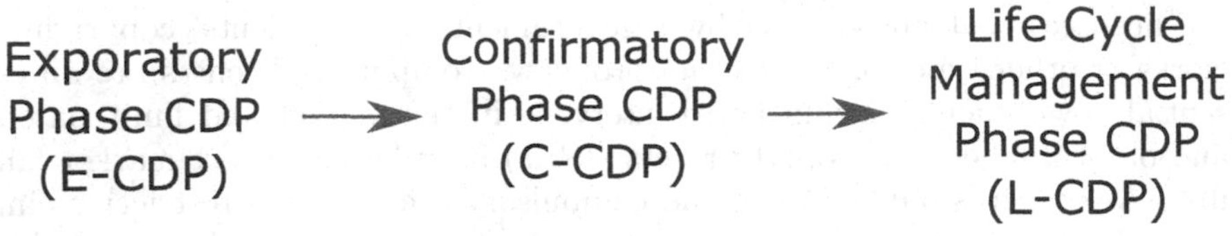

Exporatory Phase CDP (E-CDP) ⟶ Confirmatory Phase CDP (C-CDP) ⟶ Life Cycle Management Phase CDP (L-CDP)

FIGURE 2.2
Stages of Clinical Development Plan.

that allows corporate decision makers to act upon them accordingly (Namrata Bahadur, 2008).

The vision is transformed into distinct implementation phases and discrete steps, involving a series of clinical studies, each with well-defined milestones and deliverables (Namrata Bahadur, 2008)

The stages of Clinical Development Plan typically involve exploratory, confirmatory, and life cycle management phases (Figure 2.2). Different stakeholders may be involved at different stages of CDP. For small biotech companies, the stages of CDP are often combined to the extent possible to maximize efficiency and limit overall cost of the development program.

The CDP strategically outlines and documents the key goals metrics to assess performance, pathways of communication, and parties responsible for decision-making. The CDP requires a multidisciplinary, aspirational, innovative, and collaborative approach, while also providing the conceptual framework for the entire clinical trials program relating to the compound under investigation.

The CDP lays out a logical sequence of the scientific rationale, the commercial rationale, and the clinical trial plan that should be conducted to generate the information necessary to support the drug label claims. Only if the perspectives of all relevant disciplines are integrated into the development plan can the project truly reflect corporate goals (Namrata Bahadur, 2008). Key Components of the Clinical Development Plan may include:

1. Scientific Rationale for Development

2. Commercial Rationale for Development

3. High level Clinical Trials Design

4. Regulatory Considerations

5. Strategic Planning with Milestones

Undoubtedly, every program will experience unanticipated results and meet unexpected hurdles during its lifetime. In order to mitigate these inevitable risks and obstacles, an inclusive planning process should be undertaken to create a consensus across the organization regarding the project's

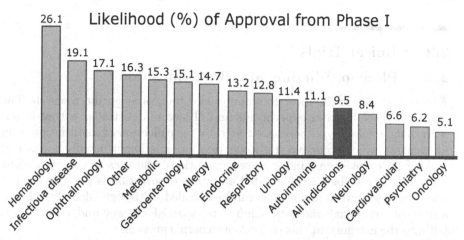

FIGURE 2.3
Likelihood of approval from Phase I (Source: BIO et al, 2016).

ultimate goals and criteria for success. The company has to evaluate their core competencies against their goals and have sensible risk mitigation plans. Of particular interest to statisticians involved in formulating the CDP, adaptive trial designs (as an example of one methodology) have recently been developed with goals to reduce both time to market and patient resources required, increase the probability of success, and deliver the right dose(s) of drug to the right patients at the right time.

Despite the significant efforts by the pharmaceutical industry, the overall success rate of bringing a drug to market is low. A recent large survey conducted by Biotechnology Innovation Organization (BIO), BiomedTracker, and AMPLION shows that the success rates from Phase 1 to drug approval ranges from 5% (oncology) to 20% (hematology) for various disease indications (Figure 2.3).

The probability of success of a clinical development program is dependent on the drug candidate, the CDP strategy and particular design of trials in each phase. As the design of both individual trials and the "collective" trials included in the CDP are the key determinant of overall success (both for approval and commercialization) of the product, it is important to examine the key elements of clinical trials (highlighting statistical considerations). Optimization of clinical development program will be discussed in the next chapter.

2.2   Clinical Trials

2.2.1   Placebo, Blinding and Randomization

Experimentation is the most commonly used tool for scientific research. The main difference between experiments and observational studies is that in observational studies hypotheses are tested by the collection of information from phenomena which occur naturally, whereas an experiment usually consists of making an event occur under known conditions where as many extraneous influences as possible are eliminated and close observation is possible so that relationships between phenomena can be revealed. Although clinical trials can also be observational, the data required to establish efficacy and safety would fall into the category in this context of experimentation.

There are three important statistical concepts in Clinical Trials: randomization, control, and blinding, which are related to the issues of confounding, placebo effect, and bias.

A *placebo* is a substance or procedure that is objectively without specific activity for the condition being treated. In medical experiments, a placebo can be pills, creams, inhalants, and injections that do not involve any active ingredients. Sham surgery, ultrasound, sham electrodes implanted in the brain, and sham acupuncture are also other examples that can all be used as placebos depending on the specific intervention under study. The placebo effect is related to the perceptions and expectations of the patient. If the substance is viewed as helpful, it can heal, but, if it is viewed as harmful, it can cause negative effects, which is known as the *nocebo effect*. Placebo effects are generally more significant in subjective measurements, such as with patient-reported outcomes, than in objective laboratory measurements such as a laboratory test (e.g., hemoglobin level) or imaging study (e.g., CT/MRI scan).

The placebo effect has been clearly established as a "real" phenomenon that needs to be accounted for in any CDP. An important task is to obtain the "true" treatment effect from the total effect by subtracting the placebo effect from the effect of the intervention. This can be done in an experiment with two groups in a clinical trial, one group treated with the test drug and the other treated with a placebo. More generally, the placebo group can be replaced with any treatment group (reference group) for comparison. Such a general group is called the control or control group. By subtracting the effect in the placebo group from the test group, we can tell the "pure" effect of the drug candidate. However, such a simple consideration of ascertaining the pure treatment effect is not appropriate because knowledge of which treatment a patient is assigned to can lead to subjective and judgmental bias by the patients and investigators. For example, patients who know they are taking a placebo may have the nocebo effect and those who are aware that they are taking the test drug may have over-reported the response. To avoid such bias, we can implement another experimental technique, called blinding.

Blinding can be imposed on the investigator, the experimental subjects, the sponsor who finances the experiment, or any combination of these participants. In a single-blind experiment, the individual subjects do not know whether they have been assigned to the experimental group or the control group. *Single-blind* experimental design is used where the experimenters must know the treatment that the patients have been randomized to (for example, when comparing sham to real surgery). However, there is a risk that subjects are influenced by interaction with the experimenter—known as the experimenter's bias. In *double-blind* experiments, both the investigator and experimental subjects have no knowledge of the group to which they are assigned. A double-blind study is usually better than a single-blind study in terms of bias reduction. In a *triple-blind* experiment, the patient, investigator, and sponsor are all blinded from the treatment group.

Randomization is a procedure to assign subjects or experimental units to a certain intervention based on an allocation probability, rather than by choice. The utilization of randomization in an experiment minimizes selection bias, balancing both known and unknown confounding factors, in the assignment of treatments (e.g., placebo and drug candidate).

Internal and external validities are also important in scientific experiments. *Internal validity* is concerned with correctly concluding that an independent variable is, in fact, responsible for variation in the dependent variable. *External validity* is concerned with the generalizability of research findings to and across populations of subjects and settings.

2.2.2 Trial Design Type

In terms of the structure or layout, experiments can be categorized into several diverse types, including: parallel, crossover, cluster, factorial, and titration trials.

In a *parallel-group design*, each participant is (usually randomly) assigned to a group to receive a specific intervention (e.g., taking the test drug or placebo). Subjects assigned to different groups will receive different interventions, e.g., different drugs or the same drug with different doses or dose schedules. A parallel design can be two or more treatment groups with one control group. Parallel designs are commonly used in clinical trials because they are simple, universally accepted, and most often applicable to both acute and chronic conditions.

Unlike a parallel-group design, in a *crossover design*, each participant is assigned (most often, at random) to a group to receive a sequence of interventions over time. Subjects assigned to a different group will receive a different sequence of interventions. There are different crossover designs, the 2 × 2 crossover design being most commonly used. In a 2 × 2 design, one group of patients first receive the treatment followed by placebo, and the other group of patients receive the placebo first, followed by the treatment.

A crossover study has two advantages: (1) a smaller sample size compared with a parallel design because in crossover design each subject serves his own reference to reduce the varibility and (2) a reduced influence of confounders because each crossover patient serves as his or her own control. There are four different effects we should be aware of: treatment, sequence, carryover, and period effects.

The *sequence effect* refers to the fact that the order in which treatments are administered may affect the outcome. An example might be that a drug with many adverse effects is given first, making patients taking a second, less harmful medicine more sensitive to any adverse effect.

The *carryover effect* between treatments refers to the situation in which the effect of treatment in the first period carries over to the second period, which confounds the estimates of the treatment effects. In practice, carryover effects can be reduced or eliminated by using a sufficiently long "wash-out" period between treatments. A typical washout period is no less than five times of the so-called half-life, the time at which the drug concentration reduces to $1/2$ of the maximum concentration in the blood.

The *period effect* refers to the situation when the same drug given at different time/period will have different effect. A period effect may exist if, e.g., period one is always in the morning or at one clinic and period two is always in the afternoon or at another clinic or home.

In a *cluster randomization trial*, pre-existing groups of participants (e.g., villages, schools) are randomly selected to receive an intervention. A cluster randomized controlled trial is a type of randomized controlled trial in which groups of subjects (as opposed to individual subjects) are randomized. Cluster randomized controlled trials are also known as *group-randomized trials*, and *place-randomized trials*.

In a *factorial design,* two or more treatments are evaluated simultaneously through the use of varying combinations of the treatments (interventions). The simplest example is the 2×2 factorial design in which subjects are randomly allocated to one of the four possible combinations of two treatments (e.g., A and B): A alone; B alone; both A and B; neither A nor B. In many cases this design is used for the specific purpose of examining the interaction of A and B. If the number of combinations in a full factorial design is too high to be logistically feasible, a fractional factorial design may be done, in which some of the possible combinations (usually at least half) are omitted.

In a *titration* or *dose-escalation* design, the dose increases over time until reaching the desired level or maximum tolerable level for that patient. There are many other designs we have not discussed here.

A recent study shows that among all clinical trials, 78% were parallel-group trials, 16% were crossover, 2% were cluster, and 2% were factorial, and 2% were others.

2.2.3 Confounding Factors

In statistics, a *confounding factor* (also *confounder, hidden variable,* or *lurking variable*) is an extraneous variable that correlates, positively or negatively, with both the dependent variable and the independent variable. Such a relationship between two observed variables is termed a spurious relationship.

A classic example of confounding is to interpret the finding that people who carry matches are more likely to develop lung cancer as evidence of an association between carrying matches and lung cancer. Carrying a match or not is a confounding factor in this relationship: smokers are more likely to carry matches and they are also more likely to develop lung cancer. However, if "carrying matches" is replaced with "drinking coffee", we may easily conclude that coffee more likely causes cancer.

For a variable to be a confounder in a clinical trial it must satisfy three conditions:

1. It must be associated with the treatment (the main factor).

2. It must be a predictor (not necessarily a cause) of the outcome being measured.

3. It must not be a consequence of the treatment (the main factor) itself.

A factor is not a confounder if it lies somewhere on the causal pathway between the variables of interest. Such a factor can be a surrogate or direct cause. For example, the relationship between diet and coronary heart disease may be explained at least in part by measuring serum cholesterol levels. Cholesterol is a surrogate, but not a confounder because it may be the causal link between diet and coronary heart disease. In lung cancer caused by smoking cigarettes, the carcinogens in the cigarette are the direct cause of the cancer.

Bias creates an association that is not true, while confounding describes an association that is true, but potentially misleading. Confounders are usually more of a problem in observational studies, where the exposure of a risk factor is not randomly distributed between groups. In evaluating treatment effects from observational data, prognostic factors may influence treatment decisions, producing the so-called confounding-by-indication bias. Controlling for known prognostic factors using randomization can reduce such a bias, but it is always possible that unknown confounding factors were not balanced even when a randomization procedure is used.

In a clinical trial, some adverse reactions (ARs) may occur randomly and depend on the length of the follow-up period. The longer the follow-up is, the more ARs one is likely to see. When two drugs in evaluation have different dose schedules (e.g., one is given in a week, the other is given in two weeks), it may lead to a different observational period and/or frequency for ARs, and artificially make one drug appear to be safer than the other, even if in fact they have a similar safety profile. Likewise, consider the case when drug effectiveness is measured by the maximum response during the treatment period. If two drugs in evaluation, one given once a week, the other given 5 times a week, have their effects on patients measured in clinic each day the drug is administered, the difference in observational frequency can create an artificial treatment difference simply because drug effects include a random component, so that more frequent measurements of response are more likely to capture a maximum value.

To control confounding in an experiment design, we can use randomization, or stratified randomization. The latter will provide a better balance of confounders between intervention groups, and confounding can be further reduced by using appropriate statistical analyses such as the analysis of covariance.

2.2.4   Variability and Bias

Variations can come from different sources. *Variability within an individual* is the variation in the measures of a subject's characteristics over time. *Variability between individuals* concerns the variation from subject to subject. Instrumental variability is related to the precision of the measurement tool. Other variabilities can be attributed to the difference in experimenter or other factors.

Variability in measurements can be either random or systematic. By increasing sample size, we can reduce the variability or increase the precision of the estimations such as treatment effect. *Bias* is a systematic error in a study that leads to a distortion of the results (Figure 2.4). Human perception occurs by a complex, unconscious process of abstraction, in which certain details of the incoming sense data are noticed and remembered, and the rest forgotten. What is kept and what is thrown away depends on an internal model or representation of the world that is built up over our entire lives.

There are other sources of bias, such as selection bias, ascertainment or confirmation bias, and publication bias.

Selection bias refers to a subject selection process or sampling procedure that likely produces a sample not representative of the population, or produces samples that result in systematical (probabilistic) imbalance of confounding variables between comparison groups.

For instance, a student is conducting an experiment to test a chemical compound's effect on mice. He knows that inclusion of a (placebo) control and randomization are important, so he randomly catches a half of the mice from the cage and administers the test compound. After days of observations, he finds that the test compound has a negative effect on mice. However, he might overlook an important fact: the mice he caught were mostly physically weaker and thus they were easily caught. Such selection bias can also be seen in the capture-recapture method due to physical differences in animals.

Another example would be the following: A clinical trial investigator might use her knowledge to assign treatments to different patients, say, sicker patients go to the new treatment group and less sick patients to the control group. Such a treatment assignment procedure may exaggerate or understate

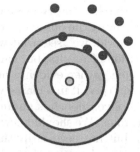 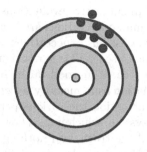

Large Bias, Large Variability   Large Bias, Small Variability

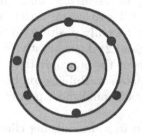 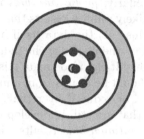

Small Bias, Large Variability   Small Bias, Small Variability

Bias Versus Variability in Shooting A Target

FIGURE 2.4
Variability versus Bias in Shooting A Target.

the treatment difference. Selection bias can occur in surveys too. For instance, in an Internet survey, selection bias could be caused by Internet accessibility or by the differences in familiarity with computer. Randomization can reduce bias but cannot completely prevent it, especially when there are a larger number of potential confounding factors.

Confirmation bias is a tendency of people to favor information that confirms their beliefs or hypotheses. Confirmation bias is best illustrated using examples in clinical trials. When knowledge of the treatment assignment can affect the objective evaluation of treatment effect and lead to systematic distortion of the trial conclusions, we have what is referred to as observer or ascertainment bias.

A patients' knowledge that he is receiving a new treatment may substantially affect the way he feels and his subjective assessment. If a physician is aware of which treatment the patient is receiving, this can affect the way he collects the information during the trial and influence the way the assessor analyzes the study results. Confirmation Bias happens more often and is more severe in subjective evaluations than in "objective laboratory evaluations."

Human observations are biased toward confirming the observer's conscious and unconscious expectations and view of the world; we "see what we expect or want to see". This is not deliberate falsification of results, but can happen to researchers in good faith. As a result, people gather evidence and recall information from memory selectively, and can interpret it in a biased way. How much attention the various perceived data are given depends on an internal value system, which judges how important it is to us. We should know that one can tell the truth, and nothing but the truth, but not necessarily the "whole truth". For example, one might only talk about the things on the positive side of the ledger.

Similarly, *publication bias* is the tendency of researchers and journals to more likely publish results that appear positive. There are (at least) two issues with this – 1) the data itself may or may not be truly positive (to be determined by the merits of the individual study), and 2) if the negative data isn't published it can also create misperceptions about the appropriate conclusions that should be drawn from a more complete data set. Publication bias can be avoided or reduced by r that all relevant data is published, particularly for drugs that are still in development.

Operational bias results when information from an ongoing clinical trial causes changes to the participant pool, investigator behavior or other clinical aspects that affect the conduct of the trial in such a way that conclusions about important efficacy or safety parameters are biased.

Missing observations or *incomplete data* can also cause bias in data analysis, especially when the missing mechanism is not random. Consider, for example, that in clinical trials, missing data often results from patients' early termination, due to ineffectiveness of the treatment or to safety issues. Missing data can distort data and make statistical analysis difficult. When encountering missing data, or patients' noncompliance to the study protocol (e.g. a patient who takes too little or too much of a drug), the experimenter may choose to exclude some data. Such subjective exclusion of data can also introduce bias.

Model selection can introduce bias too. People tend to select a simpler model even when a complicated model explains things a little better. The selection of a simpler model can be made in the name of Parsimony or mathematical simplicity. This could lead to a special type of bias—Parsimony or *model selection bias*.

There are other sources of bias. For instance, when multiple screenings are used to qualify subjects for an experiment, bias can be introduced because the qualifying screening value may just happen to be lower than it should be and after subjects are entered in the study, the value can come back to the natural status without any intervention. Such a phenomenon is called *regression to the mean*. Such bias can be removed by adding a control group and randomization.

In statistics, the bias of an estimator for a parameter is the difference between the estimator's expected value and the true value of the parameter being estimated. It is a common practice for a frequentist statistician to look for the minimum unbiased estimator. However, it is not always feasible to do so, and unbiased estimators may even exist. Therefore, we have to balance between variability and bias.

2.2.5 Randomization Procedure

Randomization is a procedure to assign subjects or experimental units to a certain intervention based on an allocation probability, rather than by choice. For example, in a clinical trial, patients can be assigned one of two treatments available with an equal chance (probability 0.5) when they are enrolled in the trial.

The utilization of randomization in an experiment minimizes selection bias, balancing both known and unknown confounding factors, in the assignment of treatments (e.g., placebo and drug candidate). In a clinical trial, appropriate use of the randomization procedure not only ensures an unbiased and fair assessment regarding the efficacy and safety of the test drug, but also improves the quality of the experiments and increase the efficiency of the trial. Bise caused the imbalance of measured confounders may be reduced using an appropriate statistical model with covariate-adjustment, but such an imbalance will reduce the efficiency of model.

Randomization procedures that are commonly employed in clinical trials can be classified into two categories: conventional randomization and adaptive randomization.

Conventional randomization refers to any randomization procedures with a constant treatment allocation probability. Commonly used conventional randomization procedures include simple (or complete) randomization, stratified randomization, cluster randomization, and block randomization.

A *simple randomization* is a procedure that assigns a subject to an experimental group with a fixed probability. Such a randomization probability can be different for different groups, but the sum of the randomization probabilities should be one. For example, in a clinical trial, patients can be assigned to one of two experiment groups with probability 0.5. Such a trial is said to have balanced design because the sample sizes (number of subjects) in the two groups are expected to be the same. Practically, it is also common to have an unbalanced design in which patients are randomized, e.g., in 2:1 ratio to the test and placebo groups in order to have the maximum exposure to the test drug for a given sample size.

Like simple randomization, a *stratified randomization* is a randomization with a fixed allocation probability. When there are important known covariates (confounding factors), stratified randomization is usually recommended to reduce treatment imbalances. For a stratified randomization, the target population is divided into several homogenous strata, which are usually determined by some combinations of covariates (e.g., patient demographics or patient characteristics). In each stratum, a simple randomization is then employed.

Cluster randomization is another conventional randomization. In certain trials, the appropriate unit of randomization may be some aggregate of individuals. This form of randomization is known as cluster randomization or group randomization. Cluster randomization is employed by necessity in trials in which the intervention is by nature designed to be applied at the cluster level such as with community-based interventions.

In practice, conventional randomization procedures could result in severe imbalance in the sample size or in confounding factors between treatment groups at some time point during the trial. When there is a time-dependent heterogeneous covariance that relates to treatment responses, it could induce a bias in the results. A *block randomization* is used to reduce the imbalance over time in treatment assignments, which may occur when a simple randomization is used. In block randomization, the allocation probability is a fixed constant before either of the two treatment groups reaches its target number. However, after the target number is reached in one of the two treatment groups, all future patients in the trial will be assigned to the other treatment group.

Adaptive randomization is a randomization technique in which the allocation of patients to treatment groups is based on the observed treatment effect: The treatment group showing a larger effect will have a larger probability of assigning newly enrolled subjects. In this way, the probability of a new subject being assigned the better treatment will gradually increase. A commonly used response-adaptive randomization is the so-called randomly-play-the-winner (Chang 2014).

In the RPW model, it is assumed that the previous subject's outcome will be available before the next patient is randomized. At the start of the clinical trial, an urn contains a_0 balls representing treatment A and b_0 balls representing treatment B, where a_0 and b_0 are positive integers. We denote these balls as either type A or type B balls. When a subject is recruited, a ball is drawn and replaced. If it is a type A ball, the subject receives treatment A; if it is a type B ball, the subject receives treatment B. When a subject's outcome is available, the urn is updated as follows: A success on treatment A (B) or a failure on treatment B (A) will generate an additional a_1 (b_1) type-B balls in the urn. In this way, the urn builds up more balls representing the more successful treatment (Figure 2.5).

Theoretically, adaptive randomization can cause the so-called accrual bias, whereby volunteers may try to be recruited later in the study to take advantage of the benefit from previous outcomes. Earlier enrolled subjects have higher probabilities of receiving the inferior treatment than later enrolled subjects.

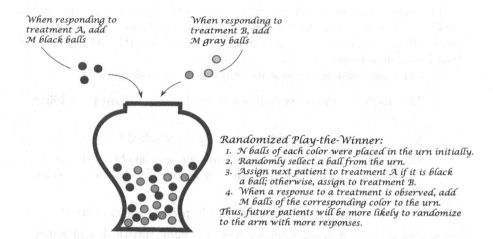

When responding to treatment A, add M black balls

When responding to treatment B, add M gray balls

Randomized Play-the-Winner:
1. *N balls of each color were placed in the urn initially.*
2. *Randomly sellect a ball from the urn.*
3. *Assign next patient to treatment A if it is black a ball; otherwise, assign to treatment B.*
4. *When a response to a treatment is observed, add M balls of the corresponding color to the urn.*
Thus, future patients will be more likely to randomize to the arm with more responses.

FIGURE 2.5
Randomized Play-the-Winner.

2.2.6 Clinical Trial Protocol

A clinical trial protocol, developed by the sponsor and approved by an investigational review board (an external expert panel that provides an independent review to ensure subject/patient safety) and in some instances FDA, is a document which outlines the trial design and conduct. To protect the trial validity and integrity, Good Clinical Practice (GCP) requires that all study investigators should adherence the protocol in conducting the clinical trial (FDA, 2018).

The protocol describes the scientific rationale, objective(s), disease indication, unmet medical needs, active ingredient of test drug, mechanism of action, previous study results, dose regimen and justifications, randomization, assessment schedule, data collection, target population defined by inclusion/exclusion criteria, type of design, study duration, primary, secondary, and sometimes exploratory efficacy and/or safety endpoints, choice of control, efficacy, laboratory and safety data collection, randomization, preservation of blinding, hypothesis test, statistical methods, analysis populations, missing data handling, and power or sample size calculation. The protocol contains a precise study plan for executing the clinical trial, not only to assure safety and health of the trial subjects, but also to provide an exact template for trial conduct by investigators to perform the study in a consistent way. This harmonization allows data to be combined collectively from all investigators. The protocol also gives the study monitors as well as the site team of physicians, nurses and clinic administrators a common reference document for site responsibilities during the trial.

The format and content of clinical trial protocols sponsored by industry in the United States, European Union, Japan, or Canada should follow the ICH (International Conference on Harmonization) guidelines. IHC release Clinical Trial Protocol Template in 2017 (NIH, 2017).

Following are some common statistical questions in design a trial:

1. How to pick the primary endpoint to achieve the highest probability of success?

2. Given a target power, what sample size is required?

3. Given sample size, how much information can be obtained (power, confidence interval, the smallest difference that can be detected, etc.)?

4. How can the potential outcome help in planing the next step?

5. What is the minimal observed effect to claim statistical significance on the primary endpoint?

6. How can the effect size be most appropriately estimated? How can risks be mitigated without unnecessarily increasing the sample size?

7. The test drug may have a different effect size on different patient populations, what is the best design to handle the uncertainty?

8. What alpha should be chosen for the trial? Should a precision approach, hypothesis approach, Bayesian Approach, or some other approach be used to determine alpha?

2.2.7 Target Population

It should be noted that the results of a clinical trial can only be generalized to patients who are similar to the study participants. The specific condition a drug is intended to treat is referred to as that drug's indication. Drug developers sometimes conduct clinical trials for drugs that have already been approved by the FDA in order to determine whether or not they can be used for additional indications or populations. When patients exhibit heterogenous efficacy, targeting at general patient population may increase the benefitted population, but the average effect of the drug over the population may be smaller or larger than that for a smaller well-defined population depending on how the drug performs in the smaller more restricted population. There is a trade-off between target patient population size and average effect of the drug for the target population. Biomarker enrichment designs may be considered to adaptively select the best suitable target population at an interim analysis. However, it is important to ensure that the diagnostic tool for the biomarker is available and also that the cost of diagnosis/screening is affordable.

2.2.8 Endpoint Selection

A clinical trial should have clear objectives that are measured by an outcome measure or endpoints. An endpoint is a direct or indirect measurement of a clinical effect in a clinical trial, required to be able to make an effective claim regarding the intervention under investigation. The goal of a clinical trial is to assess the effect of treatment on these outcome measures. A primary endpoint is used to address the primary objective of a study, whereas a secondary endpoint is related to the secondary objectives. The primary endpoint will be used as the primary efficacy evidence for the drug approval, whereas secondary endpoints are positioned as supportive efficacy evidences and often used in labeling to help doctors more appropriately prescribe the medication.

A clinical trial endpoint is defined as a measure that allows one to decide whether the null hypothesis of a clinical trial should be accepted or rejected. An endpoint can be composed of a single outcome measure or a combination of outcome measures, such as death or hospitalization due to the disease. An endpoint may be based on: a binary clinical outcome indicating whether an event, such as death, has occurred, the occurrence of disease signs or symptoms, the relief of symptoms, quality of life while, the use of healthcare resources such hospitalization. A categorical variable/endpoint such a tumor response can only have a limited number of possible values: complete response (CR), partial response (PR), stable disease (SD), and progressive disease (PD). As an endpoint, the categorical variable is usually an ordinal one, meaning that the categories can be ranked from the best to the worst: CR, PR, SD, PD as in the example. A categorical variable if not ordinal, then is nominal. A ordinal variable usually has only less than 10 possible values. When the number of levels becomes large, the ordinal variable can be considered as a continual variable, such as blood pressure and weight, which can virtually take any values between an interval (strictly speaking, the smallest increment for weight might be the molecule weight).

When choosing endpoints for a clinical trial, it is important to ensure that they (Wang and Bakhai, 2006):

- are clinically meaningful and related to the disease process

- answer the main question of the trial

- are practical so that they can be assessed in all subjects in the same way

- occur frequently enough for the study to have adequate statistical power

If the endpoint to be measured consists of more than one outcome, then these outcomes should be easily differentiable from each other so that the events may be quantified independently. There is an advantage of using a composite endpoint. An endpoint with multiple outcomes means that more outcome events will be observed in total. Since the number of patients needed in the trial decreases as the number of events occurring in the control group increases, a composite endpoint allows us to reduce sample size and more comprehensively evaluate a new treatment. However, in a composite endpoint of multiple outcomes we make the assumption that all the endpoints under consideration are equal importance but in fact they are usually not. In such a case, we may use different weights for different endpoints in a composite endpoint.

Economic endpoints are becoming increasingly important to justify reimbursement for new treatments. Since the primary economic question is how to get the most benefit from health expenditure, a US panel on cost-effectiveness has recommended using a quality-adjusted life year (QALY) analysis where possible in order to be able to make comparisons across diseases (Garber and Phelps, 1997; Gold et al. 1996.). By calculating the cost per QALY gained for different treatments, healthcare providers can compare where best to invest their limited resources. Since estimating health-economic endpoints alongside clinical trials is a relatively recent concept with many assumptions, the data analysis is less robust. Economic analyses might not be easily transferable across countries since the cost of care can be very different internationally, and clinical results are dependent on local practice patterns and the availability of facilities (Wang and Bakhai, 2006).

FDA has specific guidance on the selection endpoints for many different therapeutic areas and diseases. One example is for cancer trials (FDA, 2005, 2007, 2017b).

2.2.9   Proof of Concept Trial

After the initial value proposition, endpoint selection, and target population are determined, one important thing we want to know is: does the drug has any efficacy effect in humans? The so-called proof of concept (PoC) trial is often used to answer the question. PoC clinical trials are early phase clinical trials to establish the safety of drug candidates in the target population and explore the relationship between the dose and desired activity, as either measured directly or by means of surrogate or pharmacodynamic markers. PoC trials often link between Phase-I and dose ranging Phase-II studies. These small-scale studies are designed to detect a signal that the drug is active on a pathophysiologically relevant mechanism, as well to provide preliminary evidence of efficacy in a clinically relevant endpoint. Sponsors may also use these studies to estimate whether their compound might have clinically significant efficacy in other disease states for which the pathophysiology/mechanism of action may be applicable.

2.2.10   Sample Size and Power

Blinding and randomization can reduce confirmation bias and selection bias, while appropriate sample size can reduce the random variation, provide adequate precision of the estimated treatment effect and/or sufficient power to

TABLE 2.2

Type-I and Type-II Errors (Probabilities).

	Truth	
	H_0	H_a
Reject H_0	Type-I error (α)	Correct rejection $(1 - \beta)$
Accept H_0	Correct acceptance $(1 - \alpha)$	Type-II error (β)

detect the treatment effect. Power and sample-size calculations are one of the major tasks for biostatisticians designing clinical trials. We illustrate sample-size calculation using a two-group trial design.

To prove effectiveness of a test drug, a commonly used approach in clinical trial, especially in late phase trials, is hypothesis testing. When testing a null hypothesis $H_0 : \delta = 0$ against an alternative hypothesis $H_a : \delta = \varepsilon$, where δ is the treatment effect (difference in response). A hypothesis can either be true or false and a hypothesis test can lead either a rejection or acceptance of (failure to reject) the null hypothesis. Therefore, the are four possible situations as summarized in Table 2.2.

The type-I error rate is the probability of false rejection of H_o when H_0 is true:

$$\alpha = \Pr\{\text{reject } H_0 \text{ when } H_0 \text{ is true}\}.$$

The type-II error rate is the probability of failing to reject H_o when H_a is true:

$$\beta(\varepsilon) = \Pr\{\text{fail to reject } H_0 \text{ when } H_a \text{ is true}\}.$$

Power is the probability of detecting treatment difference $\delta = \varepsilon$, defined as

$$Power\,(\varepsilon) = 1 - \beta\,(\varepsilon).$$

We keep ε in the formulation to emphasize that power is a function of assumed treatment effect $\delta = \varepsilon$ in the alternative hypothesis H_a. The power can be visually represented by the shaded area under the alternative distribution of the test statistic, $pdf\,(H_a)$, beyond the critical value $z_{1-\alpha}$ (Figure 2.6).

For a large trial with two parallel group design with a normal endpoint, the power can be expressed as

$$Power\,(\varepsilon) = \Phi\left(\frac{\sqrt{n}\varepsilon}{2\sigma} - z_{1-\alpha}\right), \tag{2.1}$$

where $z_{1-\beta}$ and $z_{1-\alpha}$ are the percentiles of the standard normal distribution, and Φ is cdf. of the standard normal distribution.

From (2.1), the total sample-size can be obtained as

$$n = \frac{4\,(z_{1-\alpha} + z_{1-\beta})^2\,\sigma^2}{\varepsilon^2} \tag{2.2}$$

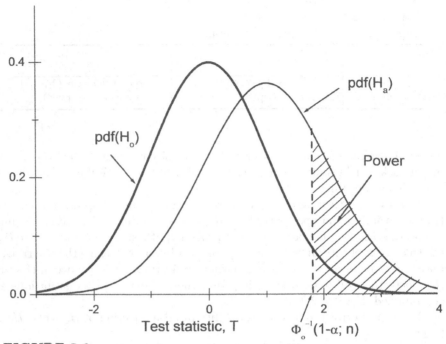

FIGURE 2.6
Power Represented by the Shaded Area.

2.2.11 Bayesian Power for Classical Design

We are going to use an example to illustrate some differences between Bayesian and frequentist approaches in trial design.

Consider a two-arm parallel design comparing a test treatment with a control. Suppose that, based on published data from 3 clinical trials of similar size, the prior probabilities for effect size are 0.1, 0.25, and 0.4 with 1/3 probability for each.

For the 2-arm trial, the power is a function of effect size of ε, given by (2.1). Considering the uncertainty of ε, i.e., prior $\pi(\varepsilon)$, the expected power

$$P_{\exp} = \int \Phi\left(\frac{\sqrt{n}\varepsilon}{2} - z_{1-\alpha}\right)\pi(\varepsilon)\,d\varepsilon. \qquad (2.3)$$

For instance, given one-sided $\alpha = 0.025$, $z_{1-\alpha} = 1.96$, and the prior

$$\pi(\varepsilon) = \begin{cases} 1/3, & \varepsilon = 0.1, 0.25, 0.4 \\ 0, & \text{otherwise,} \end{cases}$$

we conventionally use the mean of the effect size $\bar{\varepsilon} = 0.25$ to design the trial and calculate the sample-size. For the two-arm balanced design with $\beta = 0.2$ or *power* = 80%, the total sample is given by

$$n = \frac{4(z_{1-a} + z_{1-\beta})^2}{\varepsilon^2} = \frac{4(1.96 + 0.842)^2}{0.25^2} = 502.$$

However, if Bayesian approach is used, the expected power from (2.3) is

$$P_{\exp}$$
$$= \frac{1}{3}\left[\Phi\left(\frac{0.1\sqrt{n}}{2} - z_{1-\alpha}\right) + \Phi\left(\frac{0.25\sqrt{n}}{2} - z_{1-\alpha}\right) + \Phi\left(\frac{0.4\sqrt{n}}{2} - z_{1-\alpha}\right)\right]$$
$$= 66\%.$$

With the Bayesian approach that considers the uncertainty of the effect size, the expected power with a sample-size of 252 is the average of the three powers calculated using the 3 different effect sizes (0.1, 0.25, and 0.4), which turns out to be 66%, much lower than 80% as the frequentist approach claimed. Therefore, to reach the desired power, it is necessary to increase the sample-size.

This is an example of a Bayesian-frequentist hybrid approach, i.e., the Bayesian approach is used for the trial design to increase the probability of success given the final statistical criterion being p-value $\leq \alpha = 0.025$.

2.3 Summary

Determining the unmet medical need that may be met by a compound proposed for development is the starting point for a pharmaceutical company to decide whether or not to advance the drug candidate to clinical development. Understanding the competitive landscape analysis is equally important in making the final go or no-go decision. The sponsor has to evaluate on an ongoing basis the company's drivers of value, intellectual property, expertise and competence against its competitors in the dynamic drug market. There is a large amount of relevant information about prescription drugs for different indications available online (e.g., www.centerWatch and BiomedTracker). Value proposition of a drug candidate (or portfolio of candidates) is the key determinant of profitability of a drug maker. Prescription drug pricing policies worldwide can greatly affect a pharmaceutical company's decision on which clinical development programs to pursue, how to price their compounds most competitively, and overall value proposition of their portfolios. All of these variables inform how all the stakeholders (Clinical Research, Biometrics, Commercial & Marketing, Clinical Operations, Regulatory Affairs, and Manufacturing) work together in a streamlined fashion, contributing their knowledge and intelligence to the Clinical Development Plan.

Despite great effects, the average successful rate for a compound advancing from phase 1 to drug approval is low, approximately 10%. Good clinical trial designs and clinical development plan cannot make the drug candidate better, but will increase the probability of success for an effective drug candidate and reduce the cost when the drug candidate is ineffective. The gold standard

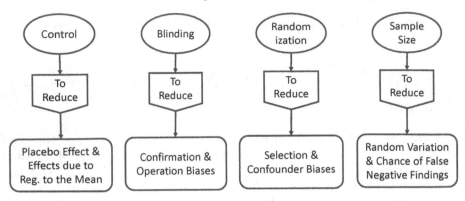

FIGURE 2.7
Control, Blinding, Randomization, and Sample Size.

of trial design should include three essential elements: Control, blinding and randomization. The primary purpose of a control as comparison group is to remove the placebo effect and effect caused by regression to the mean as might be observed in a single-group study, and the blinding procedure is critical for removing or reduce the confirmation and operational bias. The purpose of randomization is to reduce the selection bias and bias caused by the imbalance of potential and hidden confounders between the two treatment groups. Adequate sample size is an effective way to reduce the random variabilities, ensure the precision of statistical results, and reduce the probability of false negative findings or increase the power to detect treatment difference (Figure 2.7).

Clinical Trial Protocol documents detail the trial design and conduct. It is a critical document required by regulatory agencies to ensure compliance with regulations and guidance associated with good clinical practice (GCP), as well as to ensure safety of subjects/patients and standardization of data collection and analysis. The selections of the target patient population, trial design type, primary and secondary clinical endpoints, randomization procedure, and statistical analysis methods will all contribute to the success, the timing and cost of the clinical trials and consequently the entire clinical development program. Equipped with the background information, the next chapter will review how best to optimize the clinical development program.

Bibliography

Bio et al. (2016). Clinical Development Success Rates 2006-2015. www.bio.org/sites.

Chang, M. (2014). Adaptive Design Theory and Implementation Using SAS and R. 2nd Edition. Chapman & Hall/CRC, Taylor & Francis. Boca Raton, FL.

Cello Health (2017). The value of pharmaceutical competitor analysis. www.cellohealth.com/pharmaceutical-competitor-analysis/

Centerwatch, 2018. www.centerwatch.com/drug-information/fda-approved-drugs/therapeutic-areas

Duolao Wang, Ameet Bakhai, (2006). Clinical Trials - A Practical Guide to Design, Analysis, and Reporting. Remedica Publishing.

FDA, 2007. Guidance for Industry Clinical Trial Endpoints for the Approval of Cancer Drugs and Biologics, May 2007

FDA, 2005. Clinical Trial Endpoints for the Approval of NonSmall Cell Lung Cancer Drugs and Biologics, April 2005

FDA, 2017b. Multiple Endpoints in Clinical Trials Guidance for Industry (draft), Jan, 2017

FDA. 2017a. https://www.fda.gov/drugs/developmentapprovalprocess/ucm079031.htm

FDA, 2018. www.fda.gov/scienceresearch.

Friedrich Mittermayer, et al. (2015). Addressing Unmet Medical Needs in Type 2 Diabetes: A Narrative Review of Drugs under Development. Current Diabetes Reviews, 2015, 11, 17-31.

Garber AM, Phelps CE. Economic foundations of cost-effective analysis. Journal of Health Economics. 1997;16:1–31.

Gold MR, Siegel JE, Russell LB, et al. Cost-Effectiveness in Health and Medicine. New York: Oxford University Press, 1996:72–3.

Grossman, G. and Lai, E. (2008). Parallel Imports and Price Controls. RAND Journal of Economics, 2008, vol. 39, issue 2, pages 378-402.

Namrata Bahadur (2008). http://www.ich.org/.

NIH, 2017). https://osp.od.nih.gov/clinical-research/clinical-trials/

Social.eyeforpharma.com. 2017. http://social.eyeforpharma.com/

3

Clinical Development Optimization

3.1 Benchmarks in Clinical Development

In this chapter, we first study industry benchmarks in clinical development. These benchmarks will serve as guidance in determining parameters for modeling clinical development programs. In the second part we will study the optimization of clinical development programs using stochastic decision process (SDP). The benchmarks include

1. The industry standard net present value (NPV) and risk-adjusted net present value (rNPV) calculations

2. Success rates in clinical trials in different stages/phases by disease indication

3. Failure rates by reason

4. Cost of clinical trial by disease indication

5. Time-to-next phase, clinical trial length and regulatory review time

6. Rates of competitors emerging

These benchmarks can only serve as guidance. The NPV, the success rates and costs of clinical rials, the intellectual property expiration date, and time-to-market are all dependent on the profiling (efficacy, safety, therapeutic index, mechanism of action, dose-response relationship) of the drug candidate, which are characterized from preclinical studies.

3.1.1 Net Present Value and Risk-Adjusted NPV Method

Drug development costs within the pharmaceutical and biotechnology industry are known to be capital intensive, associated with a lot of risks, as well as long timelines. As a result, small biotech companies often need to raise capital at multiple points along their development path and might adopt a licensing or co-development strategy. All these events require a thorough valuation at various stages along the development spectrum. A survey conducted by Biostrat Biotech Consulting in 2011 showed that discounted cash flows approaches such as NPV and rNPV are the standard valuation methods within the industry and a standard tool used for company's internal decision-making on

TABLE 3.1
Discount Rate (Mean and 80% Interval) for NPV and rNPV.

Valuation Method	Number of Companies	Early-stage (%)	Mid-stage (%)	Late-stage (%)
NPV	88	40.1 (15-70)	26.7 (12-40)	19.5 (10-30)
rNPV	105	18.5 (12-28)	16.0 (10-22)	13.5 (9-20)

Source: Villiger, 2011

developing a drug candidate (Ralph Villiger, 2011). Understanding the NPV and rNPV methods is a way for statisticians to understand how their statistical contributions to the development program ontribute to help to achieve the ultimate corporate ? goal and provides a foundation for them to construct valid and impactful statistical models for the clinical development program.

In the NPV method, future cash flows are calculated and discounted depending on when they are predicted to occur. The discount rate should account for the time value of money and for the uncertainty or risk of the cash flows. In rNPV valuations, the cash flows are multiplied by? the probability of success to obtain the expected value and are then discounted for risk aversion. While in NPV the development risks are included in the discount rate, in rNPV these risks are addressed with the risk-adjustment of the cash flows. In the rNPV method, all cash flows get adjusted by the probability that they occur. Consequently, a large portion of the risk is already incorporated into this risk-adjustment. Therefore, it is expected that discount rates will be lower for the rNPV method (Table 3.1). In both NPV and rNPV methods, earlier-stage companies are discounted at a higher rate than later-stage companies.

The survey results suggest that rNPV is the standard method within the biotech and pharma community. However, the discount rate has a wide-range of differences, while a small difference can make an enormous difference in the calculated value.

Many biotech/pharma companies have large pipelines with individual candidates at different stages of development. Thus, for our modeling purpose, we treat these discount rates for mid- and late-stage companies as if they were for early and late phases in the clinical development program, respectively. Early stage companies are mostly in the drug discovery phase, which is outside the scope of this book.

A survey conducted in 2013 (Avance, 2008) show that discount rates for different companies: Genentech 16%-19% , Lilly 18.75%, Arpida 18%, Jerini 15%, Actelion 15%, Schering 14.25%, Schering 13.5%, CAT 12.5%, MedImmune 11.3%, Berna Biotech 9.9%, AstraZeneca 8%, and Merck KGaA 7%-7.6%. Further discussions on net present value approaches for drug discovery are available elsewhere (Svennebring and Wikberg, 2013).

These surveys and data in Table 3.1 allows for a better understanding of this important parameter and provide useful information for building a valid Stochastic Decision Process (SDP) model later. However, the purpose of using NPV as utility function in this book is somewhat different from how the commercial group might view the valuation of a preclinical product or drug candidate. In current practice, NPV is primarily used by pharmaceutical or venture capital companies for their investment decisions. The NPV and rNPV methods are oversimplified and are far from correct because they are usually considered independent of clinical trial designs within the clinical development program. The SDP model of NPV in this book will be used to evaluate the efficiency of a clinical development program, while recognizing the different success rate for different trial designs (including optimization of same) and clinical development programs. To this end, the NPV rate discount will be broken down into (1) controllable or partially controllable variables such as the probability of successfully progressing rom one phase to the next, which are in part dependent on CDP and clinical trial designs, and (2) uncontrollable ones such as commodity inflation and risk aversion due to the concern of unexpected/unidentified risks. We will use clinical trial designs to manage the controllable factors for the purpose of optimization. For uncontrollable factors, we should evaluate them on case-by-case basis under the guidance of industry benchmarks.

3.1.2   Clinical Program Success Rates

One of the important factors that impacts success of a pharmaceutical company and attraction for investors is the general success rate for both the "overall" drug pipeline and the disease-specific success rate. Another important consideration is the success rate of progression from one phase of trials to the next phase. Biotechnology Innovation Organization (BIO), BiomedTracker, and AMPLION recently conducted a research to study clinical drug development success rates (BIO et al., 2016) and generated to date the most comprehensive analysis yet ofbiopharmaceutical R&D success (Table 3.2). They analyzed a total of 9,985 clinical and regulatory phase transitions from 7,455 development programs, across 1,103 companies over the last decade, 2006-2015 in the Biomedtracker database. Phase transitions occur when a drug candidate advances into the next phase of development. They published the overall phase-transition probabilities and the transitional probabilities by therapeutic area, drug modalities and other attributes.

The report shows that the overall likelihood of approval (LOA) from compounds entering Phase I for all developmental candidates was around 10% for all indications outside of Oncology. Chronic diseases with large populations had lower LOA from Phase I than average. Of the 14 major disease areas, Hematology had the highest LOA from Phase I (26.1%) and Oncology had the lowest (5.1%). Sub-indication analysis within Oncology revealed hematologic cancers had a 2× higher LOA from Phase I than solid tumors. Oncology drugs had a 2× higher rate of first cycle approval than Psychiatric drugs, which had the lowest percent of first-cycle review approvals. Oncology drugs

TABLE 3.2

Phase Transition Probabilities of Clinical Trials.

	Test Drug	Phase 1 to Ph 2	Phase 2 to Ph 3	Phase 3 to NDA*	NDA* to Appr	Phase 3 to Appr
Hematology	86	73.3%	56.6%	75.0%	84.0%	63.0%
Infectious disease	347	69.5%	42.7%	72.7%	88.7%	64.5%
Ophthalmology	66	84.8%	44.6%	58.3%	77.5%	45.2%
Other	96	66.7%	39.7%	69.6%	88.4%	61.5%
Metabolic	95	61.1%	45.2%	71.4%	77.8%	55.5%
Gastroenterology*	41	75.6%	35.7%	60.6%	92.3%	55.9%
Allergy	37	67.6%	32.5%	71.4%	93.8%	67.0%
Endocrine	299	58.9%	40.1%	65.0%	86.0%	55.9%
Respiratory	150	65.3%	29.1%	71.1%	94.6%	67.3%
Urology	21	57.1%	32.7%	71.4%	85.7%	61.2%
Autoimmune	297	65.7%	31.7%	62.2%	86.0%	53.5%
Neurology	462	59.1%	29.7%	57.4%	83.2%	47.8%
Cardiovascular	209	58.9%	24.1%	55.5%	84.2%	46.7%
Psychiatry	154	53.9%	23.7%	55.7%	87.9%	49.0%
Oncology	1222	62.8%	24.6%	40.1%	82.4%	33.0%
All Indications	3582	63.2%	30.7%	58.1%	85.3%	49.6%

* Include both new drug and biologic license Applications (NDA & BLA)
Data source: Biotechnology Innovation Organization, et al., (2016)

were also approved the fastest of all 14 disease areas. Phase II clinical programs continue to experience the lowest success rate of the four development phases, with only 30.7% of developmental candidates advancing to Phase III. Rare disease programs and programs that utilized selection biomarkers had higher success rates at each phase of development than average. There are reportedly 7,000 rare diseases and most do not have an approved therapeutic treatment (ref: Global Genes Rare Disease Facts: http://globalgenes.org/rare-diseases-facts-statistics).

The phase transition probabilities by disease area are summarized in Table 3.2, sorted by xx. The transition probabilities characterize, in terms of success probability, the profile of the clinical development program in general. A stochastic process can be used to model the clinical development process with phase transition probabilities. Stochastic process is a sequence of random variables $X_1, X_2, ..., X_n$ with the associated probability of moving to the next state. Markov Chain (discrete) is a simple stochastic process, in which the probability of moving to the next state depends only on the present state and not on the previous states. Figure 3.1 is an illustration of the model for the probability of success of a clinical development candidate based on all disease, where P_{ij} is the transition probability from state i to state j.

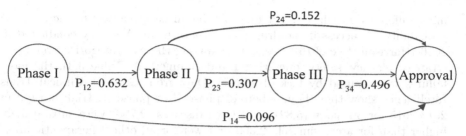

FIGURE 3.1
Markov Chain for Clinical Development Program.

Using the phase-transition probabilities of Markov Chain, we can easily calculate the probability of transiting from Phase I to Approval, i.e., the product of the 4 transition probabilities: $0.632 \times 0.307 \times 0.496 = 0.096$. The success probability from Phase 2 to approval increases to $0.307 \times 0.496 = 0.152$ and further increases to 0.496 from Phase 3. In general, the transition probability from state i to state $i+k$ is the product of transition probabilities in between, that is,

$$P_{i,i+k} = P_{i,i+1} P_{i,i+2} \cdots P_{i+k}. \tag{3.1}$$

From the above formulation, one may have the question: should decision rules simply be changed to increase early phase transition probabilities? There a good reason for it: when a drug candidate is ineffective or too toxic, the desire is to discontinue (or "kill") the program as early as possible. Unfortunately, there is usually a trade-off between the true positive discovery rate and true negative discovery rate. An increase in one will often decrease the other. From the data from Table 3.1, a test drug with a higher transitional Probability from Phase 1 to 2 may not necessarily have a higher probability going forward than other drugs that have lower early-phase transition probabilities. Similarly, a test drug with a larger transitional probability from Phase 2 to 3 may not necessarily have a larger probability going forward.

3.1.3 Failure Rates by Reason

Understanding the reasons for clinical failure is essential not only for decreasing attrition in clinical development, but also for the SDP model-building. Many factors, including but not limited to complexity and heterogeneity of the patient population, the difficulties of patient recruitment, the duration of the study, the number of sites, global international study versus national study, the limitation of patient resource, and the complexity of treatment procedures, can all affect the probability of success. The breakdowns of failure reasons can help us to effectively develop risk mitigation strategies and increase the probability of success of the clinical development program. For instance, a sample size increase may increase the power of detecting a treatment difference in efficacy, but may not be an effective way to increase the probability of success if the drug has a safety issue. A survey conducted in 2016 (Harrison, Dec 2016) reveals that among the five categories evaluated: strategy, efficacy, safety, operational and commercial (Table 3.3), the most failures were caused by lack of efficacy Data from Cortellis Clinical Trials Intelligence show that the numbers of phase II or phase III trials started in 2013-2015 for oncology (5,821) and CNS diseases (2,796) were substantially higher than for approximately 2,000 or fewer for all other therapeutic areas for the same time period. During the 12-year period, there were 218 reported failures between phase II (including phase I/II) and submission (each drug indication combination is considered as a separate record and both new active substances and new indications of marketed drugs are included in the analysis). Of these failures, 174 had stated the reason for the failure and these were used in the subsequent analysis (Harrison, 2016).

The second main reason for failures were due to safety issues (24%), where safety includes those failures that were due to an insufficient therapeutic index, followed by strategy (15%), Commercial (6%), and Operational (3%).

In considering further the breakdown by phases, failures due to efficacy are higher in phase III than in phase II, suggesting that false discovery rate in phase II is still high and partially due to a possible patient population shift from Phase II to Phase III for some of the development programs. Failures due to safety is lower for phase III trials than for phase II trials, which suggests that efforts to remove unsafe agents earlier in the development cycle are paying off. Failures for strategic reasons such as a change in therapeutic focus or being discontinued owing to mergers/acquisitions represent 21% of all phase II terminations and 14% of all phase III terminations. This may reflect the increase in mergers and acquisitions occurring in the industry during the period. The observation that only 3% of phase II failures as opposed to 10% of all phase III failures are for commercial reasons suggests that the lower cost of phase II trials outweighs the commercial risks, but the increased cost of phase III trials requires a more stringent cost-to-benefit analysis (Harrison, 2016).

For the SDP modeling purpose, the failure rates (presented in Table 3.3) for a given phase is not very informative. Failure probability of clinical trials by phase is more informative. The failure probabilities can be estimated by

TABLE 3.3

Reasons for Failures of Clinical Trials 2013-2015.

Reason	Strategy	Efficacy	Safety	Operational	Commercial
Phase 2	21%	48%	25%	3%	3%
Phase 3	14%	55%	14%	7%	10%
Total	15%	52%	24%	3%	6%

Source: Richard K. Harrison, Dec 2016

TABLE 3.4

Failure Probability of Clinical Trials 2013-2015.

Reason	Strategy	Efficacy	Safety	Operational	Commercial	Total
Phase 2	14.6%	33.3%	17.3%	2.1%	2.1%	69.4%
Phase 3	7.1%	27.6%	7.1%	3.6%	5.0%	50.4%

the proportion of failed trial for a reason among all trials instead of among only failed trials. Thus, the failure probabilities can be calculated using the failure rates in Table 3.4 multiplying the total failure rate, $1 - 0.307 = 0.693$ for Phase 2 and $1 - 0.496 = 0.504$ for Phase 3 (Table 3.2).

There is a 24.1% probability a phase II trial fails due to efficacy, and a 26.2% probability that the trial fails due to "other" reasons and, combined, these represent 50.3% of all phase II failures. Similarly, there is a slightly higher probability (27.6%) of failures in a phase II trial due to efficacy reason and 22.8% probability of failures due to other reasons and, combined, these represent 50.4% of phase III trials that didn't get market authorization. The failures due to efficacy can be reduced to a certain degree through a good trial design, which is the focus of the book. The other risks are also important and need to be estimated for the modeling, but less relevant to the design.

3.1.4 Costs of Clinical Trials

Accurately estimating the costs of clinical trials is critical for the optimization of a clinical development program. The costs for different trials are different; statisticians should work with Clinical Operations to obtain the estimates. Industry-wise, average per patient cost by indications were studied by Cutting Edge Information (Table 3.5).

As expected, in terms per patient cost, the most expensive indication is oncology, around $60,000 to $70,000 per patient per phase. The least costly

TABLE 3.5

Estimated Per Patient Costs ($) by Disease Area.

Disease Area	Phase 1	Phase 2	Phase 3
Oncology	57,500	67,500	69,000
CNS/Brain/Pain	34,000	39,500	40,500
Others	29,500	34,500	35,000
Raspiratory	26,000	30,500	31,000
Hematology	26,000	30,000	31,000
CV/Circulatory	21,500	25,000	26,000
Diabetes/Metabolic/Nutrition	16,000	18,500	19,000
Infectious	15,000	17,500	18,000

Source: Battele, based on survey data from Cutting Edge Information

TABLE 3.6
Inflation-Unadjusted Average Cost, 2004-2012.

Disease Area	Phase 1	Phase 2	Phase 3	Total
Pain and Anesthesia	1.4	17.0	52.9	71.3
Ophthalmology	5.3	13.8	30.7	49.8
Anti-infective	4.2	14.2	22.8	41.2
Respiratory System	5.2	12.2	23.1	40.5
Oncology	4.5	11.1	22.1	37.7
Central Nervous System	3.9	13.9	19.2	37.0
Hematology	1.7	19.6	15.0	35.7
Genitourinary System	3.1	14.6	17.5	35.2
Immunomodulation	6.6	16.0	11.9	34.5
Cardiovascular	2.2	7.0	25.2	34.4
Gastrointestinal	2.4	15.8	14.5	32.7
Endocrine	1.4	12.1	10.0	23.5
Dermatology	1.8	8.9	11.5	22.2

Source: Sertkaya, et al. 2016. in million US$

trial is infectious disease, around $15,000 to $18,000 per patient per phase and the total per-patient cost for the program is $50,500. In general, per patient cost increases from an early phase to later phase. Compared phase 1 to phase 3, there is approximately 20% increase in per patient cost this is because phase 3 trials usually have a longer duration, more procedures, and more data collection points. The per patient cost for phase 2 is less than but close to the cost for phase 3.

Another study shows the breakdowns of average cost center for Phase 3 CNS Trials are: Administrative staff, 23.2%, Clinical procedure, 22.5%, Data management, 0.4%, Data management, 3.1%, Patient retention, 0.2%, Physician, 8.0%, RN/CRA, 9.4%, Site monitoring, 16.2%, Site recruitment, 3.9%, Site retention, 13.0%. Total cost was $19,200,000.

The data on average cost per phase of trials by therapeutic area are reported by Sertkaya et al (2016) and summarized in Table 3.6, sorted by total cost. The most expensive clinical development program costs (including phases 1 - 3) is for pain and anesthesia, $71.3 million, of which $52.9 million is the phase 3 cost. For oncology studies, although per patient cost is high, the clinical development cost ranks number 5, just below $40 million due to a smaller number of patients that are required to be included in these trials to establish safety and efficacy. Surprisingly, among 13 disease areas, 4 of them have the cost of phase 2 more than that of phase 3: hematology, Immunomodulation, Gastrointestinal, and Endocrine.

Clinical trial costs, by cost component and phase are also reported for trials conducted between 2004 and 2012 (Table 3.7). Those data can be useful

TABLE 3.7

Clinical Trial Costs by Cost Component and Phase, 2004-2012.

Cost Component	Phase 1	Phase 2	Phase 3	Total
Per-patient costs	**1059**	**3280**	**5181**	
Patient recruitment	37	161	309	507
Patient retention	6	15	25	46
Nurse & Associates	178	441	940	1559
Physician	110	382	806	1298
Clinical Procedure	476	1,476	2,252	4,204
Central Lab	252	805	849	1906
Per-site Costs	**683**	**3781**	**5647**	
Site recruitment	52	224	395	671
Site retention	194	1,127	1,305	2,626
Administrative staffs	238	1,347	2,322	3,907
Site monitoring	199	1,083	1,625	2,905
Per-study costs	**2,058**	**6,271**	**10,063**	
Data management	50	60	39	149
Per IRB approval	12	60	114	186
IRB amendments	1.1	1.7	1.9	4.7
Source data verification	326	406	400	1132
Other costs	1669	5743	9508	16920
Total	**3,800**	**13,352**	**19,891**	37,043

Source: Sertkaya, et al. 2016. The amounts are in thousand US$.

in estimate cost for trial planning and modeling purposes. For instance, the trial cost C can be estimated using the following formulation:

$$C = \text{Per-study costs} + (\text{Per-site costs}) \times (\text{number of sites})$$
$$+(\text{Per-patient costs}) \times (\text{number of patients})$$

That is,

$$\begin{cases} C = 2059 + 683M + 1059N, & \text{for Phase 1} \\ C = 6271 + 3781M + 3280N, & \text{for Phase 2} \\ C = 10063 + 5647M + 5181N, & \text{for Phase 3} \end{cases} \quad (3.2)$$

where M is the number of sites and N is the sample size.

The category, other costs, including data analysis, report writing, etc., will not vary significantly with sample size and number of sites , and are treated as a constant in the CDP modeling. The decompositions of the cost are useful to consider in clinical development and clinical trial optimization since different designs often will require a different number of patients and sites. However, it would be more useful if data in Table 3.7 were broken down by disease area. The statistician should work with Clinical Operations closely to obtain accurate estimation of the cost for each trial design option, and should also work with the team to develop study designs that include the least number of patients over the shortest duration required to meet the study/program objectives.

TABLE 3.8

Average Time-to-Next Phase.

Testing Phase	Mean Phase Length (month)	Mean time to next Phase (month)
Phase 1	33.1	19.8
Phase 2	37.9	30.3
Phase 3	45,1	30.7

Source: Dimasi et al., Journal of Health Economics (2016)

3.1.5　Time-to-Next Phase, Clinical Trial Length and Regulatory Review Time

Time-to-market has a great impact on the NPV valuation and outcome of CDP modeling, therefore it is important to look into the allocation of time for a clinical development program. We can divide the time allocation according to the following milestones for the purpose of our CDP modeling:

1. IND, Trials design, approval (IRB, regulatory)

2. Trial execution (trial length)

3. Statistical analysis of Clinical Trial results and Clinical Summary Report (3 to 6 months)

4. Regulatory Review of NDA

We can further simplify the time into two categories: Trial Phase Length and Time-to-next Phase as summarized in Table 3.8 for all indications according to a survey.

The time-to-market will also depend on the regulatory approval time. The FDA published (FDA, 2017) the CDER approval times for priority and standard NDAs and BLAs approvals from 1993 through 2016. Data in Table 3.9 are extracted from the FDA website (FDA, 2017).

Examining FDA's median approval time (8 month for priority review and 10 months for standard review) in recent years, it is very much hit the target time. However, the mean time from filling to approval is somewhat longer. Biotechnology Innovation Organization et al. (2016) conducted a large study, showing that the average time from filing BLA/NDA to approval1.1 year for oncology and 2 years for neurology. On average 1.6 years for all disease (Table 3.10). The probability of approval following the first review ranges from 37% (Psychiatry) to 79% (oncology). The ultimate approval rate ranges from 73% for Ophthalmology to 94% for Respiratory.

TABLE 3.9

FDA Review and Approval Times (2007-2016).

Year of Approval	Priority Review		Standard Review	
	Number of Approvals	Median FDA approval time	Number of Approvals	Median FDA approval time
2007	23	6	55	10.4
2008	18	6	70	13.1
2009	19	12	78	13.0
2010	16	9	76	12.0
2011	26	6.9	68	10.8
2012	23	6	77	10.0
2013	16	6.2	82	10.1
2014	34	8	84	12.0
2015	37	8	84	12.0
2016	24	8	70	10.1

Source: CDER Approval Times NDAs and BLAs (FDA 2017)

3.1.6   Rates of Competitor Emerging

The market share of a drug very much depends on market dynamics as well as the competitive landscape. It also depends on the commercial strategies and marketing tactics employed. The relationship between market share and number of competitors can be approximately modeled by

$$\text{Market Share} = \frac{\text{Market potential}}{1 + b \times (\text{Number of competitors})}. \tag{3.3}$$

The market share decreases when the number of competitors increases. For example, if the constant in the model (3.3), $b = 0.25$, the first drug will get all the potential market without competitors. The market share "generally" will drop to 80% if there is one competitor, to 67% if two competitors, to 57% if three competitors, and so on. The relationship between the market share and number of competitors does not have to be in equation format, but an equation like (3.3) will be convenient in the later CDP modeling. For simplicity, assume the time value of a drug candidate at the time of marketing will also follow Eq.(3.3).

To estimate the average number of competitors over time, we can use the number of new drugs approved each to obtain the rate of competitors that may emerge. Table 3.10 provides a new drug approval rate over years by indication (extracted form CenterWatch website). However, two drugs in the same disease area do not mean necessarily they are competitors because some diseases area such as oncology has broad coverage including, Bladder Cancer, Breast Cancer, Colon and Rectal Cancer, Endometrial Cancer, Kidney Cancer, Leukemia, Liver Lung Cancer, Melanoma, Non-Hodgkin Lymphoma, Pancreatic Cancer, Prostate Cancer, Thyroid Cancer. This is just a list of common cancers that are diagnosed with the greatest frequency in the United States, excluding nonmelanoma skin cancers: To be considered a competitor

TABLE 3.10

Probability of Approval on Reviews and Time to Approval.

Disease Area	% Approved on 1st Review	% Approved on 2nd Review	% Final Approved	Years from Filing to Approval
Oncology	79	89	89	1.1
Allergy	71	93	93	1.3
Respiratory	71	94	94	1.6
Cardiovascular	69	83	85	1.4
Infectious	69	86	92	1.4
Urology	64	73	82	1.7
Autoimmune	63	82	86	1.6
Metabolic	63	83	83	1.5
Ophthalmology	62	69	73	1.3
Hematology	60	76	90	1.6
Gastroenterology	56	84	92	1.8
Endocrine	56	77	83	1.8
Neurology	45	70	81	2.0
Psychiatry	37	70	91	1.6
All diseases	61	80	86	1.6

Data source: Bio, et al., (2016)

it has to be specific to the indication. Equation (3.3) will be used in the CDP modeling. Because of the large variability in the number of new drugs approved, a 5-year and 10-year average yearly rate of new drugs emerging for each very specific indication is more useful in CDP modeling.

3.2   Optimization of Clinical Development Program

3.2.1   Local Versus Global Optimizations

From a business perspective, the goal of maximizing the success of clinical development program includes optimizing both the probability of success and the magnitude of success, that is the maximization of the NPV. Such maximization is called clinical development program optimization (CDPO). CDPO is different from a single trial optimization (STO), STO is a local optimization, whereas CDPO is global optimization. STO does not deal with the optimal allocations of resources among different development stages, but CDPO does. In addition, CDPO also include STO as a part of its optimization process. This chapter will mainly discuss the framework of CDPO, whereas next several chapters will deal with trial optimization include adaptive designs under framework of CDPO.

To perform the optimization, the first thing is to define the objective function, i.e., NPV, the factors or parameters that will affect the outcome/NPV, and constraints. Then, in light of the cumulative information that is developed over time, the next step is to determine what sequence of actions should be taken or more precisely, what set of action rules should be followed for the optimization. The sequence of action rules that maximize the expected utility or NPV is called "optimal policy in theory of stochastic decision process (SDP)".

The optimization problem faces several challenges: (1) the available knowledge of the efficacy and safety profiles of a drug candidate has great uncertainties, which can be characterized by a prior distribution based on aggregated efficacy and safety information prior to conducting an experiment, (2) each action among a large set of options (such as trial design, sample size, go no-go decision rules) will have an associated cost and probabilistic consequences or outcomes, (3) every action taken will have a great impact on the downstream outcomes in the development process, and (4) thus an adaptive approach with a risk-mitigation mechanism is desirable. Since clinical development is a very costly and time-consuming proposition, it is crucial to predict as accurately as possible the outcomes associated with different actions or CDP design options. In this regard, computer simulations play a vital role.

To model the CDP, SDP will be used to determine the optimal policy in clinical development process to maximize the success or expected NPV under practical constraints such as the cost, timing, regulatory requirements, operational obstacles, and competitors. The actions here refer to clinical trial design, and include the design type (classical, adaptive, etc.), go and no-go decision rules, and adaptations (especially for adaptive trials).

In what follows, we will first discuss how to construct a SDP, from a stochastic process, for the clinical development program by adding action options to each of the action points and the associated gain in terms of NPV when each milestone is achieved. We will outline the steps for the SDP construction using public data for an oncology indication as example.

3.2.2 Stochastic Decision Process for Drug Development

A Stochastic Decision Process is similar to Stochastic Process such as Markov chain, but there are also a decision or action (a_i), associated cost (c_i) at state i, and associated probability of reach next state, $p_{i,i+i}$ and gain (g_{i+1}) if the state $i + 1$ is reached successfully (Figure 3.2). SDP provides a powerful mathematical framework for modeling the decision-making process in situations where outcomes are partly random and partly under the control of the decision-maker. The optimization is to determine the set of actions or action rules (often called policy) that maximize the expected gain. The commonly used algorithm to find the optimal solution is the backward induction method when the SDP is a Markov Decision Process. Backward induction algorithm derived from the Bellman's optimality principle can be found elsewhere (Chang, 2010). Bellman's Optimality Principle can be stated: An optimal policy has the property that, whatever the initial state and initial decisions are,

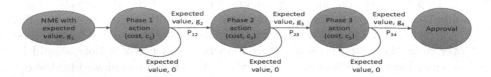

FIGURE 3.2
Actions = trial designs with decision-rules.

the remaining decisions must constitute an optimal policy with regard to the state resulting from the first decision.

The expected future reward at stage i with action a_i can be expressed as

$$g_i = p_{i,i+1}g_{i+1} - C_i \qquad (3.4)$$

When action a_i (trial design) is different, then the associated cost C_i and the transition probability $p_{i,i+1}$ will be different. The transition probability is mainly a function of the safety and efficacy profile of the drug and trial design. The drug profile is the fixed properties of the drug candidate, but efficacy and safety of an intended dose regimen can vary dependent on which dose regimen is chosen. An important consideration here is that different designs can lead to different recommendations of dose regimen(s) to be carried forward. The transition probability will be discussed in detail in consideration of both classical and adaptive trial designs conceptually and through simulations.

Monetary-wise, future discounts for commodity inflation need to be considered. A 3% commodity inflection rate might be a reasonable number. The gain g_4 can be as expressed as time value, the value of the drug at time of approval for marketing. For convenience, the cost C_i should also be determined as the time value at time of approval for marketing, using a inflation factor, $(1+r)^t$, where r is the discount rate and t is the time-to-market from decision point i, that is $C_i \rightarrow C_i(1+r)^t$.

When g_4 is calculated, g_3, g_2, and g_1 can be recursively calculated from (3.4) and no adjustment for inflation or deflation is needed because even though, e.g., g_3 is calculated for decision timepoint i, it can only be realized through g_4. No value can be realized at decision point i or beginning of Phase i. Even when it is decided to out-license the NME, the buyer has to consider that the value g_3 can only be realized at the future decision point $i = 4$ through g_4. Similar arguments for no inflation or deflation are applicable to g_2 and g_1.

Example 3.1: Stochastic Decision Process for a Cancer CDP (Figure 3.3)

Suppose the time value of a cancer drug candidate is $g_4 = \$1,000$ million at time of approval, which is provided by commercial group of the biotech company. The drug candidate is believed to be of somewhat "promise". Thus , the phase transition probabilities from Table 3.1 are used in the SDP diagram (Figure 3.4). The cost for each trial will depend on the disease indication,

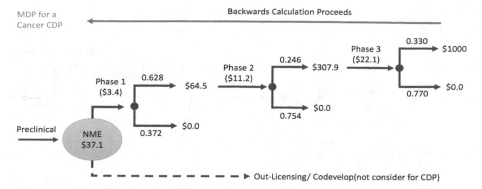

FIGURE 3.3
Stochastic Decision Process for a Cancer CDP.

trial design, patient recruitment, etc. However, the average costs (the industry benchmark from Table 3.2) will be used for cancer trials in this exercise and assume the costs are converted/inflated to the time value at the time when g_4 is valued. The expected NPV (time value at g_4 is valued) will be calculated at each decision point using backward induction.

- Step 1: At the beginning of Phase 3, for example, a decision is made to conduct the Phase 3 trials at a cost of $22.1 million. There will be a 0.33 probability that the trial will be successful and the drug will be approved for marketing with NPV $g_4 = \$1000$ million after adjusted for future discounts or the commodity inflation. Otherwise, if the drug didn't get marketing-authorization it will worth nothing. Therefore, the expected value at the beginning of the phase 3 is $g_3 = 0.33 \times 1000 + 0.77 \times 0.0 - 22.1 = \$307.9$ million.

- Step 2: The estimated cost for a Phase 2 oncology trial is $11.2 million. The probability of moving from Phase 2 to Phase 3 is 0.246 with the expected value at the end of Phase 2 is $307.9 million. If it failed, it will be worth nothing. The expected value at the end of Phase 1 or the beginning of Phase 2 is $g_2 = 0.246 \times 307.9 + 0.754 \times 0 - 11.2 = \$64.5$ million.

- Step 3: The estimated cost for Phase 1 oncology trial is $3.4 million. The probability of moving from Phase 1 to Phase 2 is 0.628 with the expected value at the end of Phase 1 is $64.5 million. If it failed, it will worth nothing. The expected value at the end of Preclinical phase or the beginning of Phase 1 is $g_1 = 0.628 \times 64.5 + 0.372 \times 0 - 3.4 = 37.13$ million.

In reality, each trial design has different probabilities of success and associated time and cost, thus the optimization is to select the design with maximum NPV, or g_i at the decision point i.

In general, the Stochastic Decision Process for the classical clinical development program can be outlined as follows (See Figure 3.4):

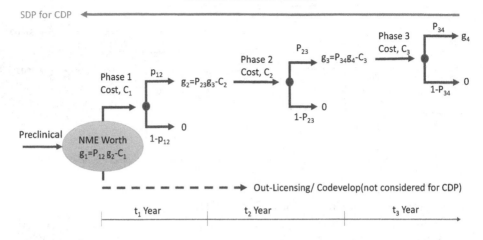

FIGURE 3.4
General CMP for Clinical Development Program.

- Step 1: Starting the beginning of Phase 3, if we conduct the phase 3 trials the cost will be C_3. There will be a P_{34} probability that the drug will obtain marketing authorization with an inflation-adjusted NPV g_4 dollars. Otherwise, if the drug didn't get marketing-approval it will be worth nothing. Therefore, the expected value at the beginning of the phase 3 is $g_3 = P_{34}g_4 - C_3$.

- Step 2: The cost for Phase 2 is C_2. The probability of moving from Phase 2 to Phase 3 is P_{23} with the expected value at the end of Phase 2, g_3. If it failed, it will be worth nothing. Therefore, the expected value at the end of Phase 1 or the beginning of Phase 2 is $g_2 = P_{23}g_3 - C_2$.

- Step 3: The cost for Phase 1 is C_1. The probability of moving from Phase 1 to Phase 2 is P_{12} with the expected value at the end of Phase 1, g_2. If it failed, it will be worth nothing. Therefore, the expected value at the end of Preclinical phase or the beginning of Phase 1 is $g_1 = P_{12}g_2 - C_1$.

The transition probability p_{ij} is a function of study design, including design type (parallel, crossover, adaptive, etc.), sample size, and Go/No-Go decision rules, while the cost is a function of the design type and the sample size . As an example, with the same (average) sample size a crossover design may have a higher probability of rejecting the null hypothesis than a two-arm parallel design and have a higher transition probability. However, a crossover design will not fit situations: the crossover trial will take longer time to finish than a parallel trial and a longer washout period might need to eliminate the carryover effect, especially when the drug has a long PK half-life.

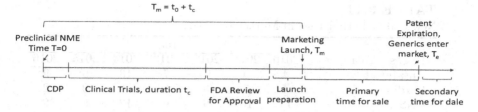

FIGURE 3.5

Milestones in Clinical Development and Commercialization.

3.2.3 Time Dependent Gain g_4,

Two major timepoints will affect the value of a new drug. (1) the time-to-market (T_m) and (2) the patent expiration date or time-to-expiration (T_e). The time required to develop CDP is approximately 3 months, time from filing to FDA/regulatory approval is approximately 12 months (Tables 3.9 and 3.10), launch preparation requires 3 months or so. These three different times combined together is approximately $t_0 = 18$ months. See Table 3.8 for the benchmarks of clinical trial durations.

The time required for to design and execute the clinical trial will include protocol design, trial execution, statistical analysis of trial data, and report writing. There is usually a time interval of 20-30 months between different phases in the traditional clinical development paradigm and 3-6 months for report writing. See the benchmarks for time-to-next phase in Table 3.8.

The time-to-market from Preclinical, T_m, can be decomposed into two parts: time required for conducting clinical trials t_c and the rest t_0, $T_m = t_0 + t_c$ (Figure 3.5). Primary time (duration) for sale $= T_e - T_m$. Denote r the commodity inflation rate, inflation-adjusted V_p is the annual net income drug sales without competitors. Strictly speaking, the V_p is smaller when t_c is larger because of a longer time for inflation discount. However, for simplicity we consider V_p is a constant. V_p is the market capacity subtracted by the commercial cost. The net profit for secondary time after patent expiration is denoted by $G_{\max}$ (commodity inflation adjusted). Considering the potential loss of the market shares due to competitors, if the program is successful and the drug is approved, the fair market value can be modeled by

$$g_4 = \left[\int_{T_m}^{T_e} \frac{V_p}{1 + bR_c t} dt \right] + G_{\max} \tag{3.6}$$

where R_c is the yearly or monthly expected competitors on the market, $\frac{1}{1+0bR_cT}$ is the reduction factor for V_p due to R_cT competitors at time t. After carrying out the integration, (3.6) becomes

$$g_4 = \frac{V_p}{bR_c} \ln \frac{1 + bR_c T_e}{1 + bR_c T_m} + G_{\max} \tag{3.7}$$

TABLE 3.11

New and Generic Drugs in Market by Year.

Disease Area	Year						
	2010	2011	2012	2013	2014	2015	2016
Anti-infective	4	9	13	7	13	9	9
Cardiovascular	4	5	3	6	2	9	2
CNS	14	10	9	6	12	6	9
Dermatology	3	6	4	7	9	6	3
Endocrine	3	4	12	5	10	4	3
Gastrointestinal	4	7	9	3	5	7	1
Hematology	1	6	8	11	10	6	5
Immunomodulation	8	11	7	7	12	5	6
Oncology	6	12	19	12	10	21	11

Source: http://www.centerwatch.com

Choosing $b = 0.25$ for a first-to-market drug, (3.7) becomes

$$g_4 = \frac{V_p}{0.25R_c} \ln \frac{1 + 0.25R_cT_e}{1 + 0.25R_cT_m} + G_{\max} \tag{3.8}$$

When there is no competitor, reduction factor $= 1$; one competitor, reduction factor $= 1/(1 + 0.25) = 0.8$; two competitors, $1/(1 + 0.5) = 0.667$; three competitors, $1/(1 + 0.75) = 0.571$. The discount constant $b = 0.25$ to 0.3 is based on the consensus that the first to market will take 75%~80% of the market share. If the drug is expected the second in market, b should be 3 to 3.5 or still use $b = 0.25$ but adjust V_p.

All the parameters can be calculated or estimated: V_p and G_{max} from the Commercial/Marketing group, T_m from Clinical Operation group, T_e is known, R_c from the Regulatory group. Those values should be checked again the industry benchmarks to make sure the estimations are reasonable.

Example 3.2: Calculation of NPV g_4 If a Drug is approved

Suppose in developing a oncology CDP, the NME patent will expire in 15 years, $T_e = 180$ months. The proposed Phase 1 trial needs 30 patients, 10 months, the Phase 2 trial, 60 patients, 14 months, and the Phase 3 trial, 900 patients, 36 months; the total time for clinical trials is $t_c = 10 + 14 + 36 = 60$ months. CDP development and FDA review time are estimated to be $t_0 = 24$ months. Thus, the time-to-market is $T_m = 60 + 24 = 84$ months. The estimated annual net income from sales for the drug without competitor is $V_p = \$200$ million. The number of approved new oncology drugs annually is about 12 (Table 3.11). However, since cancer includes a wide range of indications, , an assumption is made that 2% of the newly approved cancer drugs may become competitors. Therefore, $R_c = 12/12 \times 0.02 = 0.02/\text{month}$, meaning on average every 5 years, there will be a competitor. It is estimated that

$G_m = \$500$ million. From these, we can calculate the expected value g_4 using formula (3.7)

$$g_4 = \frac{200/12}{0.25\,(0.02)} \ln \frac{1 + 0.25(0.02)180}{1 + 0.25(0.02)84} + 500 = \$1470.7.$$

That is, with potential competitors, $g_4 = \$1470.7$ million. If without competitor, the expected value would be $g_4 = 200(180 - 84)/12 + 500 = \$2,100$ million; We can see that the number of anticipated competitor has a significant impact on g_4 by reducing the portion of sales before the expiration of the intellectual property.

3.2.4 Determination of Transition Probabilities

The transition probabilities determine the probability of success of clinical development program. The probabilities can break down into three different probabilities in terms of efficacy, safety, and unspecified factors such as merger and acquisition, funding issues, and competing patient resources.

Risk aversion due to the concern of unexpected risks and the fear of the uncertainty about the estimated probability (uncertainty). These unexpected risks are independent of the drug profile and are assumed to be independent of the trial design. The probability of stopping a trial for such reasons is denoted by p_{iu} at state i. The probability of stopping due to lack of efficacy at stage i, p_{ie}, can be calculated for each trial design based on Bayesian power of the study. The stopping probability due to safety is denoted by p_{is}, which depends on the safety profile of the NME. We assume that for a given dose regiment, stopping for efficacy and stopping for safety are independent (a patient who has drug benefit may not be more likely to have a safety issue), though both can be dependent on dose. The probabilities due to efficacy and safety are both dependent on the decision rules for the trial. Therefore, the probability of a trial continuing from decision point i to the next decision point $i + 1$, is

$$P_{i,i+1} = 1 - (p_{ie} + p_{is} + p_{iu}) + (p_{ie}p_{is} + p_{ie}p_{iu} + p_{is}p_{iu}) - p_{ie}p_{is}p_{iu} \quad (3.9)$$

The probability of p_{ie} is a function of unknown treatment effect δ and the trial designs, while the probability of p_{is} is a function of unknown safety profile of the drug and the trial designs, p_{iu} is the estimated probability of stopping due to unspecified reasons.

For a phase 3 trial, $1 - p_{ie}$ is actually the Bayesian power of the hypothesis test for the primary efficacy endpoint or the probability passing the statistical test for efficacy. When calculating p_{ie}, we have to consider the possible range (usually include H_0 and H_a) or the distribution of effect size δ. The probability of stopping for safety p_{is} can be estimated from previous data. The estimation may not be accurate but will become more accurate as the data accumulates.

Example 3.3: Calculation of Transition Probability

Suppose a parallel two-group randomized phase 2 cancer trial design has an (Bayesian) average power of 45% over a range of possible effect size (See Section 2.10 Bayesian Power for Classical Trial). Thus the stopping probability due to lack of efficacy is $p_{2e} = 1 - 0.45 = 0.55$. The safety profile is average with $p_{2s} = 0.07$ (see Table 3.5 for the benchmark, $p_{2s} = 6.7\%$) and the probability of stopping for unspecified risks is estimated to be $p_{2u} = 0.20$ (see Table 3.5 for the benchmark, $p_{2u} = 26.8\% - 6.7\% = 20.1\%$) Thus, the transition probability from phase 2 to phase 3 can be calculated from Eq. (3.9):

$$P_{23} = 1 - (0.55 + 0.07 + 0.20) + (0.55 \times 0.07 + 0.55 \times 0.20 + 0.07 \times 0.20)$$
$$-0.55 \times 0.07 \times 0.20 = 0.335,$$

which is slightly larger than the industry benchmark 30.7% for "all indications" in Table 3.1.

The stopping probability is very much dependent on the go/no-go decision rules. However, a decision rule that make easy to transit to the next phase may not necessarily lead to a better design since by doing so we can make a larger type-I error.

3.2.5   Example of CDP Optimization

Considering an NME for oncology indication, phase 1, traditional 3+3 dose-escalation trial, 7 dose levels, trial simulations using *ExpDesign Studio*^{TM} (Appendix 3.1) shows that an average of 18 patients will needed based on logistic toxicity model: $logit\ p = -5.294 + 0.028 \times Dose$. The phase 1 require 10 months to complete (oncology trial length is usually shorter than the benchmark in Table 3.2). The estimated cost (including a 4 million overhead cost to pay company employee) is $C_1 = 18 \times 57500 + 4,000,000 = \$5,035,000$ (\$57500/patient from Table 3.5). The transition probability is estimated to be $P_{12} = 0.63$.

In the Phase 2 trial, patients are dosed with the identified MTD from the Phase 1 trial, the prior response rate is assumed to follow a beta distribution $\theta \sim beta(\beta_1 = 1.5, \beta_2 = 8.3)$. $E(\theta) = \frac{\beta_1}{\beta_1 + \beta_2} = 15.3\%$. For simplicity in practice, the prior distribution is approximated using a discrete distribution: $\pi(\theta) = 1/3$ when $\theta = 0.06, 0.2$, and 0.25; otherwise $\pi(\theta) = 0$.

Based on an optimistic view as we often do, the hypothesis test is specified for the trial as $H_0 : 0.1$ versus $H_a : \theta = 0.25$. Simon's two stage single-arm optimal design with 90% power and $\alpha = 10\%$ requires a sample size of $N = 50$. The stopping rules are: at stage 1, stop for futility if response $\leq 2/21$; otherwise the trial continues to the second stage. At stage 2, stop for efficacy if responses $\geq 8/50$, reject the null hypothesis. For this design, when $\theta = 0.06$, 0.15, and 0.25, the expected sample size are 25, 39, and 48, respectively. The average power for detecting the three values of θ is $(0.006 + 0.0.408 + 0.90)/3 =$

0.30 (see Appendix 3.2 for the SAS simulation program). That is, given the prior θ, the average of the expected sample sizes is $(25 + 39 + 48)/3 = 37$ and average power is 54%.

The estimated average time to conduct the trial with the average sample size of 37 is 13 months, costing \$67,500/patient (from table 3.5). It is estimated from Table 3.4 that there is approximately a 20% probability of stopping at phase 2 due to toxicity and 10% probability of stopping due to other unspecified reasons. Thus, the phase transition probability can be calculated from (3.9):

$$P_{23} = 1 - (0.7 + 0.2 + 0.1) + (0.7 \times 0.2 + 0.7 \times 0.1 + 0.2 \times 0.1)$$
$$-0.7 \times 0.2 \times 0.1 = 21.6\%$$

The probability is slightly lower than the benchmark 24.6% for the transition probability from phase 2 to phase 3 for oncology in Table 3.1.

Considering the cost for the phase 2 trial including the estimated \$8 million overhead (payment for company employees, etc.), $C_2 = 39 \times 67500 + 8,000,000 = \$10,632,500 = (\$67500/\text{patient from Table 3.5})$.

Phase 3 trial designs:

To explain the optimization process, two two-group parallel design options are considered with 80% and 90% power for the phase 3 trial. For simplicity, assume possible prior hazard ratios are 1, 0.8, and 0.7 with an equal probability of 1/3.

Design Option 1: For a 90% power, median survival time 10 and 7 months for the test and control groups, respectively (hazard rates are $\ln(2)/10 = 0.0693$ and $\frac{\ln(2)}{7} = 0.099$, hazard ratio, $HR = 0.7$), enrollment rate $= 43$ patients/month, recruitment time $= 10$ months, total study duration $= 24$ month, and one-sided $\alpha = 0.025$, the sample size required is 215 per group (total 342 events) based on a logrank test. The time required for running the trial and analysis/report/NDA package is estimated to be 36 months.

If the hazard ratio $HR = 0.8$ and median survival times are 10 and 8 months for the test and control groups, the design with the same sample will provide a 52% power (assume we don't prolong study duration, otherwise, it will impact the cost and g_4). If the test drug has no effect, $HR = 1$, power (probability of rejection) will be 0.025. Thus, average power $= (0.9 + 0.52 + 0.025)/3 = 0.482$. The estimated probability of stopping due to lack of efficacy is $1 - 0.482 = 0.518$.

The estimated trial cost is \$67,500/patient (from table 3.5). There is an estimated 15% probability of stopping at phase 3 due to toxicity (Table 3.4) and a 5% probability of stopping due to other unspecified reasons. The phase transition probability is calculated from (3.9) with $p_{ie} = 0.518$, $p_{is} = 0.15$, $p_{iu} = 0.05$, and $i = 3$: $P_{34} = 0.38922$. This transition probability (Phase 3 to Approval) is slightly better than the industry benchmark for oncology 33.0%.

Assuming the patent will expire in 15 years, $T_e = 180$ months, the design option requires 430 patients and the cost, including an estimated of \$35 million of overhead, $C_3 = 430 \times 69000 + 35,000,000 = \$64,670,000$ (\$69000/patient from Table 3.5). The total time for phase 1-3 trials is $t_c = 10 + 13 + 36 = 59$ months. CDP development and FDA review are estimated to be $t_0 = 24$ months. Therefore, the time-to-market is $T_m = 59 + 24 = 83$ months. Annual net sales from the drug without further competitor is $V_p = \$200$ million and competitor emerge rate $R_c = 0.1$. It is estimated that $G_m = \$500$ million. From (3.7) and (3.4), we can obtain the expected values at different decision points:

$$\begin{cases} g_4 = \frac{200/12}{0.25(0.1)} \ln \frac{1+0.25(0.1)180}{1+0.25(0.1)83} + 500 = \$887.63 \text{ million} \\ g_3 = P_{34}g_4 - C_3 = 0.38922\,(887.63) - 64.67 = \$280.81 \text{ million} \\ g_2 = P_{23}g_3 - C_2 = 0.216\,(280.81) - 10.6325 = \$50.02 \text{ million} \\ g_1 = P_{12}g_2 - C_1 = 0.63\,(50.02) - 5.035 = \$26.48 \text{ million} \end{cases}$$

Even though our estimates for the overhead cost are approximate, we still want to keep many decimal points in the results for the purpose of comparison between different design options.

Design Option 2: keep all the parameters the same (including the same number of patients) except to reduce the total study duration from 24 to 19 months so that the time required for running the trial and analysis/report will reduce to 31 months. As a result, the trial will reduce to 85.5% power when $HR = 0.7$. If $HR = 0.8$, median survival time 10 and 8 months, power will be 0.46 and power $= 0.025$ if $HR = 1$. Thus, the average power $= (0.855 + 0.46 + 0.025)/3 = 0.44667$. The probability of stopping due to lack of efficacy is $1 - 0.44667 = 0.55333$. The phase transition probability can be calculated from (3.9) with $p_{ie} = 0.55333$, $p_{is} = 0.15$, $p_{iu} = 0.05$, and $i = 3$: $P_{34} = 0.35769$.

If the design option 2 is chosen with 116 patients/group and 31 months in study length, the total duration for clinical trials will be $t_c = 10 + 13 + 31 = 54$ months. Assume the same amount time required for CDP development and FDA review, $t_0 = 24$ months, the time-to-market is $T_m = 54 + 24 = 78$ months. Because this design option has a 5-month shorter duration, the cost reduces approximately by 15%, that is $C_3 = 0.85 \times 64670000 = \$54,970,000$. The estimated annual sales for the drug without competitor is $V_p = \$200$ million. $R_c = 0.1$. The estimated sales after the patent expiration is $G_m = \$500$ million. From (3.7), we obtain all the expected values at different decision points:

$$\begin{cases} g_4 = \frac{200/12}{0.25(0.1)} \ln \frac{1+0.25(0.1)180}{1+0.25(0.1)78} + 500 = \$915.30 \text{ million} \\ g_3 = P_{34}g_4 - C_3 = 0.35769\,(915.30) - 54.97 = \$272.42 \text{ million} \\ g_2 = P_{23}g_3 - C_2 = 0.216\,(272.42) - 10.6325 = \$48.21 \text{ million} \\ g_1 = P_{12}g_2 - C_1 = 0.63\,(48.21) - 5.035 = \$25.34 \text{ million} \end{cases}$$

The summary of the outcomes of the two CDP options are presented in Table 3.12.

TABLE 3.12

Comparison of Two Clinical Development Plans.

Phase i	CDP 1 ($g_1 = 26.48$)				CDP 2 ($g_1 = 25.34$)			
	t_c	C_i	$P_{i,i+1}$	g_{i+1}	t_c	C_i	$P_{i,i+1}$	g_{i+1}
3	59	64.67	0.39	887.63	54	64.67	0.36	915.30
2	12	10.63	0.22	280.81	12	10.63	0.22	272.42
1	10	5.04	0.63	50.02	10	5.04	0.63	48.21
Preclin				26.48				25.34

In practice, there are many CDP options and the optimal CDP options is the one with largest expected return at decision point i. In the above example, at the end of preclinical, Phase1, and Phase 2, we will choose CDP 1 since it gives a larger expected gain than CDP 2. At the end of Phase 3, CDP2 has a larger expected gain g_4 than CDP1, but the study is finished and there are no longer options that we could take. This seems to be a paradox, in that CDP 1 appears to be a better option in the early stages of development, however as the program progresses it is a worse option than CDP 2. When the situation is inspected closely, the paradox can be resolved: although CDP 2 has a potential larger gain g_4 than CDP 1 if the drug is approved, the probability of getting the drug approved? is lower for option 2 than option 1.

Optimal Policy:

During a stochastic decision process, at decision point i, for each option k, the total time for going-forward trials t_{ci}, the cost C_i, the transition probability $P_{i,i+1}$, $G_{\max}$, and the expected gain g_{i+1} are calculated. The optimal decision $\breve{a}_i$ (CDP design option) to be taken at decision time-point i will be the one with the largest expected value g_{i+1}. The sequence of decisions $\{\breve{a}_i, \breve{a}_{i+1}, ..., \breve{a}_K\}$ will constitute the optimal action set, while the corresponding set of decision rules constitute the optimal policy.

For capitalization or return on investment (ROI) per dollar per year, NPV/year may also be used to compare with other opportunities.

3.2.6 Updating Model Parameters

In the previous section, the expected gains, g_1, g_2, g_3, and g_4 are calculated for all the decision points in the clinical development program. However, when a decision point is passed, e.g., finishing phase 1, we only need to recalculate all the expected gains going forward, i.e., g_2, g_3, g_4, based on updated information such as time to market, t_m, time to patent expiration t_e, Annual sale for the drug without further competitor, V_p, time and costs for future trials, t_{c2}, t_{c3}, C_2, and C_3, and transition probabilities P_{23} and P_{34} that are dependent on the updated efficacy and safety profile or the posterior distributions.

Efficacy and safety parameters are updated as the data accumulate. Frequentist's point estimates are often used, but not sufficient for CDP optimization since parameters under different possible situations need to be considered, e.g., posterior distributions of efficacy and safety parameters.

Let's denote prior distribution by $\pi(\theta)$, and the sample distribution by $P(x|\theta)$. Bayesian posterior distribution can be calculated as

$$\pi(\theta|x) = \frac{P(x|\theta)\,\pi(\theta)}{\int P(x|\theta)\,\pi(\theta)\,d\theta}, \tag{3.10}$$

The simplest class of prior is so-called conjugate prior. If model $X \sim N(\theta, \sigma^2)$ with know σ, the conjugate priors for θ is $\pi(\theta) = N(\theta_0, \sigma_0^2)$, specifically, the posterior is

$$\theta \sim N\left(\theta_0 + \bar{x}, \sigma_0^2 + \hat{\sigma}^2\right) \tag{3.11}$$

where mean $\bar{x} = \frac{1}{n}\Sigma_{i=1}^n x_i$ and variance $\hat{\sigma}^2 = \frac{1}{n-1}\Sigma_{i=1}^n (x_i - \bar{x})^2$.

For binormal model $X \sim Bin(N, p)$, the conjugate priors for θ is $\pi(\theta) = Beta(\alpha, \beta)$ (interpreted as $\alpha - 1$ successes and $\beta - 1$ failures), In other words, if x successes/responses are observed out of N observations, the posterior is

$$\theta \sim Beta(\alpha + x, \beta + N - x) \tag{3.12}$$

In addition to these models for a fixed treatment, a dose-response model is often interesting to consider, which establishes the relationship between efficacy/toxicity and the dose regimens (dose levels, schedules, different drug combinations).

Drug toxicity can be measured differently for disease indications. Generally, drug toxicity is considered as tolerable if the toxicity is manageable and reversible. For oncology, the standardization of the level of drug toxicity is the Common Toxicity Criteria (CTC) developed by the United States National Cancer Institute (NCI). Any adverse event (AE) related to treatment of CTC category of Grade 3 and higher is often considered a dose-limiting toxicity (DLT). The maximum tolerated dose (MTD) is defined as the maximum dose with a DLT rate that is no more frequent than a predetermined value. The initial dose given to the first patients in a phase I study should be low enough to avoid severe toxicity. The commonly used starting dose is the dose at which 10% mortality (LD_{10}) occurs in mice.

The measures of efficacy signals can be a biomarker such as a pharmacodynamic marker in early phases of clinical development. Whether it is for modeling efficacy or safety, commonly used models are logistic (Figure 3.6) and Emax model. In addition, the so-called skeleton models are often used (Chang, 2014).

Let x be the dose and $P(x|\theta)$ be the probability of response or response rate. The logistic model is defined as

$$P(x|\theta) = [1 + b\exp(-ax)]^{-1}, \tag{3.13}$$

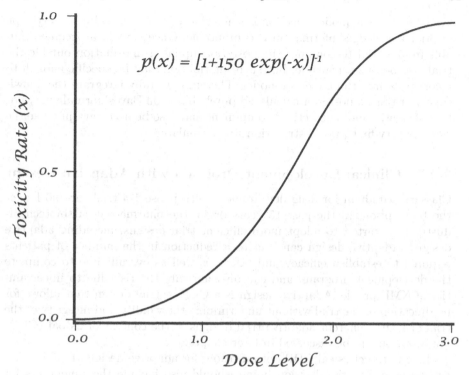

$$p(x) = [1+150 \; exp(-x)]^{-1}$$

FIGURE 3.6
Logistic Model.

where $\theta = \{a, b\}'$, b is usually a predetermined constant and a is a parameter
to be updated based on observed data.

Unspecified Risk

The stopping probability due to unspecified reasons can be modeled by
logistic model of time:

$$p_s(t) = [1 + b \exp(-at)]^{-1}, \tag{3.14}$$

where t is the duration under consideration. The longer the duration, the
more likely the unspecified risk will occur. However, a parametric model is
not necessary because the probability of stopping for unexpected reasons can
just be estimated at the decision points without any model.

Because the knowledge of the efficacy and safety profile and other relevant
information is constantly updated, these transition probabilities are constantly
updated at various decisions points (e.g., at the end of a phase, at interim analysis, etc.). For this reason, Bayesian posterior distribution of the parameters
can be an effective tool. In practice, the updated information does not have
to be the posteriors based on Bayes' formulation; it can be somewhat ad hoc.
The reason is that when formulating a prior we may use some historical data

available, but the model selection is somewhat subjective, and not every type of prior knowledge/information is computable. Once new data become available from a trial to compute the posterior, updated information outside the trial also becomes available, but such information may be specific enough to incorporate into the Bayesian model. Therefore, to fully integrate the knowledge over time, a posterior calculated purely based on Bayes' formula may not be sufficient, some "subjective" component may also be necessary just like the way the very first prior distribution was formulated.

3.2.7   Clinical Development Program with Adaptive Design

Classical paradigm for drug development with phase 1-4 trials are no longer the best option. In the past 15 years or so, the pharmaceutical/biotech industry has started to adopt more efficient trial designs, including adaptive designs. Adaptive design can lead to a reduction in the number of patients required to establish efficacy and safety as well as overall time to complete the development program, and can also mitigate the risk due to uncertainties of NME profile. Adaptive design is a CDP or trial design that allows for modification to the trial without undermining the validity and integrity of the trial or CDP. Different adaptive trial designs in the context of global (CDP) optimization will be discussed in later chapters.

Like in the classical CDP optimization, for adaptive design of CDP, SDP can be used, but the decision points should also include the timepoints for the interim analyses in addition to the design timepoints. However, at this moment, regulatory authorities require adaptations and its decision rules have to be specified at beginning of the trial. Therefore, the same stochastic decision model can be used for CDP even if it includes adaptive trials. In fact, a simple adaptive design, Simon's two-stage design has already been used in a previous example.

Adaptive design can combine two trials from different phases such as phase 1-2 seamless design or phase 2-3 seamless design. When a combination happens, the decision points for the clinical development program may reduce, but the calculation procedures are the same. Adaptive design will impact the expected gain g_i through affecting the power, the transition probability, the trial-length, the sample size, the cost of the trial, and the time-to-market. The statistical complexity of an adaptive trial requires clinical trial simulations (CTS) and more up-front planning. These topics will be discussed in the coming chapters.

Clinical trial simulations (CTS) are important in adaptive trial design and CDP optimization, this is because: (1) the statistical theory of adaptive design is complicated with limited analytical solutions available under certain assumptions; (2) the concept of CTS is very intuitive and easy to implement; (3) CTS can be used to model complicated situations to validate the type-I error rate; (4) CTS can be used not only to simulate the power of an adaptive design, but also to generate many other important operating characteristics such as expected sample-size, and conditional power, (5) CTS can used to evaluate the robustness of an adaptive design in different hypothetical clinical settings, or with protocol deviations; (6) CTS can be used to monitor trials, project outcomes, anticipate problems, and suggest remedies before it is too late; (7) CTS has minimal cost associated with it and can be done in a short time. In summary, clinical trial simulation is a useful tool for adaptive designs and CDP optimization

3.3 Summary

Various pharmaceutical industry benchmarks of clinical trials and clinical development programs are studied. Those benchmarks can serve as the guidance for constructing the Stochastic Decision Process in CDP optimization. CDP optimization is a global optimization, a better optimization than a local optimization for individual adaptive trials.

The stochastic model used for CDP optimization requires calculations or estimations of the time-to-market (T_m), the time and cost for each phase, the rate (R_m) at which market competitors emerge, and the probability of success or transition probabilities. All these depend on the sequence of trial designs in a CDP, the power of the trials and the ability to mitigate the risk. The three key formulae for the calculations in the CDP stochastic model are

$$\begin{cases} g_4 = \frac{V_p}{0.25R_c} \ln \frac{1+0.25R_cT_e}{1+0.25R_cT_m} + G_{\max} \\ P_{i,i+1} = 1 - (p_{ie} + p_{is} + p_{iu}) + (p_{ie}p_{is} + p_{ie}p_{iu} + p_{is}p_{iu}) - p_{ie}p_{is}p_{iu} \\ g_i = p_{i,i+1}g_{i+1} - C_i \end{cases}$$

The steps for the CDP optimization are (calculations should be based on the most updated information):

1. Estimate V_p, R_c, T_m for each CDP option and calculate g_4 (for simplicity, let $G_{max} = 0$ or any constant for the purpose optimization).

2. For each CDP option, calculate the Bayesian power and the probability of stopping due to lack of efficacy, p_{ie}, for Phase i ($i = 1, 2, 3, 4$), and estimate the stopping probability p_{is} due to safety and the stopping probability p_{iu} due to unspecified reasons. Then use them to calculate the transition probability $P_{i,i+1}$.

3. For each CDP option, estimate the cost C_i (the inflated cost at time when the drug is on market, $i = 1, 2, 3, 4$) and g_4 to backwards calculate g_3, g_2, and g_1.

4. Choose the CDP option with maximum g_i at decision point i or the beginning of Phase i. At decision point i, all quantities before that time point are irrelevant and don't need to be recalculated.

As the clinical development progresses, we move from one decision point to the next. At decision point i (the beginning of Phase i), the optimal design/action is simply the one with the maximum value of g_i, and has nothing to do the previous gain $g_1, ...,$ and g_{i-1} or the amount money and efforts that have already spent, $C_1, ...,$ and C_{i-1}.

It is worthwhile to mention that every time we move to the next decision point $i + 1$, we should recalculate the future expected gains, $g_{i+1}, ...,$ and g_4 based on updated information using Bayesian or frequentist approach and choose the design option that has the largest gain increase $g_{i+1} - g_i$. Furthermore, in the clinical development process, the future design options can be changed or expanded from the initial CDP options. It is important to keep in mind that CDP optimization must protect a range of parameter and not just a fixed value for treatment effect because we don't know the true effect size. In other words, the optimization maximizes the expected NPV at the decision point under posterior distribution of the parameters.

The NPV at a decision point will be compared to other investment options before making a go-decision. That is, the opportunity loss has to be considered in decision-making.

Bibliography

Avance (2008). http://www.avance.ch/newsletter/docs/discount_1.pdf

Bio et al. (2016). Clinical Development Success Rates 2006-2015. https://www.bio.org/sites/.

Chang, M. (2010). Monte Carlo Simulation for the pharmaceutical industry. Chapman & Hall/CRC, Boca Raton, FL

FDA (2017). CDER Approval Times for Priority and Standard NDAs and BLAs Calendar Years 1993 – 2016.

FDA (2017). https://www.fda.gov/downloads/Drugs/DevelopmentApproval Process/

Harrison, R.K (2016). Phase II and phase III failures: 2013–2015. Nature Reviews Drug Discovery, 15, 817-818, 2016

Ralph Villiger, R. and Nielsen, N.H. (2011). Discount rates in drug development. http://www.avance.ch/avance_biostrat_discount_survey.pdf.

Sertkaya, A., et al. (2014). Examination of clinical trial costs and barries for drug development. https://aspe.hhs.gov/report/examination-clinical-trial-costs-and-barriers-drug-development

4

Globally Optimal Adaptive Trial Designs

4.1 Common Adaptive Designs

As mentioned in Chapter 1, an adaptive design is a clinical trial design that allows adaptations or modifications to aspects of the trial after its initiation without undermining the validity and integrity of the trial. In a recent investigation on the use of different adaptive trial designs, it is reported that among all adaptive trials evaluated, 29% were group sequential design (GSD), 16% sample-size reestimation (SSR), 21% Phase-I/II or Phase-II/III seamless designs, and 41% dose-escalation, dose-selection and others (Hatfield et al., 2016). Commonly used adaptive designs here include group sequential design, sample-size re-estimation, and drop-loser design (pick-winner design).

A group sequential design (GSD) is an adaptive design that allows a trial to stop earlier based on the results of interim analyses. For a trial with a positive result, early stopping ensures that a new drug product can be available to the patients sooner. If a negative result is indicated, early stopping avoids wasting resources and reduces the unnecessary exposure to the ineffective drug. Sequential methods typically lead to savings in sample-size, time, and cost when compared with the classical design with a fixed sample-size. GSD is probably one of the most commonly used adaptive designs in clinical trials. Well-known early research on GSD include papers by Pocock (1977), O'Brien & Fleming (1979), Lan & DeMets (1983), Wang & Tsiatis (1987), Whitehead & Stratton (1983), and Lan & Demets (1989). The book, Group Sequential Design for Clinical Trials by Jennison and Turnbull (2000) made a significant on the application of GSD in the pharmaceutical industry.

A sample-size reestimation (SSR) design refers to an adaptive design that allows for sample-size adjustment or re-estimation based on the review of interim analysis results (Figure 4.1). The sample-size requirement for a trial is sensitive to the treatment effect and its variability. An inaccurate estimation of the effect size or its variability could lead to an underpowered or overpowered design, neither of which is desirable. An underpowered trial will have low ability to detect a small but clinically meaningful difference, and consequently could prevent a potentially effective drug from being delivered to patients. On the other hand, an overpowered trial can lead to unnecessary exposure of many patients to a potentially harmful compound when the drug, in fact, is not effective. In practice, it is often difficult to estimate the effect size and

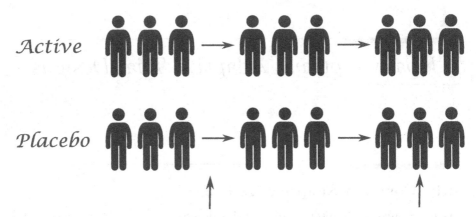

Active

Placebo

Interim results may indicate additional patients required to preserve the power

FIGURE 4.1
Sample-Size Reestimation Design.

variability because of many uncertainties during protocol development. Thus, it is desirable to have the flexibility to re-estimate the sample-size at some point during the trial.

There are two types of SSR procedures, namely, SSR based on blinded data and SSR based on unblinded data. In the first scenario, the sample adjustment is based on the pooled variance at the interim analysis to recalculate the required sample-size, which does not require unblinding the data. In this scenario, the impact of SSR on the Type-I error rate is practically negligible; in fact, FDA and other regulatory agencies typically regard this type of sample size adjustment to be unbiased and without any statistical penalty. In the second scenario, both the effect size and its variability are re-assessed during the trial, and sample-size is adjusted based on the updated information. The statistical method for adjustment can be based on the observed effect size (Cui, Wang, Hung, 1999) or the calculated conditional power (Chang, 2014). Chen, DeMets, & Lan (2004) and Mehta & Pocock (2011) proposed another Promising-Zone method. The idea behind the method is that if at interim analysis, the effect size is very small, below the clinically meaningful difference, there is no reason to increase sample size to increase the power; if the effect size is close to the initially estimated sample size, the power would be sufficiently high, no sample-size adjustment is necessary; otherwise, the observed effect size falls within a promising zone but power might be lower than planned, therefore, increasing sample size to protect the power will be beneficial.

The classical multiple-arm dose response study has been studied since the mid 1970s, Dunnett's test (1955, 1964) and Dunnett & Tamhane (1992) based on the multivariate normal distribution is most often used and Rom, Costello, Connell (1994) proposed a closed set test procedure. A recent addition to the adaptive design arsenal are multiple-arm adaptive designs. A typical multiple-arm confirmatory adaptive design (variously called drop-the-loser, drop-arm, pick-the-winner, winner, adaptive dose-finding, or Phase II/III seamless designs) consists of two stages: a selection stage and a confirmation stage. For the selection stage, a randomized parallel design with several doses and a control group is employed. After the best dose (the winner) is chosen based on numerically "better" observed responses, the patients of the selected dose group and control group continue to enter the confirmation stage (Figure 4.2). New patients are recruited and randomized to receive the selected dose or control. The final analysis is performed with the cumulative data of patients from both stages (Chang 2014). Recently, Chang and Wang (2014) derived the distribution of test statistics for $K + 1$ arm winner design.

Bretz et al. (2006) studied confirmatory seamless Phase II/III clinical trials with hypothesis selection at the interim analysis. Huang, Liu, and Hsiao (2011) proposed a seamless design to allow pre-specifying probabilities of rejecting the drug at each stage to improve the efficiency of the trial. Posch, Maurer, and Bretz (2011) described two approaches to control the Type I error rate in adaptive designs with sample size reassessment and/or treatment selection. Shun, Lan and Soo (2008) considered a study starting with two treatment groups and a control group with a planned interim analysis. The inferior treatment group would be dropped after the interim analysis. Such an interim analysis can be based on the clinical endpoint or a biomarker. They proposed a normal approximation approach to calculate the Type-I error, the power, the point estimate, and the confidence intervals. Heritier, Lô and Morgan (2011) studied the Type-I error control of seamless unbalanced designs, issues of noninferiority comparison, multiplicity of secondary endpoints, and covariance adjusted analyses. Further extensions of seamless designs that allow adaptive designs to continue seamlessly either in a subpopulation of patients or in the entire population on the basis of data obtained from the first stage of a Phase II/III design have also been developed. Jenkins, Stone, and Jennison (2011) proposed design adds extra flexibility by also allowing the trial to continue in all patients but with both the subgroup and the full population as coprimary populations when the Phase II and III endpoints are different but correlated time-to-event endpoints.

In general, there are four major components of adaptive designs in the frequentist paradigm: (1) type-I error rate or α - control: determination of stopping boundaries, (2) type-II error rate β: calculation of power or sample-size, (3) trial monitoring: calculation of test statistics or p-values against stopping boundaries and conditional power, and (4) analysis after the completion of a

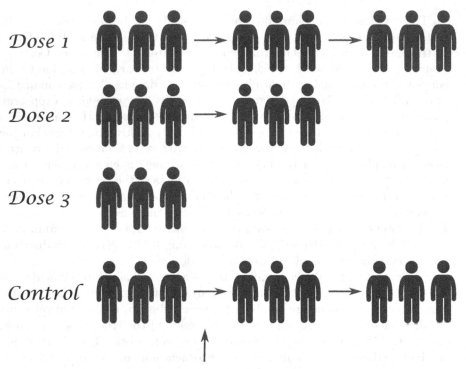

**Interim results indicate some doses are
inferior and can be dropped from the study**

FIGURE 4.2
Drop-Loser Design.

trial: calculations of adjusted p-values, unbiased point estimates, and confidence intervals.

For each type of adaptive designs, there are design parameters (sample size, power, interim analysis time, stopping rules) need to be determined. A different set of design parameters will lead to different operating characteristics (probabilities of early efficacy and futility stopping, power, ability of protect power for a smaller treatment difference, average and maximum sample sizes, probability of selecting the best dose group). So far, researchers and industry statisticians are focusing on local optimization based on maximizing the power or minimizing the sample size instead of considering a trial as an integral part of the clinical development program. The question is: if there are two options with the same cost or total sample size, (1) a smaller phase 2 study and larger phase 3 study and (2) a larger phase 2 study and a smaller phase 3 trial, which option is better one? This question can be adequately addressed through CDP optimization.

In the previous chapter, we studied the optimization of clinical development programs in a "traditional" clinical development paradigm. In this chapter, we review commonly used adaptive trial design methods and adaptive trial simulations, and discuss the adaptive trial designs based on global optimization through a case study.

4.2 Group Sequential Design

4.2.1 Test Statistics

There are three different types of GSDs: early efficacy stopping design, early futility stopping design, and early efficacy or futility stopping design. If we believe (based on prior knowledge) that the test treatment is very promising, then an early efficacy stopping design may be used to potentially shorten the time-to-market. If we are concerned that the test treatment may not work, an early futility stopping design may be employed to have resource savings. If we are not certain about the magnitude of the effect size, a GSD permitting both early stopping for efficacy and futility should be considered. In practice, if we have reasonable knowledge regarding the effect size, then a classical design with a fixed sample-size could be a good option.

The statistical determination of drug efficacy in a Phase-III trial is typically through hypothesis test:

$$H_0 : \delta = 0 \text{ (drug is ineffective) vs } H_a : \delta > 0 \text{ (drug is effective)}. \quad (4.1)$$

Controlling family-wise Type-I is the minimal statistical requirement for the internal validity of a Phase-III clinical trial. Such error control is realized in practice through the so-called stopping boundaries in an adaptive design.

The test statistic T_k at the kth interim analysis (IA) is a combination of the data from the first k stages. As an example, the test statistic at the second stage is

$$T_2 = \sqrt{\tau_1}z_1 + \sqrt{\tau_2}z_2, \quad (4.2)$$

where z_1 and z_2 are the common stagewise z-statistics formulated based on data collected from statges 1 and 2, respectively (not cumulative data), and τ_1, τ_2 are the information times (bounded by 0 and 1) or sample size fractions at stages 1 and 2, respectively.

Since $\sqrt{\tau_1}$ and $\sqrt{\tau_2}$ are predetermined constant or are independent of data z_1 and z_2, $\sqrt{\tau_1}z_1$ and $\sqrt{\tau_2}z_2$ in the test statistic T_2 are independent. As a result, the probability distribution of T_2 is uniform on $[0,1]$ under null hypothesis H_0.

The stopping rules of a GSD can be specified as

$$
\begin{array}{lll}
\text{Reject } H_0 \text{ (Stop for efficacy)} & \text{if } T_k \geq \alpha_k, \\
\text{Accept } H_0 \text{ (Stop for futility)} & \text{if } T_k < \beta_k, & (4.3) \\
\text{Continue trial to the next stage} & \text{if } \alpha_k > T_k \geq \beta_k,
\end{array}
$$

TABLE 4.1
Stopping Boundary α_2 on p-scale.

τ_1	α_1					
	0.0000	0.0025	0.0050	0.0100	0.0150	0.0200
1/4	0.0250	0.0233	0.0212	0.0168	0.0120	0.0064
1/3	0.0250	0.0235	0.0217	0.0174	0.0126	0.0071
1/2	0.0250	0.0240	0.0225	0.0188	0.0143	0.0086
3/4	0.0250	0.0247	0.0241	0.0219	0.0184	0.0130

Note: One-sided $\alpha = 0.025$ and 1,000,000 simulation runs

where the stopping boundary $\alpha_k > \beta_k$ $(k = 1, ..., K - 1)$, and $\alpha_K = \beta_K$ are determined so that the Type-I error rate is controlled at the nominal level α. For convenience, α_k and β_k are called the efficacy and futility boundaries, respectively.

The stopping rules (4.3) can be written on p-scale,

$$\begin{aligned} &\text{Reject } H_0 \text{ (Stop for efficacy)} &&\text{if } p_k \leq \alpha_k^*, \\ &\text{Accept } H_0 \text{ (Stop for futility)} &&\text{if } p_k > \beta_k^*, \\ &\text{Continue trial to the next stage} &&\text{if } \alpha_k^* < p_k \leq \beta_k^*, \end{aligned} \qquad (4.4)$$

where $p_i = 1 - \Phi(T_i)$ and α_k^* and β_i^* are the associated efficacy and stopping boundaries. As for non-normal endpoints, Lehmacher-Wassmer (1999) proposed so-called inverse-normal method for different endpoints for the GSD method (Chang, 2014).

The stopping boundaries can be determined using numerical integrations or simulations. Examples of stopping boundaries for a two-stage design are presented in Table 4.1.

In theory, the critical value α_2 is a function of efficacy stopping boundary α_1 and futility stopping boundary β_1, but practically efficacy stopping boundaries are independent of futility boundaries This is because of the so-called non-binding futility currently adopted by regulatory agencies. Regulatory authorities believe the current practice in the pharmaceutical industry is that sponsors do not necessarily follow the prespecified futility boundaries. Therefore, to be conservative, the efficacy stooping boundaries have to be determined based on the worst scenario that the futility stopping rules are not followed. This is called non-binding futility rule.

4.2.2   Commonly Used Stopping Boundaries

In classical group sequential design (GSD), the stopping boundaries are usually specified as a function of stage k. Commonly used functions are the Pocock and O'Brien-Fleming boundary functions. Wang and Tsiatis (1987) proposed a family of two-sided tests with a shape parameter Δ, which includes Pocock's and O'Brien-Fleming's boundary functions as special cases. The Wang-Tsiatis boundary on z-scale is defined by $c\tau_k^{\Delta-1/2}$ ($\Delta = 0$ for Pocock's and $\Delta = 1/2$ for O'Brien-Fleming's), where $\tau_k = \frac{k}{K}$ or $\tau_k = \frac{n_k}{N_K}$ (information time) and c (dependent on K, α,and Δ) is determined to ensure that the familywise error rate is α.

Practically, interim analysis (IA) time can be different from the initially planned due to different availability of Independent Monitoring Committee (DMC) members. Such a change in timing of IA is allowed (will not cause a type-I error inflation) as long as the change does not depend on the trial data and the stopping boundaries are recalculated at the actual information time following the prespecified error-spending function (ESF) – a cumulative error function since stage 1 of GSD. A popular error-spending function is power function family:

$$\pi(t) = \alpha t^\theta, \theta > 0. \tag{4.5}$$

The power function covers broad spending functions including an approximation to O'Brien-Fleming function,

$$\pi(\tau_k) = \begin{cases} 2\left[1 - \Phi\left(\frac{z_{1-\alpha/2}}{\sqrt{\tau_k}}\right)\right], & \tau_k > 0 \\ 0, & \tau_k = 0 \end{cases} \tag{4.6}$$

and Pocock's error-spending function (Kim and DeMets,1992),

$$\pi(\tau) = \alpha \log[1 + (e - 1)\tau] \tag{4.7}$$

The error-spending function can be any monotonically non-decreasing function $\pi(\tau)$ with a range of $[0, \alpha]$. When the error-spending function $\pi(\tau)$ is prefixed and the determination of interim analysis time does not depend on the observed data from the trial, then the overall type-I error rate is controlled because $\Sigma_{k=1}^{K}[\pi(\tau_k) - \pi(\tau_{k-1})] = \pi(1) - \pi(0) = \alpha$. This is true even when both the number of analyses K and the timing of the analyses τ_k are not predetermined. Figure 4.3 is an illustration of different error-spending functions.

The stopping boundary can either determined using numerical integration or simulations. To determine stopping boundaries $\alpha_1, \alpha_2, ..., \alpha_K$ based on selected error-spending function or $\pi_1, \pi_2, ..., \pi_K$, a recursive algorithm can be used. The key idea to determine the stopping boundaries based on an error-spending function is that the rejection probability at stage i must be equal to the error-spending at the ith stage, $\pi_i - \pi_{i-1}$, that is,

$$\Pr(T_1 > \alpha_1, T_2 > \alpha_2, ..., T_{i-1} > \alpha_{i-1}, T_i \le \alpha_i) = \pi_i - \pi_{i-1} \tag{4.8}$$

knowing $\alpha_1 = \pi_1$ and π_2, we can solve α_2 numerically based on $\Pr(T_1 > \alpha_1, T_2 \le \alpha_2) = \pi_2 - \pi_{i-1}$ using numerical integration (Chang, 2014)

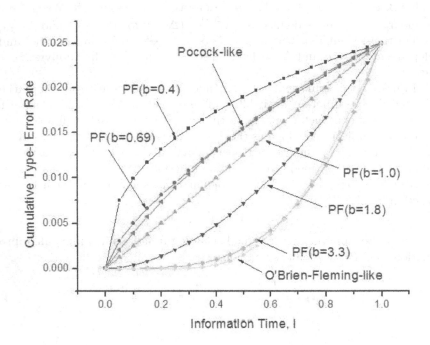

FIGURE 4.3
Error-spending functions.

or simulation. Recursively, knowing α_1, α_2, π_2, and π_3 we can use (4.8) to solve α_3 numerically. For the simulation approach, the algorithms are outlined as follows:

1. Determine the number of analyses K and interim analysis time τ_i $(i = 1, 2, ..., K)$

2. Follow a error-spending function (e.g., $\pi(\tau) = \alpha\tau^{1.8}$), calculate, $\pi_1, \pi_2, ..., \pi_{K-1}$, $\pi_K = \alpha$ for all the stages.

3. Calculate error-spending at each stage, $\pi_{i+1} - \pi_i$, $i = 1, 2, ..., K - 1$.

4. Given α_1 and try different values of α_2 in the simulations until efficacy stopping probability at stage 2 equals $\pi_2 - \pi_1$

5. Given α_1 and α_2, and try different values of α_3 in the simulations until efficacy stopping probability at stage 3 equals $\pi_3 - \pi_2$

6. ......

7. Given α_1, α_2, ...,α_{K-1}, and try different values of α_K in the simulations until efficacy stopping probability at stage K equals $\pi_K - \pi_{K-1}$

A set of four SAS macros for two-stage GSD with different endpoints are developed (See Appendix 4.1) to be used for the determination the stopping boundaries and power or sample size. To simulate the GSD trials with normal, binary, Poisson, or survival endpoint, simply invoke the corresponding SAS macro with appropriate parameters.

As an example, for a two-stage GSD with a normal endpoint, testing a mean effect 0.4 versus 0.95 between placebo and the test groups with a common standard deviation of 1.2, we can choose an interim analysis performed on 50 patients per group for efficacy claim only ($\alpha_1 = 0.0025$ and $\beta_1 = 1$, implies no interim futility stopping) and the final analysis performed on 100 patients per group with $\alpha_2 = 0.024$ (from Table 4.1) and invoke the following macro to check the type-I error rate:

%GSDNormal(nSims=1000000, ux=0.4, uy=0.4, sigma=1.2, N1=50, N2=50, alpha1=0.0025, beta1=1, alpha2=0.024);

and simulate the power by invoking the following macro:

%GSDNormal(nSims=1000000, ux=0.4, uy=0.95, sigma=1.2, N1=50, N2=50, alpha1=0.0025, beta1=1, alpha2=0.024);

The simulation results include interim futility stopping probability ($FSP = 0$), interim efficacy stopping probability ($ESP = 0.30295$), average sample size ($AveN = 84.8526$), and power ($Power = 0.89786$).

Similarly, if the primary endpoint is a binary response with response rates in the two groups being 0.5 and 0.6, sample size 300 per group at interim analysis and 600 per group in the final analysis, we will invoke the following SAS code to obtain power and other operating characteristics:

%GSDBinary(nSims=1000000, px=0.5, py=0.6, N1=300, N2=300, alpha1=0.0025, beta1=1, alpha2=0.024);

The simulation results include interim futility stopping probability ($FSP = 0$), interim efficacy stopping probability ($ESP = 0.3731$), average sample size ($AveN = 488.07$), and power ($Power = 0.93556$).

If we want to compare two Poison processes with parameter $\lambda_1 = 0.4$ versus $\lambda_2 = 0.6$, the power simulation code will be as follows:

%GSDPoisson(nSims=1000000, Lamdax=0.4, Lamday=0.6, N1=125, N2=125, alpha1=0.0025, beta1=1, alpha2=0.024);

The simulation results include interim futility stopping probability ($FSP = 0$), interim efficacy stopping probability ($ESP = 0.28153$), average sample size ($AveN = 214.808$), and power ($Power = 0.8858$). The sample size and stopping boundaries can be changed as necessary to obtain desired operating characteristics.

Trial Example 4.1: Adaptive Design for Oncology Trial

In designing a two-arm comparative oncology trial with the primary efficacy endpoint, time-to-progression (TTP), an exponential survival distribution is assumed with a 8-month median TTP (hazard rate 0.0866) for the control group and 10-month (hazard rate 0.0693) for the test groups. The common used logrank test will be used with a one-sided significance level $\alpha = 0.025$. Given a uniform enrollment with an accrual period of 12 months and a total study duration of 24 months, the classical design will require a sample-size of 494 patients per group or total 733 events for 85% power, which is obtained from running the following simulation code.

%GSDSurvival(nSims=1000000, tStd=24, tAcr=12, Lamdax=0.0693, Lamday=0.0866, N1=247, N2=247, alpha1=-1, beta1=1, alpha2=0.025);

For a GSD with an interim analysis performed on 50% of total patients, $\alpha_1 = 0.0025$, $\beta_1 = 0.5$ ($\beta_1 = 0.5$ implies the observed treatment effect must be positive to continue the trial), and $\alpha_2 = 0.024$ from Table 4.1. We first checking the type-I error control by invoking the following macro:

%GSDSurvival(nSims=1000000, tStd=24, tAcr=12, Lamdax=0.0866, Lamday=0.0866, N1=250, N2=250, alpha1=0.0025, beta1=1, alpha2=0.024);

Since the simulation results show that power or rejection probability under H_0 is 0.0249, very close to the significance level $\alpha = 0.025$, the efficacy stopping boundaries are correct ($\beta_1 = 1$ instead of 0.5 is used because of non-binding futility rule). To obtain operating characteristics under H_a, we invoke the following SAS code:

%GSDSurvival(nSims=1000000, tStd=24, tAcr=12, Lamdax=0.0693, Lamday=0.0866, N1=250, N2=250, alpha1=0.0025, beta1=0.5, alpha2=0.024);

With maximum 500 patients per group (a 6 patient increase from the classical design), the simulation results show that interim futility stopping probability ($FSP = 0.017$), interim efficacy stopping probability ($ESP = 0.251$), the total number of events ($nEvents = 742$) (if the trial continues to the second stage, average number of events ($AvenEvents = 643$), and power ($Power = 0.850$). Therefore, the GSD will have $733 - 643 = 90$ events savings on average. Furthermore, the futility stopping boundary beta1=0.5 will cut down the number of events required from 733 to 584 when H_0 is true from, which can be obtained the following simulations:

%GSDSurvival(nSims=1000000, tStd=24, tAcr=12, Lamdax=0.0866, Lamday=0.0866, N1=250, N2=250, alpha1=0.0025, beta1=0.5, alpha2=0.024);

The simulation results include early futility stopping probability ($FSP = 0.5$), average number of events required (AvenEvents = 584), and rejection probability (Power = 0.0246). This suggests that if the futility boundary is always followed, the type-I error rate will be 0.0246, smaller than $\alpha = 0.025$.

4.3   Sample Size Reestimation Design

4.3.1   Test Statistic

The main statistical challenge of SSR compared to GSD is that unlike in GSD, in which the $\sqrt{\tau_1}z_1$ and $\sqrt{\tau_2}z_2$ in the test statistic T_2 are independent, in SSR, because $\sqrt{\tau_2}$ is a function of the second stage sample size n_2 that depends on the observed treatment difference or z_1 from the first stage data, z_1 and z_2 are not independent. Therefore, the joint distribution of T_1 and T_2 is much more complicated than in GSD. Several solutions have been proposed, including (1) the fixed weight method in forming the test statistic (Cui, Hung, Wang, 1999, Wassmer, 1999), (2) the method of adjusting stopping boundary through simulations or numerical integration (Chang, 2014), and (3) promising-zone methods (Chen, DeMets, and Lan, 2004; Mehta, Pocock, 2011).

In the fixed weight method, the test statistic is defined as a linear combination of two statistics of subsamples from the two stages.

The weights w_1 and w_2 can be any positive values, satisfying $w_1^2 + w_2^2 = 1$ (Wassmer, 1999). As a special case, if $w_1^2 = \tau_0 = \frac{n_1}{N_0}$ and $w_2^2 = 1 - w_1^2$, where n_1 is sample size and N_0 is the original cumulative sample size, it becomes Cui-Wang-Hung's test statistic (1999),

$$T_2 = \sqrt{\tau_0} z_1 + \sqrt{1 - \tau_0} z_2. \tag{4.9}$$

The weighted Z-statistic approach with (4.9) is flexible in that the decision to increase the sample size and the magnitude of sample size increment are not mandated by pre-specified rules.

Chen, DeMets, and Lan (2004) proposed the Promising-Zone method, where the unblinded interim result is considered "promising" and eligible for SSR if the conditional power is greater than 50 percent, equivalently, the sample size increment needed to achieve a desired power does not exceed a prespecified upper bound. The Promising-Zone method may be justifiable to effectively put resources on drug candidates that are likely effective or that might fail only marginally at the final analysis with the original sample size, based on the information seen at the interim analysis.

Chen, DeMets, and Lan use a conservative test statistic for the second stage:

$$T_2 = \min \left\{ \sqrt{\frac{n_1}{N_0}} z_1 + \sqrt{\frac{N_0 - n_1}{N_0}} z_2, \sqrt{\frac{n_1}{N}} z_1 + \sqrt{\frac{N - n_1}{N}} z_2 \right\} \tag{4.10}$$

where z_1 and z_2 are the usual Z-statistic based on the subsamples from stages 1 and 2, respectively. n_1 is the sample size at the interim analysis, N_0 is the original final sample size and N is the new final sample size after adjustment based on the interim analysis. Using this modified test statistic, the authors proved that when the conditional probability based original sample size is larger than 50%, then adjusted sample size, i.e., increasing the sample size when the unblinded interim result is promising will not inflate the type I error rate.

Mehta and Pocock (2011) simplified Chen-Demets-Lan's method, using the same test statistic as in GSD:

$$T_2 = \sqrt{\frac{n_1}{N}} z_1 + \sqrt{\frac{N - n_1}{N}} z_2 \tag{4.11}$$

They define the promising zone as the interim p-value p_1 between 0.1587 ($z_1 = 1.206$) and 0.0213 ($z_1 = 2.027$). They chose these values because when one-sided p-value p_1 is larger but close to 0.1 at the interim analysis with information time $\tau = 0.5$, the trial is likely to marginally fail to reject H_0 at the final analysis with p-value around 0.06 to 0.15. Those drug candidates are likely clinically effective, thus we want to "save" those trials and allow them a better chance to show statistical significance by increasing the sample size. If the p_1 is, say, larger than 0.2 (0.4 for two-sided p-value), we will stop the trial earlier at the first stage. For practical purposes, we recommend the following approach: combine the futility boundary with the upper bound of the promising zone and recommend using $\beta_1 = 0.2$ for the one-sided p-value at the interim analysis with information time 0.5. The promising zone can be defined differently as long as the type-I error rate is controlled it is usually is statistically valid method. The promising zone method is generally more efficient than Cui-Wang-Hung's method because the latter down-weights the second stage data, making an sample size increase less effective regarding the power increase.

4.3.2   Rules of Stopping and Sample-Size Adjustment

The stopping rules for efficacy and futility are similar to a group sequential design, but there is an additional sample size reestimation rule at the interim analysis:

$$
\begin{array}{lll}
\text{Reject } H_0 \text{ (stop for efficacy)} & \text{if } T_k \geq \alpha_k, & \\
\text{Accept } H_0 \text{ (Stop for futility)} & \text{if } T_k < \beta_k, & \\
\text{Continue to stage 2 with SSR} & \text{if } b_L > T_k \geq b_U, & (4.12) \\
\text{Continue to Stage 2 without SSR} & \text{other wise} &
\end{array}
$$

where the stopping boundary $\alpha_k \geq b_U \geq b_L > \beta_k$ ($k = 1, 2$), and $\alpha_2 = \beta_2$.

The commonly used approach is to adjust sample size based on the target conditional power. The conditional power p_c can be expressed as (Mehta et al., 2016)

$$
p_c = \Phi \left(z_1 \sqrt{\frac{n_2}{n_1}} - \frac{z_{1-\alpha}\sqrt{n_1 + n_{02}} - z_1\sqrt{n_1}}{\sqrt{n_{02}}} \right)
\tag{4.13}
$$

Let p_c be the target conditional power $1 - \beta$ and solve it for new sample size at stage 2, we obtain

$$
n_2 = \frac{n_1}{z_1^2} \left(\frac{z_{1-\alpha}\sqrt{n_1 + n_{02}} - z_1\sqrt{n_1}}{\sqrt{n_{02}}} + z_{1-\beta} \right)^2.
\tag{4.14}
$$

4.3.3   Simulation Examples

SAS macros (Appendix) are developed for different endpoints with Mehta-Pocock promising-zone method. Examples of simulations are provided below.

The titles indicate the purposes of simulations and most input parameters are self-explanatory, Target Power is the target conditional power, the promising-zone is based on p-scale. The stopping boundaries can be (but don't have to be) the same as those for GDS and the promising zone lower and upper bounds can be modified as long as the type-I error is no more than α. The SAS macros can also be used for GSD simulations if the second stage sample size is fixed, i.e., N2max=n2. To simulate a classic design, set alpha1 = 0, alpha2 = alpha, beta1=1, and N2Max = n2.

For normal endpoint with two group designs, following are some simulation examples:

Title "Type-I error checking for 2-group SSR promising-zone design with normal endpoint under non-binding futility rule";

%SSRTwoGroupDesignNormal(n1=100, n2=100, N2max=150, u0=1, u1=1, sigma=1.2, alpha=0.025, TargetPower=0.9, alpha1= 0.0025, alpha2=0.024, beta1=1, PromisingL=0.0213, PromisingU=0.214);

The simulation outcomes show the rejection probability (power) is 0.0250, matching the significance level α.

Title "Power Simulation for 2-group SSR promising-zone design with normal endpoint and futility stopping ";

%SSRTwoGroupDesignNormal(n1=100, n2=100, N2max=150, u0=1, u1=1.4, sigma=1.2, alpha=0.025, TargetPower=0.9, alpha1= 0.0025, alpha2=0.024, beta1=0.6, PromisingL=0.0213, PromisingU=0.214);

The simulation outcomes include: early futility stopping probability (FSP=0.005), early efficacy stopping probability (ESP=0.326), power (power=0.939), and average sample size per group (AveN=180).

Title "Power Simulation for classical design with normal endpoint ";

%SSRTwoGroupDesignNormal(n1=100, n2=100, N2max=100, u0=1, u1=1.4, sigma=1.2, alpha=0.025, alpha1= 0, alpha2=0.025, beta1=1);

The simulation outcomes show power = 0.915 for sample size 200/group.

Title "Power Simulation for 2-group GSD (without SSR) with normal endpoint and futility stopping ";

%SSRTwoGroupDesignNormal(n1=100, n2=100, N2max=100, u0=1, u1=1.4, sigma=1.2, alpha=0.025, alpha1= 0.0025, alpha2=0.024, beta1=0.5);

The simulation outcomes include: early futility stopping probability (FSP=0.009), early efficacy stopping probability (ESP=0.326), power (power=0.912), and average sample size per group (AveN=166).

For binary endpoint with one or two groups, the following are some examples of trial simulations.

Title "Power Simulation for one-group SSR promising-zone design with binary endpoint and futility stopping";

%Mehta_PocockSSROneGroupDesign(n1=100, n2=100, N2max=200, p0=0.4, p1=0.5, alpha=0.025, TargetPower=0.9, alpha1= 0.002, alpha2=0.024, beta1=0.8, PromisingL=0.0213, PromisingU=0.214);

The simulation outcomes include: early futility stopping probability (FSP=0.002), early efficacy stopping probability (ESP=0.184), power (power=0.877), and average sample size per group (AveN=215).

Title "Power Simulation two-group SSR promising-zone design with binary endpoint, without futility stopping";

%Mehta_PocockSSRTwoGroupDesign(n1=100, n2=100, N2max=100, p0=0.15, p1=0.25, alpha=0.025, TargetPower=0.9, alpha1= 0.00153, alpha2=0.02454, beta1=0.8, PromisingL=0.0213, PromisingU=0.214);

The simulation outcomes include: early futility stopping probability (FSP=0.005), early efficacy stopping probability (ESP=0.123), power (power=0.715), and average sample size per group (AveN=187).

4.4 Pick-Winner-Design

4.4.1 Shun-Lan-Soo Method for Three-Arm Design

In the case of three group design with normal endpoint, interim winner selection is based on the larger observed mean between two active groups, and the final test statistic is defined as

$$T = \frac{\bar{x}_{si} - \bar{x}_{0i}}{\hat{\sigma}/\sqrt{n/2}}, \text{ arm } s \text{ is the winner and n is the final sample size per group.}$$

(4.15)

where $\bar{x}_{01}, \bar{x}_{11}$, and $\bar{x}_{21}$ are the final observed means for the control, active groups 1 and 2, respectively

Shun, Lan and Soo (2008) found that under the global null hypothesis, the statistic T from the winner group is approximately normal distributed with mean $E(T) = \sqrt{\frac{\tau}{2\pi}}$, τ = information time at the interim analysis, n_1/n, and $var(T) = 1 - \frac{\tau}{2\pi}$. Therefore, a modified test statistic is proposed:

$$Z^* = \frac{T - \sqrt{\frac{\tau}{2\pi}}}{\sqrt{1 - \frac{\tau}{2\pi}}},$$

(4.16)

which has approximately the standard normal distribution.

The approximate p-value can be easily obtained: $p_A = 1 - \Phi(Z^*)$. The exact p-value, based on the exact distribution of Z^w, is given by $p = p_A + 0.0003130571(4.444461^\tau) - 0.00033$.

4.4.2 K-Arm Pick-Winner Design

Suppose in a K-group trial, the global null hypothesis is that all arms have the same effect, that is, $H_G : \mu_0 = \mu_1 = \mu_2 \cdots \mu_K$ and the hypothesis test between the selected arm (winner) and the control is written as

$$H_G : \mu_0 = \mu_s, \ s = \text{selected arm}. \tag{4.17}$$

Chang (2014) derived formulations for the two-stage pick-the-winner design with any number of arms. The design starts with all doses under consideration, at the interim analysis, the winner with the best response observed is selected and will continue to the second stage as well as the control group.

Suppose a trial starts with K dose groups (arms) and one control arm (arm 0). The maximum possible sample size for each group is N. The interim analysis will perform on N_1 independent observations per group, x_{ij} from $N(\mu_i, \sigma^2)$ $(i = 0, .., K; j = 1, ..., N_1)$. The active arm with maximum response at the interim analysis and the control arm will be selected and additional $N_2 = N - N_1$ subjects in each arm will be recruited at the second stage. Denoted by $\bar{x}_i$ the mean of the first N_1 observations in the ith arm $(i = 0, 1, ...K)$, and $\bar{y}_i$ the mean of the additional N_2 observations y_{ij} from $N(\mu_i, \sigma^2)$ $(i = 0, S; j = 1, ..., N_2)$. Here, winner arm S is the active arm selected for the second stage. Let $t_i = \frac{\bar{x}_i}{\sigma}\sqrt{N_1}$ and $\tau_i = \frac{\bar{y}_i}{\sigma}\sqrt{N_2}$, so that, under the H_G, t_i and τ_i are the standard normal distribution with pdf and cdf ϕ and Φ, respectively.

The maximum statistic at the end of stage 1 is

$$T_1 = \max(t_1, t_2, ..., t_K). \tag{4.18}$$

If t_i are drawn independently from an identical cdf $F(t)$, then the cdf of T_1 is $F_{T_1}(t) = [F(t)]^K$ and the pdf is $f_{T_1}(t) = K[F(t)]^{K-1} f(t)$. Here $f(t)$ is the pdf associated with the $F(t)$. Therefore, under the H_G, the pdf of T_1 can be written as

$$f_{T_1}(t) = K[\Phi(t)]^{K-1} \phi(t). \tag{4.19}$$

At the final stage, using all data from the winner, we defined the statistic

$$T_2 = T_1\sqrt{\tau} + \tau_i\sqrt{1-\tau} \text{ if } i = S \text{ (arm } i \text{ is selected)} \tag{4.20}$$

where $\tau = \frac{N_1}{N}$ is the information time at the interim analysis.

Let the indicator $\delta_i = 1$ when $i = S$ (i.e., arm i is selected); otherwise, $\delta_i = 0$. From (15.4), it is convenient to define the cdf of T_2 as

$$F_{T_2}(t) = \sum_{i=1}^{K} P\left(\delta_i = 1 \cap T_1\sqrt{\tau} + \tau_i\sqrt{1-\tau} < t\right). \tag{4.21}$$

Under the H_G, the three variables δ_i, T_1 and τ_i are mutually independent, therefore,

$$\begin{aligned}
F_{T_2}(t) &= \frac{1}{K}\sum_{i=1}^{K}\int_{-\infty}^{\infty}\int_{-\infty}^{\frac{t-\tau_i\sqrt{1-\tau}}{\sqrt{\tau}}} K[\Phi(T_1)]^{K-1}\phi(T_1)\phi(\tau_i)\,dT_1 d\tau_i \\
&= \int_{-\infty}^{\infty}\left[\Phi\left(\frac{t-\tau_i\sqrt{1-\tau}}{\sqrt{\tau}}\right)\right]^{K}\phi(\tau_i)\,d\tau_i
\end{aligned} \tag{4.1}$$

The final test statistic is defined as

$$T_2^* = (T_2 - t_0)/\sqrt{2}. \tag{4.23}$$

Since $T_2^* \leq z$ is equivalent to $T_2 - t_0 \leq \sqrt{2}z$ and $T_2 - t_0$ and $T_2 + t_0$ have the same distribution under H_G, the cdf of T_2^* under H_G is given by the convolution:

$$F_{T_2^*}(z) = \int_{-\infty}^{+\infty} F_{T_2}(t) \, \phi\left(\sqrt{2}z - t\right) dt$$

$$F_{T_2^*}(z) = \int_{-\infty}^{+\infty} \int_{-\infty}^{\infty} \left[\Phi\left(\frac{t - \tau_i\sqrt{1-\tau}}{\sqrt{\tau}}\right) \right]^K \phi(\tau_i) \, d\tau_i \phi\left(\sqrt{2}z - t\right) dt \tag{4.24}$$

When the information time $\tau = 1$, (15.8) reduces to Dunnett test:

$$F_{T_2^*}(z) = \int_{-\infty}^{\infty} [\Phi(t)]^K \, \phi\left(\sqrt{2}z - t\right) dt. \tag{4.25}$$

This formulation is much simpler than the multivariate normal integration.

For simplicity, we only consider a design that rejects the null hypothesis H_0 at the final and the interim analysis is for selecting winner only. That is, if the test statistic $\hat{T}_2^* \geq c_\alpha$, the H_0 is rejected; otherwise, H_0 is not rejected. In such a case, the stopping boundary c_α can be determined using (4.25), that is, find c_α such that $F_{T_2^*}(c_\alpha) = 1 - \alpha$ for a one-sided significance level α. Numerical integration or simulation method can be used to determine the stopping boundary and power. For $\tau = 0.5$, the numerical integrations using *Scientific Workplace* give $c_\alpha = 2.352$, 2.408, 2.451, and 2.487 for $K = 4, 5, 6$, and 7, respectively, which are consistent with the results provided by the simulations in Table 4.2. The SAS Macro for the critical value and power of the pick-the-winner design is presented in Appendix 4C. When the information time $\tau = 1$ (let nStage2=0 in the Macro), it reduces to the Dunnett test.

TABLE 4.2
Critical Value c_α for Pick-the-Winner Designs.

Info Time τ	K						
	1	2	3	4	5	6	7
0.3	1.960	2.140	2.235	2.299	2.345	2.382	2.424
0.5	1.960	2.168	2.278	2.352	2.407	2.452	2.487
0.7	1.960	2.190	2.313	2.398	2.460	2.510	2.550
1.0	1.960	2.212	2.349	2.442	2.512	2.567	2.613

Note: One-sided $\alpha = 0.05$, 10,000,000 runs per scenario

Example 4.2 Seamless Design of Asthma Trial

The objective of this trial in asthma patients is to confirm sustained treatment effect, measured as FEV1 change from baseline to the 1-year of treatment. Initially, patients are equally randomized to four doses of the new compound and a placebo. Based on early studies, the estimated FEV1 change at week 4 are 6%, 12%, 13%, 14%, and 15% (with pooled standard deviation 18%) for the placebo (dose level 0), dose level 1, 2, 3, and 4, respectively. One interim analysis is planned when 60 per group or 50% of patients have the efficacy assessments. The interim analysis will lead to picking the winner (arm with best observed response). The winner and placebo will be used at stage 2. At stage 2, we will enroll 60 patients per group in the winner and control groups. The simulations are carried out by invoking the SAS macro as follows:

Title "Determine Critical Value Z_alpha for 4+1 Arms Winner Design";

Data dInput;

Array mu(4)(0, 0, 0, 0);

%WinnerDesignNormal(NumOfArms=4, mu0=0, sigma=1, Z_alpha=2.352, nStage1=100, nStage2=100);

The simulation results show the rejection probability is 0.025, therefore, the critical value $z_a = 2.352$.

Title "Determine Power for 4+1 Arms Winner Design";

Data dInput;

Array mu(4)(0.12, 0.13, 0.14, 0.15);

%WinnerDesignNormal(NumOfArms=4, mu0=0.06, sigma=0.18, Z_alpha=2.352, nStage1=60, nStage2=60);

The simulation results show the probabilities of selecting arms 1, 2, 3, and 4 are 0.0788, 0.1541, 0.2830, and 0.4845, respectively. The power is 0.951 with total sample size 420.

In general, there are two steps: (1) determine or check the critical value Z_alpha using the H_0 condition, and (2) determine the sample size to achieve the target power using H_a. For binary endpoint with large sample size, due to normality assumption, the critical points for rejection in Table 4.2 are valid. For small trials, the critical point can be determined using simulations. The samples of simulations are presented below:

Title "Determine rejection Boundary for 4+1 Arms Winner Design with Binary Endpoint";

Data dInput;

Array p(4)(0.06, 0.06, 0.06, 0.06);

%WinnerDesignBinary(NumOfArms=4, P0=0.06, Z_alpha=2.352, nStage1=100, nStage2=100);

The simulation results show the rejection probability is 0.025, therefore, the critical value $z_a = 2.352$.

Title "Determine Power for 4+1 Arms Winner Design with Binary Endpoint";

Data dInput;

Array p(4)(0.12, 0.13, 0.14, 0.15);

%WinnerDesignBinary(NumOfArms=4, P0=0.06, Z_alpha=2.352, nStage1=100, nStage2=100);

The simulation results show the probabilities of selecting arms 1, 2, 3, and 4 are 0.14, 0.21, 0.28, and 0.37, respectively. The power is 0.802 with total sample size 700.

Practically, the seamless trials require early efficacy readouts. This early efficacy assessment can be the primary endpoint or surrogate endpoint (biomarker).

4.5 Global Optimization of Adaptive Design - Case Study

We will illustrate how to design a globally optimal adaptive trial using a market drug for COPD. The actual clinical development program involves an adaptive trial, but not globally optimized. We will use the actual data from early phase trials to design later phase globally optimal adaptive trials. We will keep the true data as much as possible, but the information from trials are very rich. We will only include some key data in our designs.

4.5.1 Medical Needs for COPD

Chronic Obstructive Pulmonary Disease (COPD) is the third leading cause of death in the United States (Figure 4.4). More than 11 million people have been diagnosed with COPD, but an estimated 24 million may have the disease without even knowing it. COPD causes serious long-term disability and early death. At this time there is no cure, and the number of people dying from COPD is growing (American Lung Association, 2015, http://www.lung.org). Early signs include: Chronic cough, Shortness of breath (dyspnea), Frequent respiratory infections, Blueness of the lips or fingernail beds (cyanosis), Fatigue, Producing a lot of mucus, Wheezing. Medications Available include tiotropium (Spiriva, 2004) and formoterol (Foradil, Perforomist, 2006).

Deaths resulting from COPD in women are higher than in men. There are, according to American Lung Association, a few reasons why this happens: (1) In the late 1960s, the tobacco industry intensely targeted women. This resulted in a huge increase in women smoking. (2) Women are more vulnerable than men to lung damage from cigarette smoke and other pollutants. Their lungs are smaller and estrogen plays a role in worsening lung disease. (3) Women are often misdiagnosed. Because COPD has long been thought of as a man's disease, many doctors still do not expect to see it in women and miss the proper diagnosis (http://www.lung.org).

Spirometry (a test used to assess how well your lungs work) is the most common of the pulmonary function tests (PFTs). It measures lung function,

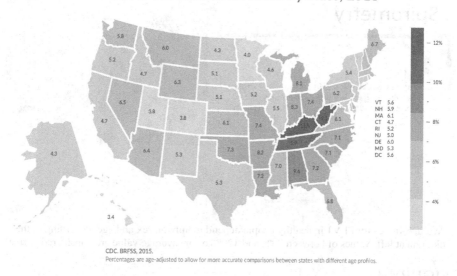

COPD Prevalence in Adults by State, 2015

VT	5.6
NH	5.9
MA	6.1
CT	4.7
RI	5.2
NJ	5.0
DE	6.0
MD	5.3
DC	5.6

CDC. BRFSS, 2015.
Percentages are age-adjusted to allow for more accurate comparisons between states with different age profiles.

FIGURE 4.4
How Serious Is COPD (American Lung Association).

specifically the amount (volume) and/or speed (flow) of air that can be inhaled and exhaled (Figure 4.5). Spirometry is helpful in assessing breathing patterns that identify conditions such as asthma, pulmonary fibrosis, cystic fibrosis, and COPD. Spirometry generates pneumotachographs, which are charts that plot the volume and flow of air coming in and out of the lungs from one inhalation and one exhalation (Figure 4.6).

4.5.2 COPD Market

According to the report, "Chronic Obstructive Pulmonary Disease (COPD) Market to 2019 - Highly-Priced New Combination Products Forecast to Capture Significant Market Share and Drive Growth", released by GBI Research, a leading business intelligence provider, "the global COPD market is estimated to currently be worth $11.3 billion, and is forecast to reach a value of $15.6 billion by 2019. Much of this growth will be fuelled by a high number of new, more efficacious and convenient products entering the market and commanding greater value compared to the therapies already in the market. The drugs driving this growth include once-daily LABA/LAMA fixed-dose combinations such as QVA-149, umeclidinium bromide/vilanterol and olodaterol/tiotropium. Despite recent patent expirations, including that of Advair Diskus (salmeterol/fluticasone propionate), a market leader, generic

Spirometry

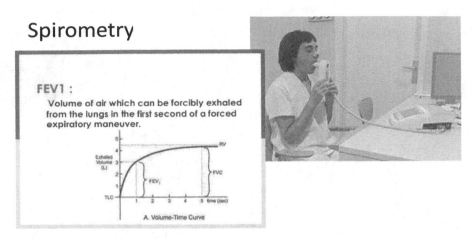

Average values for FEV1 in healthy people depend mainly on sex and age, according to the diagram at left. Values of between 80% and 120% of the average value are considered normal.

FIGURE 4.5
Spirometry for FEV measures.

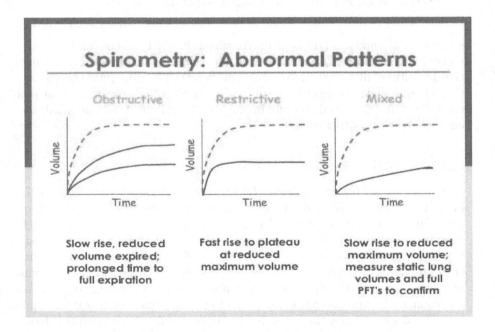

FIGURE 4.6
Spirometry: Abnormal Patterns.

Indacaterol for COPD

Molecular Formula: $C_{24}H_{28}N_2O_3$
Molecular Weight: 392.5 g/mol

FIGURE 4.7
Molecular Structure of Indacaterol for COPD.

erosion in the COPD market may not be as pronounced as that observed in other indications. This is largely down [due] to the difficulty in replicating a fixed-dose combination therapy and the associated device." "Although the COPD market is characterized by low diagnosis rates, campaigns to increase awareness of the disease in both patients and physicians has resulted in steadily rising diagnosis of COPD. Therefore, this has also contributed to market growth throughout the forecast period."

4.5.3 Indacaterol Trials

Disclaimer: Information in this case study is taken from the public domain, where it is necessary the materials might be modified slightly to meet the needs of the book. The authors have no financial associations with the product, Indacaterol.

Indacaterol was an investigational, novel, inhaled once-daily ultra-long-acting β_2-agonist for the treatment of COPD. Indacaterol was a small new molecular entity (NME, Figure 4.7) brought into clinical development around 2005, with the following profiles.

Mechanism of Action: Indacaterol inhalation powder, a long-acting beta2-adrenergic agonist. When inhaled, Indacaterol acts locally in the lung as a bronchodilator. The precise function of beta1-receptors is not known, but their presence raises the possibility that even highly selective β_2-Adrenergic agonists may have cardiac effects.

Safety Profile: The most common adverse effects in adults include skeletal muscle tremor and cramps, insomnia, tachycardia, decreases in serum potassium and increases in plasma glucose. no clinically meaningful QT-interval prolongations.

Pharmacokinetics: $T_{\max} = 15$ minutes after single or repeated inhaled doses. Steady-state was achieved within 12 to 15 days. Approximate Dose-proportionality, 40% absolute bioavailability, Major serum clearance and minor renal clearance. $T_{1/2} = 40$ to 56 hours for dosing with once daily doses between 75 mcg and 600 mcg.

Pharmacodynamics: Showed functional properties of Indacaterol against the three human β-adrenoceptor subtypes.

Two small dose range studies were completed in 2008. The initial dose range was determined based on a 2-week dose-ranging trial with 551 asthma patients. This initial dose range was confirmed with a 2-week dose-ranging trial with 51 COPD patients.

4.5.4   US COPD Phase II Trial Results

The US COPD trial results are outlined as follows (Bauwens et al., 2009).

Objective: To assess the bronchodilator efficacy, safety and tolerability of Indacaterol in COPD patients.

Study design: This crossover, double-blind, double-dummy study was conducted to evaluate the 24-h bronchodilator effect of a range of single doses of Indacaterol (150 microg, 300 microg and 600 microg), given in the morning via single-dose dry powder inhaler (SDDPI) in subjects with COPD, compared with placebo and with the daily therapeutic dose of formoterol (two 12 microg doses 12 h apart, via an SDDPI).

Primary Efficacy Endpoint: The 24-h trough FEV(1).

Key results: 51 subjects (age $\geq$ 40 year) with moderate-to-severe COPD received each of the five treatments on separate study days in randomized sequence. The 24-h trough FEV(1): mean (SD) was 1.46 (0.39) L with Indacaterol 600 microg, 1.45 (0.39) L with Indacaterol 300 microg, 1.42 (0.39) L with Indacaterol 150 microg, 1.41 (0.39) L with formoterol and 1.28 (0.39) L with placebo (Note: SD is taken from Kato M at al., 2010, screening FEV1). All treatments were significantly better than placebo. High and middle doses of Indacaterol were significantly better than formoterol. All treatments were well tolerated and there was little effect on serum potassium, blood glucose or QTc interval.

Conclusion: All doses of Indacaterol were effective in providing 24-h bronchodilation and were well-tolerated in subjects with COPD. The bronchodilator efficacy of Indacaterol (150, 300 and 600 microg) at 24 h post-dose was at least as efficacious as formoterol 12 microg twice daily

4.5.5   Optimal Design

Given the information above, the task is to design the next phase trial of Indacaterol for COPD as a pivotal trial for NDA.

TABLE 4.3

Posterior after Phase 2 Trial.

i	(δ_i, p_i)		
	$150\mu g$	$300\mu g$	$600\mu g$
1	(0, 0.2)	(0, 0.2)	(0, 0.2)
2	(0.10, 0.5)	(0.12, 0.5)	(0.13, 0.5)
3	(0.13, 0.3)	(0.14, 0.3)	(0.17, 0.3)

Note: Posterior = prior for the phase 3 trial.

To search an optimal design phase 3 trial, we not only need to have the estimate the effect size of the treatment, but also need to know the distribution of effect size or the posterior distribution of the effect size up per the data cumulated so far up to the phase 2 trials. Assume the calculated posterior is shown in Table 4.2 (the derivation will be discussed later). This posterior will serve as the prior for the pivotal trial to be designed (Table 4.3).

Safety stopping probabilities are estimated to be $P_s = 0.09$, 0.1, and 0.11 for 150, 300, and $600\mu g$ doses, respectively. Stopping probability due to unspecified reasons is assessed to be $P_u = 0.1$, the same for all three doses.

(1) Classical Design with Indacaterol 300 μg versus formoterol

Indacaterol 300 μg is chosen as the dose for phase 3 since it has a similar effect size as the high dose 600 μg, but potentially a safer profile. With a two-group parallel design, formoterol as control, a hypothesis test with the null hypothesis $H_0 : 1.28L$ for formoterol versus the alternative hypothesis H_a: $1.42L$, and a common standard deviation $0.39L$, a sample size 676 (338/group) patients will provide 95% power at one-sided $\alpha = 0.025^2 == 0.000625$ level for single pivotal trial.

From previous data, prior probabilities of the effect size are determined and presented in Table 4.3, thus the power (rejection probability) under those conditions should also be assessed. With a sample size of 700 (350/group), the trial will provide 0.0625%, 80.0%, and 93.6% power (rejection probability) for effective size $\delta = 0$, 0.12, and $\delta = 0.14$, respectively. The potential effect size and prior, and power are summarized in Table 4.4.

TABLE 4.4

Prior and Power for Dose $300\mu g$.

δ	0	0.12L	0.14L
Prior	0.2	0.5	0.3
Power	0.000625	0.800	0.936

Note: common standard deviation $\sigma = 0.39$.

The probability of success in term of the primary efficacy endpoint is the probalistically (prior distribution) weighted power, that is,

$$
\begin{aligned}
P_{suc} &= p_1 \text{Power}(\delta_1) + p_2 \text{Power}(\delta_2) + p_3 \text{Power}(\delta_3) \\
&= 0.2(0.00625) + 0.5(0.800) + 0.3(0.936) = 0.682.
\end{aligned}
$$

Thus, the probability of failing to demonstrate efficacy is $p_e = 1 - P_{suc} = 0.318$. The transition probability can be calculated using formula (3.7) with $p_e = 0.318$, $p_s = 0.1$, and $p_u = 0.1$:

$$
P_{34} = 1 - (p_e + p_s + p_u) + (p_e p_s + p_e p_u + p_s p_u) - (p_e p_s p_u) = 0.552
$$

(2) Group sequential design with Indacaterol 300 μg versus formoterol (GSD1)

This will be a two-groups GSD, Indacaterol 300 μg versus formoterol, the interim analysis (IA) performed based on 350 patients, the final analysis on 700 patients, O'Brien-Fleming efficacy stopping boundary.

The expected average sample size is

$$
E\left(\bar{N}\right) = p_1 \bar{N}_1 + p_2 \bar{N}_2 + p_3 \bar{N}_3.
$$

Similar to the classical design, the expected power is

$$
P_{suc} = p_1 \text{Power}(\delta_1) + p_2 \text{Power}(\delta_2) + p_3 \text{Power}(\delta_3).
$$

The powers and sample sizes are obtained by invoking the SAS macro for the three different effect sizes:

%GSDNormal(ux=0, uy=0, sigma=0.39, N1=175, N2=175, alpha1=0.00006, beta1=1, alpha2=0.00059);

%GSDNormal(ux=0, uy=0.12, sigma=0.39, N1=175, N2=175, alpha1=0.00006, beta1=1, alpha2=0.00059);

%GSDNormal(ux=0, uy=0.14, sigma=0.39, N1=175, N2=175, alpha1=0.00006, beta1=1, alpha2=0.00059);

The simulation results show that for a maximum sample size of 700 (350/group), the trial will provide 0.0625% ($\bar{N} = 350$), 79.7% ($\bar{N} = 321$), and 93.4% ($\bar{N} = 295$) power for effective size $\delta = 0$, 0.12, and $\delta = 0.14$, respectively. Thus, the expected average sample size is

$$
E\left(\bar{N}\right) = 2(0.2(350) + 0.5(321) + 0.3(295)) = 638
$$

The expected power is

$$
P_{suc} = 0.2(0.00625) + 0.5(0.797) + 0.3(0.934) = 0.680.
$$

The transition probability can be calculated using formula (3.7) with $p_e = 1 - 0.680 = 0.320$, $p_s = 0.1$, and $p_u = 0.1$:

$$
\begin{aligned}
P_{34} &= 1 - (0.320 + 0.1 + 0.1) + (0.320 \times 0.1 + 0.320 \times 0.1 + 0.1 \times 0.1) \\
&\quad -(0.320 \times 0.1 \times 0.1) = 0.551
\end{aligned}
$$

To compare effect of different stopping boundaries, another option of group sequential design (GSD2) is similar to GSD1, but using the Pocock instead of the O'Brien-Fleming efficacy boundary. The powers and sample sizes are obtained by invoking the SAS macro for the three different effect sizes:

%GSDNormal(ux=0, uy=0, sigma=0.39, N1=175, N2=175, alpha1=0.000332, beta1=1, alpha2=0.000332);

%GSDNormal(ux=0, uy=0.12, sigma=0.39, N1=175, N2=175, alpha1=0.000332, beta1=1, alpha2=0.000332);

%GSDNormal(ux=0, uy=0.14, sigma=0.39, N1=175, N2=175, alpha1=0.000332, beta1=1, alpha2=0.000332);

The simulation results show that for a maximum sample size of 700 (350/group), the trial will provide 0.0625% ($\bar{N} = 350$), 75.6% ($\bar{N} = 298$), and 91.4% ($\bar{N} = 266$) power for effective size $\delta = 0$, 0.12, and $\delta = 0.14$, respectively. Thus, the expected average sample size is

$$E\left(\bar{N}\right) = 2(0.2(350) + 0.5(298) + 0.3(266)) = 598$$

The expected power is

$$P_{suc} = 0.2(0.00625) + 0.5(0.756) + 0.3(0.914) = 0.653.$$

The transition probability can be calculated using formula (3.7) with $p_e = 1 - 0.653 = 0.347$, $p_s = 0.1$, and $p_u = 0.1$:

$$
\begin{aligned}
P_{34} &= 1 - (0.347 + 0.1 + 0.1) + (0.347 \times 0.1 + 0.347 \times 0.1 + 0.1 \times 0.1) \\
&\quad -(0.347 \times 0.1 \times 0.1) = 0.529
\end{aligned}
$$

To study effect of the timing of the interim analysis, GSD3 is a GSD similar to GSD2, but the IA will be conducted earlier on 250 patients (125/group). The power and average sample size can be simulated by executing the following SAS code:

%GSDNormal(ux=0, uy=0, sigma=0.39, N1=125, N2=225, alpha1=0.000324, beta1=1, alpha2=0.000324);

%GSDNormal(ux=0, uy=0.12, sigma=0.39, N1=125, N2=225, alpha1=0.000324, beta1=1, alpha2=0.000324);

%GSDNormal(ux=0, uy=0.14, sigma=0.39, N1=125, N2=225, alpha1=0.000324, beta1=1, alpha2=0.000324);

The simulation results show that for a maximum sample size of 700 (350/group), the trial will provide 0.0625% ($\bar{N} = 350$), 75.0% ($\bar{N} = 331$), and 91.2% ($\bar{N} = 286$) power for effective size $\delta = 0$, 0.12, and $\delta = 0.14$, respectively. Thus, the expected average sample size is

$$E\left(\bar{N}\right) = 2(0.2(350) + 0.5(331) + 0.3(331)) = 670$$

The expected power is

$$P_{suc} = 0.2(0.00625) + 0.5(0.750) + 0.3(0.912) = 0.650$$

The transition probability can be calculated using formula (3.7) with $p_e = 1 - 0.650 = 0.350$, $p_s = 0.1$, and $p_u = 0.1$:

$$P_{34} = 1 - (0.35 + 0.1 + 0.1) + (0.35 \times 0.1 + 0.35 \times 0.1 + 0.1 \times 0.1)$$
$$-(0.35 \times 0.1 \times 0.1) = 0.527.$$

Sample-Size Reestimation (SSR) Designs allow for increasing sample size: the SSR design is similar to GSD1, but allowed sample size re-estimation at the interim analysis with 150 patients/group. The Mehta-Pocock promising-zone method for adjusted sample size. The promising zone is obtained through simulations for the target error rate = $\alpha = 0.000625$. The average power and expected $\bar{N}$ are presented in Table 4.4, generated from the following SAS code:

%SSRTwoGroupDesignNormal(n1=150, n2=150, N2max=300, u0=0, u1=0.0, sigma=0.39, alpha=0.000625, TargetPower=0.9, alpha1= 0.00006, alpha2=0.00059, beta1=1, PromisingL=0.005, PromisingU=0.0356);

%SSRTwoGroupDesignNormal(n1=150, n2=150, N2max=300, u0=0, u1=0.12, sigma=0.39, alpha=0.000625, TargetPower=0.9, alpha1= 0.00006, alpha2=0.00059, beta1=1, PromisingL=0.005, PromisingU=0.0356);

%SSRTwoGroupDesignNormal(n1=150, n2=150, N2max=300, u0=0, u1=0.14, sigma=0.39, alpha=0.000625, TargetPower=0.9, alpha1= 0.00006, alpha2=0.00059, beta1=1, PromisingL=0.005, PromisingU=0.0356);

The simulation results show that for a maximum sample size of 900 (450/group), the IA conducted at 150 patients/group, no futility stopping at IA, the trial will provide 0.0625% ($\bar{N} = 304$), 78.1% ($\bar{N} = 321$), and 91.7% ($\bar{N} = 294$) power for effect size $\delta = 0$, 0.12, and $\delta = 0.14$, respectively. Thus, the expected average sample size is

$$E\left(\bar{N}\right) = (0.2(304) + 0.5(321) + 0.3(294)) = 620$$

The expected power is

$$P_{suc} = 0.2(0.00625) + 0.5(0.781) + 0.3(0.917) = 0.667.$$

The transition probability can be calculated using formula (3.7) with $p_e = 1 - 0.667 = 0.333$, $p_s = 0.1$, and $p_u = 0.1$:

$$P_{34} = 1 - (0.333 + 0.1 + 0.1) + (0.333 \times 0.1 + 0.333 \times 0.1 + 0.1 \times 0.1)$$
$$-(0.333 \times 0.1 \times 0.1) = 0.540$$

Beyond two-arm design, a 2-stage, 2+1-arm, Pick-Winner-Design (PWD) is simulated with the interim analysis performed on 120 patients/group for dose selection, the final analysis will be performed on two arms: the winner and control with 240 patients per arm and total sample size is 600 patients for the three arms. There are $3 \times 3 = 9$ possible combinations of effects with corresponding powers, $\text{Pow}(\delta_{300,i}, \delta_{600,j})$. The expected power is

$$P_{suc} = \sum_{i,j} p_i p_j Pow\left(\delta_{300,i}, \delta_{600,j}\right)$$

$$= 0.2^2 Pow(0,0) + 0.2(0.5)Pow\,(0, 0.13) + 0.2(0.3)Pow\,(0, 0.17)$$
$$+0.5(0.2)Pow\,(.12, 0) + 0.5^2 Pow\,(.12, 0.13) + 0.5\,(0.3)\,Pow\,(.12, .17)$$
$$+0.3\,(0.2)\,Pow\,(.14, 0) + 0.3\,(0.5)\,Pow\,(.14, .13) + 0.3^2 Pow\,(.14, .17).$$

That is,

$$P_{suc} = 0.2^2 \times 0.625 + 0.2(0.5) \times 0.598 + 0.2(0.3) \times 0.916$$
$$+0.5(0.2) \times 0.486 + 0.5^2 \times 0.664 + 0.5\,(0.3) \times 0.898$$
$$+0.3\,(0.2) \times 0.702 + 0.3\,(0.5) \times 0.763 + 0.3^2 \times 0.917$$
$$= 0.728,$$

where power, $Pow\left(\delta_{300,i}, \delta_{600,j}\right)$, is obtained through simulations. For example, $Pow(0.12, 0.17)$ is obtained by invoking the following SAS macro (the critical value z_alpha = 3.4 was obtained from simulation at $\alpha = 0.000625$):

Data dInput;
Array mu(2)(0.12, 0.17);
%WinnerDesignNormal(nSims=1000000,NumOfArms=2, mu0=0, sigma=0.39, Z_alpha=3.4, nStage1=120, nStage2=120);

The simulation results include: the winning probability is 0.161 and 0.839, respectively for the two active arms. The power of claiming efficacy is 89,8% with total 500 patients.

The stopping probability due to safety is calculated using the Winning Probabilities of doses and the stopping probabilities of the winner doses. For example, the corresponding $Power(0.12, 0.17)$, the winning probabilities are 0.16078 and 0.83922 for the 300mg ($p_s = 0.1$) and 600 mg ($p_s = 0.11$), respectively. The stopping probability for that scenario is

$$p_s^* = 0.160780 \times 0.1 + 0.83922 \times 0.11 = 0.108$$

The expectation of p_s^* can be calculated using the prior probabilities in Table 4.2, which is approximately $\bar{p}_s = 0.107$. This $\bar{p}_s$ will replace p_s is calculating p_{34}, $p_e = 1 - 0.728 = 0.272$, $p_u = 0.1$. It follows that

$$P_{34} = 1 - (0.272 + 0.107 + 0.1) + (0.272 \times 0.1 + 0.272 \times 0.107 + 0.107 \times 0.1)$$
$$- (0.272 \times 0.107 \times 0.1) = 0.585.$$

For all six different designs, P_{suc}, $E\left(\bar{N}\right)$, and P_{34} are summarized in Table 4.4. The time to market (T_m) is estimated based on the average sample size and other factors, such as complexity of trials. Clinical Operation can usually provide T_m and cost C_3 estimations for different trial designs. For the exercise, assume the expected time to market is a function of the expected sample size:

$$\bar{T}_m = 36 + 0.01 \times E\left(\bar{N}\right),$$

and the expected cost is another function of the number of sites (which is a function sample size) and the expected sample size, similar to Eq. (3.2) but including the cost of the sponsor employee's time:

$$\bar{C}_3 = 5,000,000 + 10,000 \times E\left(\bar{N}\right).$$

For selecting the optimal design, only per patient cost in $\bar{C}_3$ will affect the decision.

As discussed earlier, the COPD market value is estimated of $11.3 billion and can reach $15.6 billion in 2019. Since Indacaterol will not be the first to market, the value V_p is estimated to be 300 million/year and the value after patent expiration is $G_{max} = 500$ million. The value of G_{max} will not affect the selection of optimal design. The time to expiration is $T_e = 120$ months. The competitor rate is $R_c = 0.02$/month, meaning approximately every 5 years, there will be a new competitor.

The expected value g_4 can be calculated based on Eq.(3.8):

$$g_4 = \frac{300/12}{0.25\,(0.02)} \ln \frac{1 + 0.25\,(0.02)\,(120)}{1 + 0.25\,(0.02)\,\bar{T}_m} + 500$$

$$g_3 = P_{34}g_4 - \bar{C}_3.$$

All the operating characteristics for the designs are presented in Table 4.4. To determine the optimal design, PWD is chosen simply because it has the largest $g_3 = \$1098.7$ million, $75 million (7.3%) more than classical design. The most undesirable design is GSD3 with Pocock's stopping boundary and IA at information time $\tau = 125/350 = 0.36$, which has the expected value of $g_4 = \$980.38$ million, $12.31 million lower that GSD with the IA at information time at 0.5. Comparing design with the BO-F boundary (GSD1) versus the Pocock boundary (GSD2), the former shows $36.81 million higher in the expected value g_3, $1029.50 million versus $992.69 million. A design with sample size reestimation will gain value over the corresponding group sequential design without SSR, the SSR design has value $1010.90 million, while GSD2 has only a value of $992.69 million. Surprisingly, the classical design has value $g_3 = 1023.70$ million, ranking the 3rd best among the six. It conforms that not all but only good adaptive designs will gain more value than a classical design.

TABLE 4.5

Summary of Trial Designs.

Design	P_{suc}	$E(\bar{N})$	$\bar{T}_m$	g_4	P_{34}	$\bar{C}_3$	g_3
Classical	0.552	700	43.00	1876.3	0.552	12.00	1023.70
GSD1	0.680	638	42.38	1889.1	0.551	11.38	1029.50
GSD2	0.653	598	41.98	1897.3	0.529	10.98	992.69
GSD3	0.650	670	42.70	1882.5	0.527	11.70	980.38
SSR	0.667	620	42.20	1892.8	0.540	11.20	1010.90
PWD	0.728	600	42.00	1896.9	0.585	11.00	1098.70

Note: Time in month, $ in million.

4.6   Summary & Discussions

An adaptive clinical trial design allows aspects of the trial to be modified without undermining the integrity and validity of the trial. Commonly used adaptive trial designs include group sequential design, sample-size reestimation design, pick-winner design, and biomarker-adaptive designs. Simulation programs are provided for these adaptive designs in the Appendices.

Among different adaptive design options, power and average sample size are often the conventional criteria for selecting an adaptive design. However, such a choice is not globally optimal because the decision is not based on the clinical development program as an interconnected entity, but a minimal related individual trials. Based on the globally optimal model discussed in Chapter 3, we described the "globally optimal" Phase-III trial design using a COPD case study design.

When designing an optimal adaptive trial, Bayesian posteriors from previous studies are useful. This posterior will often serve a prior for designing the current trial. However, because, for example, the phase 3 population characteristics may shift from Phase 2, the Bayesian posterior may not reflect such a change. Therefore, the prior for the Phase-III trial may have to modify from the Bayesian posterior to incorporate such shift even if the methodology is somewhat subjective.

If we have the formulations for prior of effect-size and costs as functions of sample-size, p_s as function of dose, p_u as a function of dose, and T_m as function of dose, we can implement them in the simulation programs and simulate g_4 for each simulated trial and obtain the expected $\bar{g}_4$, $\bar{g}_3$, $\bar{g}_2$, and $\bar{g}_1$. In theory, this method will be more accurate for calculating NPV.

Lastly, other factors such as the minimal sample size required for safety evaluation should also be considered when designing an adaptive trial.

Bibliography

Bauwens, O., Ninane, V., et al. 24-hour bronchodilator efficacy of single doses of indacaterol in subjects with COPD: comparison with placebo and formoterol. Current Medical Research and Opinion 2009;25:463–70.

Bretz, F. et al. (2006). Confirmatory seamless phase II/III clinical trials with hypotheses selection at interim: General concepts. Biometrical Journal 48:4, 623–634.

Chang, M. and Wang, J. (2014). The Add-Arm Design for Unimodal Response Curve with Unknown Mode. Journal of Biopharmaceutical Statistics. Oct. 2014.

Chang, M. (2014). Adaptive Design Theory and Implementation Using SAS and R. 2nd Edition. Chapman & Hall/CRC, Taylor & Francis. Boca Raton, FL.

Charles W. Dunnett & Ajit C. Tamhane (1992). A Stepup Multiple Test Procedure. Journal of the American Statistical Association Volume 87, 1992 - Issue 417.

Chen, Y.H.J., DeMets, D.L. and Lan, K.K.G. (2004). Increasing the sample-size when the unblinded interim result is promising. Statistics in Medicine. 23:1023–1038.

Cui, L., Hung, M.J. and Wang, S.J. (1999). Modification of sample-size in group sequential trials. Biometrics, 55, 853-857.

Dunnett, C.W. (1955). A multiple comparison procedure for comparing several treatments with a control. Journal of the American Statistical Association, 50: 1096-121.

Dunnett C. W. (1964.) New tables for multiple comparisons with a control, Biometrics, 20:482–491.

Heritier, S., Lô, S.N., Morgan, C.C. (2011). An adaptive confirmatory trial with interim treatment selection: practical experiences and unbalanced randomization. Statistics in Medicine 2011 Jun 15;30(13):1541-54

Huang WS, Liu JP, Hsiao CF. (2011). An alternative phase II/III design for continuous endpoints. Pharmaceutical Statistics 2011 Mar-Apr;10(2):105-14.

Isabella Hatfield, Annabel Allison, Laura Flight, Steven A. Julious and Munyaradzi Dimairo (2016). Adaptive designs undertaken in clinical research: a review of registered clinical trials. Trials201617:150

Jenkins M, Stone A, Jennison C. (2011). An adaptive seamless phase II/III design for oncology trials with subpopulation selection using correlated survival endpoints. Pharmaceutical Statistics 2011 Jul-Aug;10(4):347-56.

Jennison, C. and Turnbull, B.W. (2000). Group Sequential Tests with Applications to Clinical Trials. Chapman & Hall: London/Boca Raton, Florida.

Lan, K.K.G. and DeMets, D. L. (1983). Discrete sequential boundaries for clinical trials. Biometrika, 70, 659–663.

Lan, K.K.G. and DeMets, D. L. (1989). Changing frequency of interim analysis in sequential monitoring. Biometrics 45, 1017–1020.

Mehta, C.R., Pocock, S.J. (2011). Adaptive increase in sample size when interim results are promising: a practical guide with examples. Stat Med. 2011 Dec 10;30(28):3267-84.

O'Brien, P.C. and Fleming, T.R. (1979). A multiple testing procedure for clinical trials. Biometrika 35, 549–556.

Pocock, S.J. (1977). Group sequential methods in the design and analysis of clinical trials. Biometrika. 64, 191–199.

Posch, M., Maurer, W., and Bretz, F. (2011). Type I error rate control in adaptive designs for confirmatory clinical trials with treatment selection at interim. Pharmaceutical Statistics, 10.96–104.

Rom, D.M., Costello, R.J., Connell, L.T. (1994). On closed test procedures for dose-response analysis. Statistics in Medicine 1994 Aug 15;13(15):1583-96.

Shun, Z., Lan, K.K., Soo, Y. (2008). Interim treatment selection using the normal approximation approach in clinical trials. Statistics in Medicine 2008 Feb 20;27(4):597-618.

Wang, S.K. and Tsiatis, A.A. (1987). Approximately optimal one-parameter boundaries for a sequential trials. Biometrics, 43, 193-200.

Wassmer, G. (1999). Multistage adaptive test procedures based on Fisher's product criterion. Biometrical Journal 41, 279–293.

Whitehead, J. and Stratton, I. (1983). Group sequential clinical trials with triangular continuation regions. Biometrics 39, 227–236.

www.statisticians.org

5

Trial Design for Precision Medicine

5.1 Introduction

Precision medicine or personalized medicine is a method of targeting patients into different groups, often based on genotypic or phenotypic characterization, so that the treatments or procedures can be tailored to the individual patient based on their predicted response and/or risk of disease. Precision medicine can potentially bring the following additional benefits to patients beyond the "traditional" approach to prescribing medicines: (1) ability to make more informed medical decisions, (2) higher probability of desired outcomes, (3) minimize the risk of side effects, (4) focus on prevention of disease rather than reaction to it, and (5) reduced healthcare costs. The ultimate goal of precision medicine is to bring the right medicine to the right person with right amount at right time for a minimal cost.

Precision medicine is a very timely and rapidly evolving topic. The book, Clinical and Statistical Considerations in Precision Medicine (Carini, Menon and Chang, 2014) explores recent advances related to biomarkers and their translation into clinical development. Leading clinicians, biostatisticians, regulators, commercial professionals, and researchers address the opportunities and challenges in successfully applying biomarkers in drug discovery and pre-clinical and clinical development.

Traditional clinical development of a novel therapy often utilizes the "one-size-fits-all" approach by testing treatment effect in the entire patient population with a specific disease. It assumes that response in the disease population is homogeneous. Recent advances in genetic engineering such as DNA sequencing and mRNA transcript profiling has made a finer taxonomy of disease possible, which enables the development of precise diagnostic, prognostic, and therapeutic paradigms for specific subsets of patients in order to achieve the ultimate goal of precision medicine. Thus, these targeted therapies may benefit only a subset of the entire patient population and may not benefit or even harm the rest of the population. However, usually the benefit observed in this targeted patient population is much greater than the "average" benefit observed in a heterogeneous patient population. Biomarkers also have the potential to provide substantial added value to current medical practice in the context of precision medicine. Biomarkers are widely used as a tool in drug discovery, to more precisely understand the mechanism of action of a drug, to investigate efficacy and toxicity signals at an early stage of pharmaceutical development, and to identify patients likely to respond to treatment.

As a result of these new opportunities and challenges, the traditional paradigm of drug development, which generally does not to take into account response heterogeneity, may be suboptimal. To embark upon the mission of precision medicine, innovative statistical designs with biomarkers should be more frequently utilized. Biomarker-adaptive design (BAD) refers to a design that allows for adaptations using information obtained from biomarkers.

The study of rare diseases fits the model of precision medicine naturally: majority of them arise from genetic variations, and show a varying degree of heterogeneity from patient to patient (Graiger, 2016). Thus, biomarker-adaptive clinical trials are useful in studying rare diseases, particularly considering that the availability of patients with rare diseases is quite limited. Biomarkers have the potential to help identify patients who are most likely to respond to the test treatment under investigation. Consequently, biomarker-adaptive designs may result in (1) smaller study sizes, (2) higher probability of trial success, and (3) enhancement of the benefit-risk relationship.

In the past decade, precision medicine and biomarker-driven clinical trials have been discussed and studied by many authors in the literature, e.g., Hawgood et al. (2015), Collins and Varmus (2015), Jameson and Longo (2015), Bayer and Galea (2015), Mirnezami et al (2012), Simon and Maittournam (2004), Mandrekar and Sargent (2009), Weir and Walley (2006), Simon (2010), and Baker et al. (2012). In practice, biomarker-driven adaptive designs are adaptive designs that allow us to select target populations based on interim data (Simon and Simon, 2013). Simon and Wang (2006) and Freidlin, Jiang and Simon (2010) studied a genomic signature design, Jiang, Freidlin and Simon (2007) proposed Biomarker-adaptive threshold design, Chang (2006, 2007), Wang et al. (2007), Wang, Hung and O'Neill (2009) and Jenkins et al. (2011) studied population enrichment design using biomarkers, which allow an interim decision on the target population to be made based on power or utility. Zhou et al (2008) studied Bayesian adaptive randomization design that provides patients with potentially more effective treatments as the conduct of the trial progresses. Song and Pepe (2004) studied markers for selecting a patient's treatment . Studies on biomarker-adaptive design were done by Beckman, Clark, and Chen (2011) for oncology trials. Recently, Wang (2013), Wang, Chang, and Menon (2014, 2015) used an adaptive design with hierarchical model to solve the mystery regarding why the first level correlation plays a limited role in biomarker-adaptive design.

A biomarker is a characteristic that is objectively measured and evaluated as an indicator of normal biologic or pathogenic processes or pharmacologic response to a therapeutic intervention (Chakraverty, 2005). A biomarker can be a classifier, prognostic, or predictive marker.

A classifier biomarker is a marker, e.g., a DNA marker, that usually does not change over the course of study. A classifier biomarker can be used to select the most appropriate target population to include in a clinical trial.

For example, a study drug is expected to have effects on a population with a biomarker, which is only 20% of the overall patient population. Because the sponsor suspects that the drug may not work for the overall patient population, it may be efficient and ethical to run a trial only for the subpopulations with the biomarker rather than the general patient population. On the other hand, some biomarkers such as RNA markers are expected to change over the course of the study. These types of markers could be either prognostic or predictive markers.

A prognostic biomarker informs the clinical outcomes, independent of treatment. It provides information about natural course of the disease in individuals with or without treatment under study. A prognostic marker does not inform the effect of the treatment. For example, Non-small cell lung cancer (NSCLC) patients receiving either EGFR inhibitors or chemotherapy have better outcomes with a specific mutation than without this mutation . Prognostic markers can be used to separate good and poor prognosis patients at the time of diagnosis. If expression of the marker clearly separates patients with an excellent prognosis from those with a poor prognosis, then the marker can be used to aid the decision about therapeutic decisions. The poor prognosis patients might be considered for clinical trials of novel therapies that will, hopefully, be more effective (Conley and Taube, 2004). Prognostic markers may also inform the possible mechanisms responsible for the poor prognosis, thus leading to the identification of new targets for treatment and new effective therapeutics.

A predictive biomarker informs the likelihood of treatment effect on the clinical endpoint. A predictive marker can be population-specific: a marker can be predictive for population A but not population B. A predictive biomarker, as compared to true endpoints like survival, can often be measured earlier, easier, and more frequently and is less subject to competing risks. For example, in a trial of a cholesterol-lowering drug, the ideal endpoint may be death or development of coronary artery disease (CAD). However, such a study usually requires thousands of patients and many years to conduct. Therefore, it is desirable to have a biomarker, such as a reduction in post-treatment cholesterol, if it predicts the reductions in the incidence of CAD.

Many biomarkers are being used in phase III clinical studies and have helped in bringing forward effective treatments to marker-defined patient populations in a timely manner. A few examples include: use of HER2 expression in the study of lapatinib plus letrozole for metastatic breast cancer; use of KRAS mutation status in the study of cetuximab plus chemotherapy for stage III colon cancer, and the use of EGFR expression in the study of erlotinib for metastatic non-small cell lung cancer. In a recent survey conducted by BIO et al. (2016), it was shown that rare disease programs and programs that utilized selection biomarkers had higher success rates at each phase of development versus the overall success rate for all drugs.

From a regulatory perspective, FDA (Oct. 2013) released a report, Paving the Way for Personalized Medicine, FDA's Role in a New Era of Medical

Product Development. The former FDA commissioner, Dr. Hamburg stated: "The report describes the ways in which FDA has worked to respond to, anticipate and help drive scientific developments in personalized therapeutics and diagnostics. For the first time, it provides a compendium of FDA's many recent efforts to advance regulatory standards, methods and tools in support of personalized medicine and to further refine critical regulatory processes and policies in order to bring about personalized medical product development. This thoughtful report should serve as a useful resource for those looking toward a future where all stages of patient care—from prevention to diagnosis to treatment to follow-up—are truly personalized."

5.2   Overview of Classical Designs with Biomarkers

5.2.1   Biomarker-enrichment Design

The biomarker-enrichment design is a randomized design involving only patients with a specific biomarker status (Freidlin et al., 2010; Sargent et al., 2005; Chang, 2006, 2007). This design is most appropriate when the mechanistic behavior of drug is known and there is compelling preliminary evidence of benefits in a subgroup of patient population defined by a specific biomarker status.

In biomarker-enrichment design, patients are screened for the presence or absence of a biomarker(s) profile. After extensive screening, only patients with the presence of a certain biomarker characteristic or profile are enrolled in the clinical trial. In principle, this design essentially consists of an additional criterion for patient inclusion in the trial (Figure 5.1) (Freidlin and Korn, 2014; Huang et al. 2015).

A recent example for the enrichment design was of mutated BRAF-kinase (Chapman et al. 2011). Almost 50% of melanomas have an activating V600E BRAF mutation. This leads to the hypothesis that inhibition of mutated BRAF kinase will have meaningful clinical benefit. Hence only patients who tested positive for V600EBRAF mutation were enrolled in the study. Patients were randomized to an inhibitor of mutated BRAF-kinase or control treatment. As hypothesized, the large treatment benefit was observed in the pre-specified subgroup.

The following considerations should be taken into account in this design – 1) during the conduct of the study, it is important to have rapid turnaround times for the assay results in order to enroll patients faster; 2) the assay testing should be consistent between different labs; 3) restricted enrollment does not provide data to establish that treatment is ineffective in biomarker negative patients; 4) a low prevalence of the marker may be challenging operationally and financially.

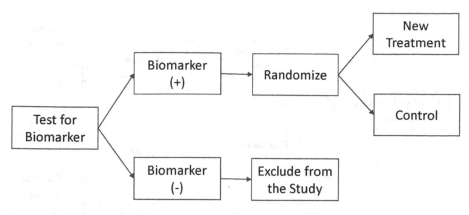

FIGURE 5.1
Biomarker-enrichment Design.

Merits & Limitations: Potential of smaller sample size, higher probability of trial success, and enhancement of benefit-risk relationship, but restricted enrollment provides no information for biomarker negative patients.

5.2.2 Biomarker-Stratified Design

In biomarker stratified design, patients are tested for biomarker status and then separately randomized according to their positive or negative status of the marker (Freidlin et al. 2010). This design is chosen when there is no preliminary evidence to strongly favor restricting the trial to patients with specific biomarker profile that would necessitate a biomarker-enrichment design.

In biomarker stratified design, randomization is done using marker status as the stratification factor; however only the patients with a valid measurable marker results are randomized (Figure 5.2). Two separate hypotheses tests are conducted to determine the treatment effects for the biomarker group and the overall population. In determining the sample size the overall power and power for detecting efficacy in the biomarker group can both be considered.

Merits & Limitations: Provide overall risk-benefit assessment in general population, and prospective marker validation, but requires rapid turnaround times for the assay results in order to randomize patients

5.2.3 Sequential Testing Strategy Design

Sequential testing strategy designs can be viewed as a special case of the classical randomized clinical trial for all comers or unselected patients. In this design, randomization is not stratified by biomarker status. Thus, sample sizes in the treatment groups within each biomarker defined subgroup should be large enough to balance important prognostic baseline factors to ensure effec-

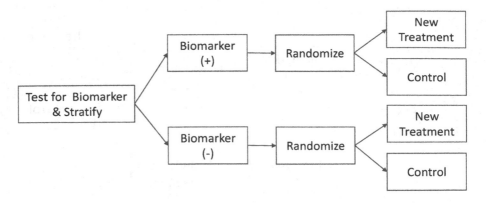

FIGURE 5.2
Biomarker Stratified Design.

tive results. Two testing strategies are frequently used: test overall difference followed by subgroup; and test subgroup followed by overall population.

(1) Test Overall Difference Followed by Subgroup

Simon and Wang (2006) proposed an analysis strategy where the overall hypothesis is tested first to see if there is a difference in the response in new treatment versus the control group in the entire patient population. If there is no difference and the response is not significant at a pre-specified significance level (for example 0.04), then the new treatment is compared to the control group in the biomarker positive patients. The second comparison uses a threshold of significance which is the proportion of the traditional 0.05 not utilized by the initial test (for example 0.01). This approach is useful when the new treatment is believed to be effective in a wider population, and the subset analysis is supplementary and used as a fall back option (Figure 5.3).

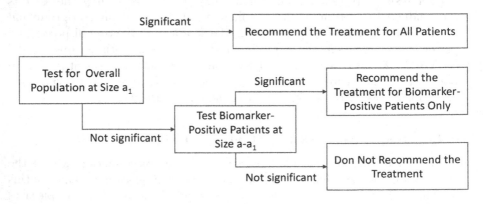

FIGURE 5.3
Test Overall Difference Followed by Subgroup.

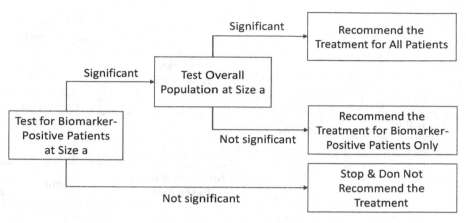

FIGURE 5.4
Test subgroup followed by the overall population.

Song and Chi (2007) later proposed a modification of the above method. Their method takes into account the correlation between the test statistics of the hypotheses of the overall population and the biomarker positive population.

(2) Test subgroup followed by the overall population

In this analysis strategy, the hypothesis for the treatment is first tested in the biomarker positive status patients and then tested in the overall population. This strategy is appropriate when there is a preliminary biological basis to believe that biomarker status positive patients will benefit more from the new drug and there is sufficient marker prevalence to appropriately power the trial. The study would be powered for effect in the biomarker positive status group and the size of biomarker negative status group could be determined separately to allow a reasonable estimate of effect in marker negative group. In this closed testing procedure, the final type I error rate is always preserved (Figure 5.4).

Merits & Limitations: Provide overall risk-benefit assessment in general population and potential of higher probability of trial success, but possibility of confounding as randomization is not stratified by biomarker status.

5.2.4 Marker-based Strategy Design

In this design, patients are randomly assigned to treatment dependent or independent of the marker status (Figure 5.5). All patients randomized to the non-biomarker based arm receive the control treatment. In the biomarker based arm, the biomarker positive patients will receive the experimental therapy while biomarker negative patients receive control treatment (Freidlin et al 2010; Sargent, 2005).

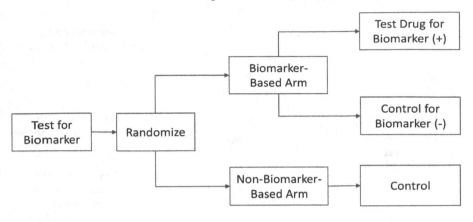

FIGURE 5.5
Marker-based Strategy Design.

The outcome of all of the patients in the marker based subgroup is compared to that of all patients in the non-marker based subgroup to investigate the predictive value of the marker. One downside of this design is that patients treated with the same regimen are included in both the marker-based and the non–marker-based subgroup, resulting in a substantial redundancy. Another disadvantage is the inability to examine the effect of targeted therapy in biomarker negative patients as none of these patients receive it. The treatment difference between the new treatment and the control treatment can be diluted by marker-based treatment selection and sometimes can be a poor choice as compared to the randomized design.

Merits & Limitations: Can be used to assess predictive value of biomarker redundancy, but inability to examine treatment effect in biomarker negative patients

5.2.5 Hybrid Design

Hybrid design should be considered when there is compelling prior evidence demonstrating the efficacy of a certain treatment for a biomarker subgroup renders it unethical to randomly assign patients with that particular biomarker status to other treatment options. In this design, only marker-positive patients are randomly assigned to treatments, whereas patients in the marker-negative group are assigned to control or standard-of-care treatment (Figure 5.6). The study is powered to detect treatment difference only in the marker-positive group. However, samples are collected from all the subjects to help testing for additional markers in the future.

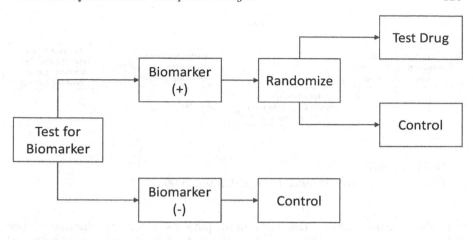

FIGURE 5.6
Hybrid Design.

Merits & Limitations: Potential of higher probability of trial success and enhancement of benefit-risk relationship, but Inability to examine treatment effect in biomarker negative patients.

5.3 Overview of Biomarker-Adaptive Designs

5.3.1 Adaptive Accrual Design

If biomarker-based subgroups are predefined, but with uncertainty on the best possible endpoint and population, an adaptive accrual design could be considered with interim analysis that may lead to modification of the patient population to accrue.

Chang (2006, 2007) proposed *Biomarker-Adaptive Winner Design.* In this design, the recruitment starts with an "overall" patient population who are then randomized into control and test groups. At the interim analysis either the biomarker-positive or the overall population is selected as the winner population and recruitment of the winner population is continued at the second stage of the trial. In the final analysis, the hypothesis test will be conducted on the winner population (test versus control). The winner can be determined based on effect sizes, the interim p-values, conditional powers, or utility functions of the population group (Figure 5.7).

Wang et al. (2007) proposed a phase III design comparing an experimental treatment with a control treatment that begins with accruing both positive and negative biomarker status patients. An interim futility analysis would be performed, and based on results of the interim analysis the decision is

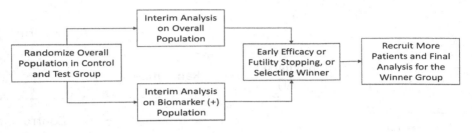

FIGURE 5.7
Biomarker-Adaptive Winner Design (Chang 2006, 2007).

made to either continue the study in all patients or only the biomarker positive patients. Specifically, the trial follows the following scheme: begin with accrual to both marker-defined subgroups; an interim analysis is performed to evaluate the test treatment in the biomarker-negative patients. If the interim analysis indicates that confirming the effectiveness of the test treatment for the biomarker-negative patients is futile, then the accrual of biomarker-negative patients is halted, and the final analysis is restricted to evaluating the test treatment for the biomarker-positive patients. Otherwise, accrual of biomarker-negative and biomarker-positive patients continues to the target sample size until the end of the trial. At that time, the test treatment is compared to the standard treatment for the overall population and for biomarker-positive patients (Figure 5.8).

Jenkins et al. (2011) proposed a similar design but with more flexibility. It allows the trial to test treatment effect in the overall population, subgroup population or the co-primary populations at the final analysis based on the results from interim analysis. Besides, the decision to extend to the second stage is based on intermediate or surrogate endpoint correlated to the final endpoint (Figure 5.9). In this design, a combination of test statistics for the final endpoint from each stage is used for hypothesis testing. The patients who

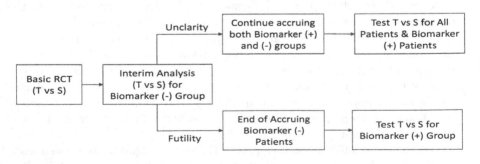

FIGURE 5.8
Adaptive Accrual Design (Wang et al. 2007).

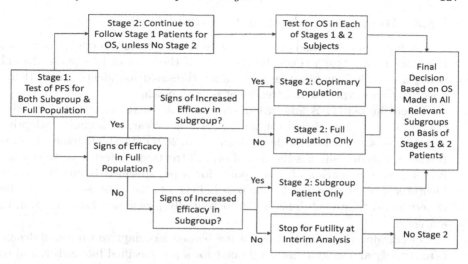

FIGURE 5.9
Adaptive Accrual Design (Jenkins et al. 2011).

start in the first stage will remain in the study and would be monitored for their long term (final) endpoint.

Merits & Limitations: Allows interim modification of patient population to accrual, higher probability of trial success, and enhancement of benefit-risk relationship, but increases complexity to avoid type I error inflation due to interim adaptations and multiplicity. The design can be used when biomarker-based subgroups could be predefined, but with uncertainty on the best possible endpoint and population.

5.3.2 Biomarker-Informed Group Sequential Design

The biomarker-informed Group Sequential Design (BIGSD) is similar to a group sequential design except that the interim analysis is conducted on the biomarker instead of the primary endpoint. The design is useful when a sufficient amount of data of the primary endpoint such as survival is not available at the interim analysis, but the biomarker can be measured earlier and is predictive. The biomarker-informed GSD can be used for early futility design, unless the biomarker is a valid surrogate, in which case the design cannot be used for early efficacy stopping.

Merits & Limitations: BIGSD can inform the treatment futility early on and can be generalized to a multiple arm drop-loser design, in which the interim results on biomarker will be used for picking the winner. However, the correlation between the biomarker at IA and the primary endpoint at the final analysis has a very limited impact on power.

5.3.3   Biomarker-Adaptive Threshold Design

To develop biomarkers and then to validate them is usually very expensive and time consuming. Often times, by the time of the start of late phase clinical trials, a reliable biomarker, as well as its threshold for identifying patients sensitive to an experimental treatment is not known.

When the marker is known but the threshold or the cut point for defining a positive or negative biomarker status is not clear, a biomarker-adaptive threshold design can be considered (Jiang et al, 2007). The biomarker-adaptive threshold design combines the test of overall treatment effect with the establishment and validation of a cut point for a pre-specified biomarker which identifies a biomarker-based subgroup believed to be most sensitive to the experimental treatment. This design potentially provides substantial gain in efficiency.

Specifically, the main purpose of the biomarker-adaptive threshold design is to identify and validate a cut-off point for a pre-specified biomarker, and to compare the clinical outcome between experimental and control treatments for all patients and for the patients identified as biomarker positive in a single study. The procedure provides a prospective statistical test of the hypotheses that the experimental treatment is beneficial for the entire patient population or that the experimental treatment is beneficial for a subgroup defined by the biomarker, and provides an estimate of the optimal biomarker cut-off point.

The statistical hypothesis test can be carried out by splitting the overall type I error rate α. First, compare the treatment response on the overall population at α_1 and if not significant then perform the second test at $\alpha - \alpha_1$. For example, if the null hypothesis of no benefit in overall population is rejected at a desired significance level of, for example, 0.04 then the testing is stopped. Otherwise, the testing is carried out at 0.01 to test the hypothesis of no benefit in identified biomarker-based subpopulation. This strategy controls overall alpha below the 0.05 level. The advantage of this procedure is its simplicity and that it explicitly separates the effect of the test treatment in the broad population from the subgroup specification. However, it takes a conservative approach in adjusting for multiplicity in combining the overall and subgroup analyses. Other strategies of combining the two statistical tests for overall and subgroup patients involve consideration of the correlation structure of the two test statistics. A point estimate and a confidence interval for the cut-off value could be estimated by a bootstrap re-sampling approach.

Merits & Limitations: Biomarker-adaptive threshold designs increase efficiency by combining the test of overall treatment effect with the establishment and validation of a cut point for a pre-specified biomarker; but also increase complexity to avoid type I error inflation due to multiplicity. The design can be used when the threshold of biomarker for defining a positive or negative biomarker status is not clear.

5.3.4 Adaptive Signature Design

The adaptive signature design (Freidlin et al 2009) is a design proposed to select the subgroup using a large number of potential biomarkers. This design is appropriate when both the potential biomarkers and the cut off are unknown, however there is some evidence that the targeted therapy may work in some of the shortlisted biomarkers.

It combines a definitive test for treatment effect in the entire patient population with identification and validation of a biomarker signature for the subgroup sensitive patient population. There are three elements in this design: (a) trial powered to detect the overall treatment effect at the end of the trial; (b) identification of the subgroup of patients who are likely to benefit to the targeted therapy at the first stage of the trial; (c) statistical hypothesis test to detect the treatment difference in the sensitive patient population based only the subgroup of patients randomized in the latter half of the trial. These elements are pre-specified prospectively.

Statistical tests should be conducted appropriately in this design to account for multiplicity. A proposed strategy is as follows: test the initial null hypothesis of no treatment benefit in overall population at a slightly lower significance level than the overall alpha of 0.05 (for example, 0.04). If the initial null hypothesis is rejected at the lower significance level, then the targeted therapy is declared superior than the control treatment for the overall population. The hypothesis testing and analysis is complete at this stage. If the first hypothesis is not rejected, then the signature component of the design is used to select a potentially promising biomarker subgroup. It is done by the following steps: split the study population into a training sub-sample and a validation sub-sample of patients. The training sub-sample is used to develop a model to predict the treatment difference between targeted therapy and control as a function of baseline covariates. The developed model is then applied to validation sub-sample to obtain the prediction for each subject in this sample. A predicted score is calculated to classify the subject as sensitive or non-sensitive. The subgroup is selected using a pre-specified cut-off for this predicted score. The second hypothesis test is conducted in this sensitive subgroup to see the benefit of the targeted therapy against the control. This test is conducted at a much lower significance (for example, 0.01).

According to Freidlin and Simon (2005), this design may be ideal to use for Phase II clinical trials for developing signatures to identify patients who respond better to targeted therapies. The advantage of this design is its ability to de-risk losing the label of broader population. However, since only half of the patients are used for development or validation, and with the large number of potential biomarkers for consideration, a large sample size may be needed to adequately power the trial.

Merits & Limitations: Adaptive signature designs have the ability to de-risk losing the label of broader population by combining the test of overall treatment effect with identification and validation of a biomarker signature for a sensitive patient population, but have increased complexity to avoid type I error inflation due to multiplicity. The design can be used when both the potential biomarkers and the cut off are unknown.

5.3.5   Cross-Validated Adaptive Signature Design

Cross-validated adaptive signature design (Freidlin et al, 2010) is an extension of the adaptive signature design, which allows use of the entire study population for signature development and validation.

Similar to the adaptive signature design, the initial null hypothesis is to test the benefit of the targeted therapy against the control is conducted in the overall population which is conducted at a slightly lower significance level α_1 than the overall α. The sensitive subset is determined by developing the classifier using the full population, which is done by the following steps

1. Test the initial null hypothesis of no treatment benefit in the overall population at α_1, which is a slightly lower significance level than the overall α. If this hypothesis is rejected, then the targeted therapy is declared superior to the control treatment for the overall population and analysis is completed. If the first hypothesis is not rejected; then the following steps for signature development and validation should be carried out:

2. Split study population into "k" sub-samples.

3. One of the "k" sub-samples is omitted to form a training sub-sample. Similar to the adaptive signature design, develop a model to predict the treatment difference between targeted therapy and control as a function of baseline covariates using training sub-sample. Apply the developed model to each subject not in this training sub-sample so as to classify patients as sensitive or non- sensitive.

4. Repeat the same process leaving out a different sample from the "k" sub-samples to form training sub-sample. After "k" iterations, every patient in the trial will be classified as sensitive or non-sensitive.

5. Compare the treatment difference within the subgroup of patients classified as sensitive using a test statistic (T). Generate the null distribution of T by permuting the two treatments and repeating the entire "k" iterations of the cross-validation process. Perform the test at $\alpha - \alpha_1$. If the test is rejected, then the superiority is claimed for the targeted therapy in the sensitive subgroup.

The cross-validation approach can considerably enhance the performance of the adaptive signature design as it permits the maximization of information contributing to the development of the signature, particularly useful in the high-dimensional data setting where the sample size is limited. Cross-validation also maximizes the size of the sensitive patient subset used to validate the signature. One drawback is the fact that the signature for classifying sensitive patients in each subsample might not be the same and thus can cause difficulty in interpreting the results if a significant treatment effect is identified in the sensitive subgroup.

Merits & Limitations: Cross-validation adaptive signature designs have the ability to use the entire study population for signature development and validation enhanced efficiency, but have increased complexity to avoid type I error inflation due to multiplicity difficulty in interpreting the significant results in sensitive subgroup. The design can be used when both the potential biomarkers and the cut off are unknown Merits.

5.4 Trial Design Method with Biomarkers

5.4.1 Impact of Assay Sensitivity and Specificity

There are several challenges in utilization of biomarkers in clinical trials: (1) the estimated effect size for each subpopulation at the design stage is often very inaccurate, (2) a cost is associated with screening patients for the biomarker, (3) the test for detecting the biomarker often requires a high sensitivity and specificity, and the screening tool may not be available at the time of the clinical trial, (4) screening patients for the biomarker may cause a burden and impact patient recruitment, and (5) in globally optimal design as discussed in Chapters 3 and 4, the net present value g_4 will be different for different designs and populations. These factors must be considered when choosing an appropriate study design.

It is informative to know how the assay sensitivity and specificity will impact the estimation of the treatment effect size for the patients in the trial. The N patients identified as biomarker $(+)$ patients consists of N_+ biomarker$(+)$ and N_- biomarker$(-)$ patients, with the following relationship:

$$N = N_+ S_e + N_- (1 - S_p),\qquad(5.1)$$

where N_+ and N_- are the sizes of patient populations with and without the biomarker, respectively; S_e is the sensitivity of the screening test, i.e., the probability of correctly identifying the biomarker among patients with the biomarker, and S_p is the specificity of the screening test, which is defined as the probability of correctly identifying biomarker-negative among patients without biomarker. The average treatment effect for diagnostic biomarker $(+)$ patients:

$$\Delta = \frac{\Delta_+ N_+ S_e + \Delta_- N_- (1 - S_p)}{N}.\qquad(5.2)$$

When the specificity increases, the target population decreases overall, however average treatment effect in the target population will increase because the misdiagnosis of biomarker-negative as positive will reduce the average treatment effect.

5.4.2   Biomarker-Stratified Design

Denote treatment difference between the test and control groups by δ_+, δ_-, and δ, for biomarker-positive, biomarker-negative, and overall patient populations, respectively. The null hypothesis for biomarker-positive subpopulation is

$$H_{01} : \delta_+ = 0. \tag{5.3}$$

The null hypothesis for biomarker-negative subpopulation is

$$H_{02} : \delta_- = 0. \tag{5.4}$$

The null hypothesis for overall population is

$$H_0 : \delta = 0. \tag{5.5}$$

Without loss of generality, assume that the first n patients have the biomarker among N patients and the test statistic for the subpopulation is given by

$$Z_+ = \frac{\sum_{i=1}^{n} x_i - \sum_{i=1}^{n} y_i}{n\sigma} \sqrt{\frac{n}{2}} \sim N(0,1) \text{ under } H_0, \tag{5.6}$$

where x_i, and y_i $(i = 1, ..., n)$ are the responses in treatment A and B.

Similarly, the test statistic for biomarker-negative group is defined as

$$Z_- = \frac{\left(\sum_{i=n+1}^{N} x_i - \sum_{i=n+1}^{N} y_i\right)}{(N-n)\sigma} \sqrt{\frac{N-n}{2}} \sim N(0,1) \text{ under } H_0. \tag{5.7}$$

The test statistic for overall population is given by

$$Z = \frac{\hat{\delta}}{\sigma} \sqrt{\frac{N}{2}} = T_+ \sqrt{\frac{n}{N}} + T_- \sqrt{\frac{N-n}{N}} \sim N(0,1) \text{ under } H_0. \tag{5.8}$$

We choose the test statistic for the trial as

$$T = \max(Z, Z_+). \tag{5.9}$$

It can be shown that the correlation coefficient between Z and Z_+ is

$$\rho = \sqrt{\frac{n}{N}}. \tag{5.10}$$

Therefore, the stopping boundary can be determined by

$$\alpha = 1 - \Pr\left(Z < z_{2,1-\alpha}, Z_+ < z_{2,1-\alpha}|H_0\right), \tag{5.11}$$

where $z_{2,1-\alpha}$ is the bivariate normal $100(1-\alpha)$-equipercentage point under H_0.

The p-value corresponding to an observed test statistic t is given by

$$p = \Pr(T \geq t | H_0). \tag{5.12}$$

The power can be calculated using

$$power = 1 - \Pr(Z < z_{2,1-\alpha}, Z_+ < z_{2,1-\alpha} | H_a). \tag{5.13}$$

The numerical integration or simulations can be performed to evaluate $z_{2,1-\alpha}$ and the power.

Multivariate normal equal percetiles can be obtained using qmvnorm function in mvtnorm package from R. For at a design with one-sided $\alpha = 0.025$, we can use the following code to obtain the critical value $z_{2,1-\alpha}$ when the interim analysis is to conduct at information time $\tau_1 = \frac{n_p}{N}$, where n_p and N are the sample size per treatment group for the biomarker positive and overall patients, respectively.

```
library(mvtnorm)
alpha=0.025; mu1=0; mu=0; np=100; N=200; rho=sqrt(np/N)
s=matrix(c(1,rho, rho, 1), 2,2)
qmvnorm(1-alpha, mean=c(0,0), sigma = s, tail = "lower")
```

The output will be the critical value $z_{2,1-\alpha} = 2.17831$. As an example for power simulation, this $z_{2,1-\alpha} = 2.17831$ is then used in the following R code to obtain power for effect size 0.8 and 0.6, respectively, for the biomarker positive (60 subjects per group) and overall populations (120 subjects per group) with IA information time =0.5.

```
library(mvtnorm)
sigma0=1.6; np=60; N=120; mup=0.8; mu=0.6; rho=sqrt(np/N)
up=mup/sigma0*sqrt(np/2); u=mu/sigma0*sqrt(N/2)
s=matrix(c(1,rho, rho, 1), 2,2)
Power= 1-pmvnorm(lower=c(-Inf, -Inf), upper=c(2.17831, 2.17831), mean=c(up, u), sigma=s)
```

The numerical integration gives 84.2% power for the trial design 120 patients per group. If the trial was to recruit all patients without using the biomarker, the power will be 83% with 120 patients per group. If the trial only enrolls biomarker positive patients (biomarker-enrichment design), the power will be 78% with 60 per group (the number of patients screened will be much larger).

If the effect size for the biomarker negative group reduces to 0, the effect for the overall population will be 0.4 and the classical design with biomarker will have 73.6% However, without biomarker, 120 patients per group will only provide 49% power if the trial is conducted for overall patients.

5.4.3 Biomarker-Adaptive Winner Design

Formulate the test statistic using data from stage 1:

$$T_1 = \max(Z_1, Z_{1+}).\tag{5.14}$$

where Z_1 and Z_{1+} are similar to Z and Z_+ in (5.6) and (5.8), but only based on Stage 1 data.

$$p_1 = 1 - \Phi(T_1).\tag{5.15}$$

The decision rules at Stage 1:

1. If $p_1 > \beta_1$ stop trial for futility

2. If $p_1 \leq \alpha_1$ claim treatment effect in overall population if $Z_1 \geq Z_{1+}$ or in biomarker positive patients if $Z_1 < Z_{1+}$.

3. If $\alpha < p_1 \leq \beta_1$ continue to the second stage. If $Z_1 \geq Z_{1+}$, the overall group is the winner and recruit n_2 additional patients (m_2 biomarker positive patients) per treatment group; otherwise the biomarker positive group is winner and recruit m_2 additional patients per arm for the placebo and the winner arm.

Calculate the final statistic Z for the winner using the combined data from stages 1 and 2 and (naive) p value:

$$p_2 = 1 - \Phi(Z).\tag{5.17}$$

The decision rule at Stage 2:

If $p_2 \leq \alpha_2$ claim efficacy for the winner arm; otherwise no efficacy can be claimed.

To control the type-I error under the global null, the efficacy stopping boundaries are determined through simulations.

TABLE 5.1
Stopping Boundaries Biomarker-Adaptive Winner Design.

α_1	.0000	.0010	.0020	.0030	.0040	.0050	.0060	.0070	.0080
α_2	.0156	.0151	.0144	.0137	.0128	.0119	.0109	.0099	.0088

Note: one-sided $\alpha = 0.025$. sample size ratio 1:2 (biomarker positive: negative), IA Info time $=0.5$. For stopping boundaries on z-scale, use transfer: $z_{1-\alpha_i}$.

SAS Macro 5.1, BMAD, is developed for simulating Biomarker-Adaptive Winner Design. The typical simulation code to determine the stopping boundaries α_1 and α_2 in Table 5.2 is:

%BMAD(nSims=10000000, nStages=2, u0p=0, u0n=0, sigma=1, np1=50, np2=50, nn1=100, nn2=100, alpha1=0.004, beta1=1,alpha2=0.0128);

To study power of the Biomarker-Adaptive Winner Design, suppose a cancer trial with two biomarker groups that might have different treatment effects on progression free survival time. Assume, after adjusted for misdiagnosis, the hazard ratio is $\theta = 0.6$ for the biomarker positive group and $\theta = 0.2$ for the biomarker negative group. The power can be obtained using the following SAS code:

%BMAD(nStages=2, u0p=-log(0.6), u0n=-log(0.9), sigma=1, np1=50, np2=50, nn1=100, nn2=100, alpha1=0.004, beta1=1,alpha2=0.0128);

The simulation results show the trial has 92.7% with an average total number of events of 378.

Note that the overall population has a mixture of exponential distribution if the two subpopulations have exponential distributions with different hazard rates.

5.4.4 Biomarker-Informed Group Sequential Design

The BIGSD is a special group sequential design, in which the biomarker response instead of the primary endpoint is used at the interim analysis for decision-making. The design is useful when the sufficient amount of data of the primary endpoint such as survival is not available at the interim analysis, but the biomarker can be measured earlier and is predictive. Here biomarker can be a binary tumor response or time-to-event such as time-to-progress.

It is well known that the logrank statistic T for a two-group test is approximately normal (Schoenfeld, 1981)

$$T \sim N\left(\log\theta\sqrt{f_1 f_2 D}, 1\right),\tag{5.18}$$

where θ is hazard rate and f_1 and f_2 are the sample size fractions for the two groups. When the two groups have the same survival, i.e., the hazard ratio $\theta = 1$, the logrank test statistic has approximately the standard normal distribution.

Suppose in a group sequential design, Z_1 and Z_2 are the logrank statistics at stage 1 and stage 2. Z_1 and Z_2 are approximately bivariate normal with means $\log\theta\sqrt{f_1 f_2 D_1}$ and $\log\theta\sqrt{f_1 f_2 D_2}$, and correlation $\sqrt{\frac{D_1}{D_2}}$, where D_1 and D_2 are the cumulative numbers of deaths at the stages 1 and 2, respectively.

Assume the primary endpoint Y and biomarker X are correlated and the corresponding test statistics $(Z_X$ and $Z_Y)$ of the variables follow a bivariate normal distribution under the large sample size assumption,

$$\begin{pmatrix} Z_X \\ Z_Y \end{pmatrix} \sim N\left(\begin{pmatrix} \nu_x \\ \nu_y \end{pmatrix}, \begin{pmatrix} 1 & \rho \\ \rho & 1 \end{pmatrix}\right)\tag{5.19}$$

If the treatment has no effect on the primary endpoint, then $\nu_y = 0$, if no effect on the biomarker, then $\nu_x = 0$.

Since the true correlation between the biomarker and the primary endpoint is not exactly known in practice, to find the critical value, we have to assume conservatively a perfect correlation between the biomarker and the primary endpoint. As a result, the same stopping boundaries as for GSD can be used with the non-binding futility rule.

The biomarker-informed design simulation is described as follows:

1. Simulate stage 1 data from bivariate normal distribution,

$$\begin{cases} Z_x = Z_1 + v_X \\ Z_y = \rho Z_1 + \sqrt{1 - \rho^2} Z_2 + v_y, \end{cases}$$

where Z_1 and Z_2 are independently drawn from the standard normal distribution.

2. At the end of Stage 1, an interim analysis of biomarker is performed and p-value $p_{1x} = 1 - \Phi(z_{1x})$ is calculated. The following decision rules are used:

   • If $p_{1x} > \beta_1$ stop trial for futility
   • If $p_{1x} \le \alpha_1$ claim efficacy (only if the biomarker is surrogate marker; otherwise α_1 must be 0)
   • If $\alpha < p_{1x} \le \beta_1$ continue to the second stage.

3. Simulate Stage 2 data from the standard normal distribution, z_{2y} (logrank test statistic of the survival data at Stage 2)

4. Formulate the final test statistic based on $z = \sqrt{\tau_1} z_{1y} + \sqrt{1 - \tau_1} z_{2y}$ and calculate the p-value, $p = 1 - \Phi(z)$.

Here z_{1x}, z_{1y} and z_{2y} can be from normal, binary, survival, or mixed endpoints with large sample size.

To control familywise error rate, we need to consider that H_0: $N(Z_x, Z_y; v_x, 0, \rho)$, where the mean for the biomarker is $v_x > 0$. Thus, if X is not a surrogate marker, then $\alpha_1 = 0$ and $\alpha_2 = \alpha$. If X is a surrogate marker, then $\beta_1 = 1$ for the nonbinding futility rule.

SAS Macro BID is developed (Appendix xx) for simulating the BIGSD. As an example for power simulation, assume a hazard ratio of 0.7 for both biomarker and survival endpoints, $\rho = 0.8$, the total sample size for the first stage $n_1 = 150$ (75 per group), and the second stage $n_2 = 150$ (75 per group). The simulation code for power is:

%BID(nSims=100000, thetax=-log(0.7), thetay=-log(0.7), rho=0.8, n1=150, n2=150, alpha1=0.0, beta1=0.25, alpha2=0.025);

The simulation results show power = 0.84. The simulation results in Table 5.2, which shows how the effect size θ and correlation ρ affect the power. We can see that the hazard ratio θ_x has a great impact on the power, while the correlation ρ has a minimal impact on the power.

In the simulation program, for a survival endpoint, the effect size $\theta_x = -\ln(\text{hazard ratio})$, where the negative sign means "a smaller hazard rate is better", the sample size is the number of total events required. For a binary

TABLE 5.2

Effects of v_x and ρ on the power.

θ_x	0.4	0.4	0.7	0.7	0.7	0.9	0.9	1.0	1.0
ρ	0.2	0.8	0.0	0.2	0.8	0.2	0.8	0.2	0.8
Power	0.87	0.87	0.81	0.82	0.84	0.44	0.47	0.23	0.25

Note: $\theta_y = 0.7, n1 = n2 = 150, \alpha_1 = 0, \beta_1 = 0.25, \alpha_2 = 0.025$

biomarker endpoint, the effect size $\theta_x = \frac{p_{2x} - p_{1x}}{\sqrt{(p_{1x}(1-p_{1x}) + p_{2x}(1-p_{2x}))/2}}$, where p_{1x} and p_{2x} are the proportions for the groups 1 and 2, respectively. For a normal endpoint, the effect size $\theta_x = \theta_x = \frac{(\mu_{2x} - \mu_{1x})}{\sqrt{(\sigma_{1x}^2 + \sigma_{2x}^2)/2}}$, where μ_{1x} (σ_{1x}) and μ_{2x} (σ_{2x}) are the means (standard deviation) for the groups 1 and 2, respectively.

The Biomarker-informed group sequential design can be generalized to multiple arm design, i.e., biomarker-informed winner design, which is similar to the standard pick-winner design, but the interim analysis is performed on biomarker X instead of the primary endpoint Y.

Let biomarker $X^{(j)}$ and primary endpoint $Y^{(j)}$ with treatment j $(j = 0, ..., K)$ have the following distributions

$$\begin{cases} X^{(j)} \sim N\left(v_j, \sigma_x^2\right) \\ Y^{(j)} = \rho X^{(j)} + \mu_j - \rho v_j + \varepsilon, \end{cases}$$

where $\varepsilon \sim N\left(0, \sigma_y^2 - \rho^2 \sigma_x^2\right)$. Therefore, $Y^{(j)} \sim N\left(\mu_j, \sigma_y^2\right)$, $X^{(j)}$ and $Y^{(j)}$ have a correlation coefficient ρ.

It is interesting that Chang (2007, 2014) showed with an example that the correlation is a "friendship" relationship: a positive correlation (ρ_{tb}) between treatment and the biomarker and a positive correlation (ρ_{bp}) between the biomarker and the primary endpoint do not guarantee a positive correlation (ρ_{tp}) between treatment and the primary endpoint. It is just like friendships: Person A is a friend of person B and B is a friend of person C, but A is not necessarily a friend of C. The correlation does not have the transitivity property.

Here is an example,

$$\begin{cases} X^{(j)} \sim N\left(jv, \sigma^2\right) \\ Y^{(j)} = X^{(j)} - jv, \end{cases}$$

We can see that $X^{(j)}$ and $Y^{(j)}$ are perfectly correlated with $\rho = 1$ within each treatment j. Furthermore, the treatment j has an effect jv beyond placebo $(j = 0)$ on biomarker X, but has no effect on the primary endpoint Y since $Y^{(j)} \sim N\left(0, \sigma^2\right)$. Because a treatment effect on a biomarker does not secure an effect on the primary endpoint, the biomarker is often just used for futility stopping.

5.5   Basket and Population-Adaptive Designs

The discovery of numerous molecular subtypes of common cancers has led tothe investigation of biomarkers potentially predictive of treatment effect of an experimental treatment, which may be relevant in multiple histologies. However, the prevalence of a putative predictive biomarker within any given histology is often low, which makes it challenging to enroll an adequate number of patients in a conventional histology-based confirmatory trial. An alternative approach is to study patients with a common biomarker signature in a "basket" trial across multiple histologies under the assumption that the fundamental etiology of cancer is molecular (Cong Chen et al. 2017; Meador et al. 2014, Lacombe et al. 2014, Sleijfer et al. 2013, Kopetz et al. 2013, Barker et al. 2009).

As pointed out by Chen and Beckman (2017), basket designs can have several benefits: patients with different tumor types will have access to a potentially effective drug earlier through the FDA accelerated approval paradigm in United States, and the conditional approval paradigm in European Medicines Agency (EMA) or other regulatory mechanisms. For sponsors, development of biomarker-driven drugs would be facilitated and overall costs would be lowered by pooling indications; and health authorities may have more robust data for risk and benefit evaluation across tumor indications. However, one of the challenges is that if the indications in a Baskets design involve more than one divisions within a regulatory agency (or multiple regulatory agencies), harmonization among them will be a very challenging task.

In the following, we will discuss FWER control approaches (numerical integration and simulation approaches) and similarity-based approach.

5.5.1   Basket Design Method with Familywise Error Control

A two-stage basket adaptive design is basically a pick-winner-design. At interim analysis, the best r arms will be selected as winners for the second stage of the trial. The observations from the n arms (corresponding to the n indicators) at the first stage is independent. However, the final test statistics for different winner arms are combination of the data from the first and second stages, which are not independent.

The FWER control methods are based on the joint distribution of the order statistics (the test statistics). You may opt to skip this section with impairing you to design basket design since you can use trial simulation approach presented later.

Assume $X_1, X_2, ..., X_n$ are independently from pdf $f(x)$ with corresponding cdf $F(x)$ and let $X_{k(1),n}, X_{k(2),n}, ..., X_{k(r),n}$ be a subset of order statistics $(X_{(1),n} \leq X_{(2),n} \leq, ..., \leq X_{(n),n})$, where $1 \leq k(1) \leq k(2) \leq \cdots \leq k(r) \leq n$. The joint pdf of the subset of the order statistics is (Chapter 2, Ahsanullah,

Nevzorov, and Shakil, 2013):

$$f_{k(1),k(2),...,k(r):n}(x_1, x_2, ..., x_r) \qquad (5.1)$$

$$= \begin{cases} C \prod_{m=1}^{r+1} (F(x_m) - F(x_{m-1}))^{k(m)-k(m-1)-1} \prod_{m=1}^{r} f(x_m), & \text{if } x_1 < x_2 < \cdots x_r \\ 0, & \text{otherwise,} \end{cases}$$

where $C = \frac{n!}{\prod_{m=1}^{r+1}(k(m)-k(m-1)-1)!}$, $k(0) = 0, k(r+1) = n+1, x_0 = -\infty$ and $x_{r+1} = \infty$.

Special case (1): if $r = 2, 1 \leq i < j \leq n$, and $x_1 < x_2$, then the bivariate joint distribution is

$$f_{i,j:n}(x_1, x_2) = \frac{n!}{(i-1)!(j-i-1)!(n-j)!} \qquad (5.2)$$

$$\times (F(x_1))^{i-1}(F(x_2) - F(x_1))^{j-i-1}(1 - F(x_2))^{n-j}f(x_1 f(x_2.))$$

Special case (2): if $k(1) = 1, k(2) = 2, ..., k(r) = r$, then the r smallest order statistics have the joint distribution of

$$f_{1,2,...,r:n}(x_1, x_2, ..., x_r) \qquad (5.3)$$

$$= \begin{cases} \frac{n!}{(n-r)!}(1 - F(x_r))^{(n-r)} \prod_{m=1}^{r} f(x_m), & \text{if } x_1 < x_2 < \cdots x_r \\ 0, & \text{otherwise,} \end{cases}$$

Special case (3): if $k(1) = n-r+1, k(2) = n-r+2, ..., k(r) = n$, then the r largest order statistics have the joint distribution of

$$f_{n-r+1,n-r+2,...,n:n}(x_1, x_2, ..., x_r) \qquad (5.4)$$

$$= \begin{cases} \frac{n!}{(n-r)!}(F(x_1))^{(n-r)} \prod_{m=1}^{r} f(x_m), & \text{if } x_1 < x_2 < \cdots x_r \\ 0, & \text{otherwise,} \end{cases}$$

Suppose in a basket design with initial n indications, at the interim analysis, and up to r winners with best efficacy results will be selected to continue on the second stage. Denote $X_1, X_2, ..., X_n$ the statistics from the first stage data and $Y_1, Y_2, ..., Y_n$ the same statistics from the second stage data (not cumulative). We define the test statistics at the final analysis as $Z_i = \sqrt{\tau_1}X_i + \sqrt{1 - \tau_1}Y_i$ for all winners. The rejection rules at the finally analysis are: reject null hypothesis H_i and claim efficacy for indication i ($i = 1, 2, ..., r$) if $Z_i \geq Z_c$; otherwise retain H_i. The critical value Z_c can be obtained from the following equation (note: Y_i only depends on x_i, not others $x_j, j \neq i$) under the global H_0,

$$
\begin{aligned}
\alpha &= \Pr\left(\cup_{i=1}^{r}\left(Z_i = \sqrt{\tau_1}X_i + \sqrt{1-\tau_1}Y_i \geq Z_c\right)\right) \\
&= \int_{-\infty}^{\infty}\int_{-\infty}^{x_r}\cdots\int_{-\infty}^{x_3}\int_{-\infty}^{x_2}\Pr\left(\cup_{i=1}^{r}Y_i \geq \frac{Z_c - \sqrt{\tau_1}x_i}{\sqrt{1-\tau_1}}|x_i\right) \\
&\quad\times f_{n-r+1,n-r+2,\ldots,n:n}\left(x_1, x_2, \ldots, x_r\right)dx_1 dx_2 \cdots dx_{r-1}dx_r \\
&= \int_{-\infty}^{\infty}\int_{-\infty}^{x_r}\cdots\int_{-\infty}^{x_3}\int_{-\infty}^{x_2}\left[1 - \Pr\left(\cap_{i=1}^{r}Y_i < \frac{Z_c - \sqrt{\tau_1}x_i}{\sqrt{1-\tau_1}}|x_i\right)\right] \\
&\quad\times f_{n-r+1,n-r+2,\ldots,n:n}\left(x_1, x_2, \ldots, x_r\right)dx_1 dx_2 \cdots dx_{r-1}dx_r
\end{aligned}
$$

Because $X_1, X_2, \ldots$, and X_n are mutually independent and $Y_1, Y_2, \ldots$, and Y_n are also mutually independent, the previous equation can be simplified as

$$
\begin{aligned}
\alpha &= \int_{-\infty}^{\infty}\int_{-\infty}^{x_r}\cdots\int_{-\infty}^{x_3}\int_{-\infty}^{x_2}\left[1 - \prod_{i=1}^{r}F\left(\frac{Z_c - \sqrt{\tau_1}x_i}{\sqrt{1-\tau_1}}\right)\right] \quad\quad (5.5) \\
&\quad\times\frac{n!}{(n-r)!}\left(F\left(x_1\right)\right)^{(n-r)}\prod_{m=1}^{r}f\left(x_m\right)dx_1 dx_2 \cdots dx_{r-1}dx_r
\end{aligned}
$$

where f and F are the pdf and cdf under the global H_0 and the information time $\tau_1 = N_1/N$. Solve critical value Z_c for given α. To carry out the integration in (5.28), the package "cubature" in R code can be used .

Alternatively, trial simulation methods can be used. The basic steps in the simulation approach is to simulate the observations for n arms (indictions) at the first stage and select r winners. Simulate the observations for the r winner arms for the second stage. (3) Combine the data from the two stages to formulate the test statistics.

Simulation approach can not only provide the stopping boundaries but also provide power for the basket design. Two SAS macro are developed: BasketDesignNormal for a normal endpoint and BasketDesignBinary for a binary endpoint. As an example, for a 5 + 1-arm design with a normal endpoint, allowing up to 3 winners, use the following code to obtain the critical value Z_alpha = 2.5690, which gives power (one-sided alpha) 0.025:

```
data dInput;
Array Sigmas(5)(1, 1, 1, 1, 1);
Array u0s(5)(0.3, 0.3, 0.3, 0.3, 0.3);
Array us(5)(0.3, 0.3, 0.3, 0.3, 0.3);
Array N1s(5)(10, 10, 10, 10, 10);
Array N2s(5)(10, 10, 10, 10, 10);
%BasketDesignNormal(nSims=10000000, NumOfArms=5, nWinners=3,
Z_alpha=2.5690);
```

The critical values for designs with different number of indications and different number of winners can be obtained either using numerical interrogations or simulations. See Table 5.3 for examples.

TABLE 5.3

Critical Value Z_alpha for Basket Design.

Number of Indications	Maximum number of Winners Allowed				
	1	2	3	4	5
2	2.2121	2.2390			
3	2.3485	2.3865	2.3905		
4	2.4418	2.4847	2.4930	2.4950	
5	2.5115	2.5600	2.5690	2.5715	2.5719

Note: 10,000,000 simulations. Interim analysis at 50% per arm patients.

Note that the basket design method can not only be used for multiple indications, but can also be used for multiple population due to different baseline characteristics (disease severity, genetics, race). It can even be used for an umbrella trial (multiple drugs for one indication) and a trial with multiple drugs for multiple indications as long as the test statistics are independent.

5.5.2 Basket Design for Cancer Trial with Imatinib

Imatinib mesylate is a small-molecule selective inhibitor of the tyrosine kinases ABL, Abl-related gene product (ARG), KIT, CSF-1R, and platelet-derived growth factor receptors α and β (Heinrich et al., 2008). Dysregulation of imatinib-sensitive tyrosine kinases is a key factor in the pathogenesis of several malignancies, and imatinib treatment dramatically benefits patients with such cancers.

An early single-arm Phase II study was conducted to evaluate the activity of imatinib in treating advanced, life-threatening malignancies expressing one or more imatinib-sensitive tyrosine kinases (Heinrich et al., 2008). One hundred eighty-six patients ($\geq$15 years old) with 40 different malignancies were enrolled (78.5% solid tumors, 21.5% hematologic malignancies). Patients were treated with 400 or 800 mg/d imatinib for hematologic malignancy and solid tumors, respectively. Treatment was continued until disease progression or unacceptable toxicity was observed. Confirmed response occurred in 8.9% of solid tumor patients (4 complete, 9 partial) and 27.5% of hematologic malignancy patients (8 complete, 3 partial). Partial responses were observed in at least 6 of 40 indications. In solid tumors, synovial sarcoma achieved 6.3% (1/16) PR and 6.3% (1/16) ORR; dermatofibrosarcoma protuberans, 33.3% (4/12) CR, 50% (6/12) PR, and 83.5% (10/12) ORR; aggressive fibromatosis, 10.0% (2/20) PR and 10.0% (2/20) ORR. In hematologic malignancies, hypereosinophilic syndrome had 35.7% (5/14) CR, 7.1% (1/14) PR, and 42.8% (6/14) ORR; myeloproliferative disorders, 42.9% (3/7) CR, 14.3% (1/7) PR, and 57.2% (4/7) ORR; systemic mastocytosis, 20% (1/5) PR, 20% (1/5) PR, and 40% (2/5) ORR.

The main conclusion of the Phase II study was that Clinical benefit was largely confined to diseases with known genomic mechanisms of activation of imatinib target kinases. Therefore, an important role for molecular characterization of tumors is to identify patients likely to benefit from imatinib treatment.

Suppose the task now is to design a Phase III Basket trial include the 4 types of tumors for which the Imatinib showed promising results in terms of ORR.

We choose a two-arm randomized basket design with above 4 indications with ORR larger than 10% and allow to pick as many as 3 winners. Assume the primary endpoint is ORR. The estimate ORR for the 4 indications are: 83.5% for dermatofibrosarcoma protuberans, 42.8% for hypereosinophilic syndrome, 57.2% for myeloproliferative disorders, and 40% for systemic mastocytosis. Further assume that the Imatinib will have around 30% improvement over the standard care for all the indications. Specifically, the control has the rates of 0.6, 0.27, 0.35, and 0.25, respectively, for 4 indications. The sample sizes are 30, 50, 40, and 60 per arm for dermatofibrosarcoma protuberans, hypereosinophilic syndrome, myeloproliferative disorders, and systemic mastocytosis, respectively.

We first use the simulation SAS code for the Basket Design with binary endpoint. Here is the code for determine the critical value:

```
data dInput;
Array p0s(4)(0.6, 0.27, 0.35, 0.25);
Array p1s(4)(0.6, 0.27, 0.35, 0.25);
Array N1s(4)(30, 50, 40, 60);
Array N2s(4)(30, 50, 40, 60);
%BasketDesignBinary(nSims=10000000, NumOfArms=4, nWinners=3,
Z_alpha=2.571);
```

The result shows the critical value Z_alpha = 2.571 will give power (one-sided type-I error 2.5%). The power for the assumed response rates of the 4 indications can be obtained using the following code:

```
data dInput;
Array p0s(4)(0.6, 0.27, 0.35, 0.25);
Array p1s(4)(0.835, 0.428, 0.572, 0.40);
Array N1s(4)(30, 50, 40, 60);
Array N2s(4)(30, 50, 40, 60);
%BasketDesignBinary(nSims=1000000, NumOfArms=4, nWinners=3,
Z_alpha=2.571);
```

The simulation results indicate that the power to claim efficacy is 95.8%, 60.2%, and 53.9% for the winners (winners can change from trial to trial) and the overall power (claim efficacy at least for one of the 4 indications) is 0.987.

5.5.3   Methods based on Similarity Principle

One possible argument against multiplicity adjustment for α is that a basket design is just a combination of several trials into one trial for operational convenience and cost-efficiency, thus no multiplicity adjustment is required. We can even argue further: not only the multiplicity adjustment is not necessary, but also the results from different indications can be combined to provide the totality evidence. However, such a totality evidence should be composed unbiasedly. We cannot just select indications with positive results to compose the so-called totality of evidence. Instead, data from all indications (negative or positive) should be used. We suggest the totality of evidence should be constructed based on the similarity principle.

Similar things will behave similarly. The similarity in behaviors will increase as the similarity between two subjects increases. This is a simple statement of the similarity principle (Chang, 2012, 2014). The principle is used everywhere, in both science and daily life. For example, a drug may have similar effects on patients of the same race, but less similar effects on patients of different races. We may believe men and women have similar longevity.

In drug discovery, the rational approach uses structure-activity relationships (SAR) to discover, optimize or even design drug candidates. Compounds with similar chemical structures are expected to have similar effects (biological, physiological, safety, efficacy). The term "drug-like" describes various empirically found structure characteristics of molecular agents, which are associated with pharmacological activities. It is not strictly defined but provides a general concept of what makes a drug a drug. Drug-likeness may be considered as an overall likelihood of a molecular agent that can be turned into a drug.

In drug development, we believe a ligand will have similar effect in animals and humans. For this reason, we conduct animal studies first, hopefully the data obtained from preclinical studies in animals study will provide useful information to consider and incorporate into clinical studies of the same compound in humans. However, it should be noted that the ability to extrapolate the results of animal studies into humans is often quite limited. The similarities between humans are much higher.

The notion of the similarity principle motivates us to the following weighting approach for data analysis in basket designs.

Suppose there are m indications of the same drug in a single trial with effect $\mu_1,...,\mu_m$. The effect of the drug for a person with disease indication k is defined as

$$\delta_k = \frac{1}{\sum_{i=1}^{m} w_{ki}} (w_{k1}\mu_1 + ... + w_{km}\mu_m), \qquad (5.29)$$

where the weight w_{ki} is defined by the similarity score (0-1) between indication k and indication i. This is because a person in group k is similar to all the groups in some way, thus the drug effect on him is the weighted average defined by (5.29). This effect is really individualized.

The effect δ_k is estimated by

$$\hat{\delta}_k = \frac{w_{k1}\bar{x}_1 + ... + w_{km}\bar{x}_m}{\sum_{i=1}^{m} w_{ki}} \qquad (5.30)$$

TABLE 5.4

An Example of Tanimoto Index.

	Property								
	A	B	C	D	E	F	G	H	I
Molecule/Indication k	0	1	1	0	0	1	1	1	0
Molecule/Indication i	1	1	1	1	0	0	0	1	1

When w_i =sample size fraction $\frac{n_i}{N}$, (5.30) is simply a pooling method. The pooling method can only be used in the indications with consistent effects or homogeneous effect cross indications.

The test statistic is defined

$$z_k = \frac{\hat{\delta}_k}{\sigma_{\delta_k}},$$

where

$$\sigma_{\delta_k}^2 = \frac{1}{\left(\sum_{i=1}^m w_{ki}\right)^2} \left(w_{k1}^2 \sigma_{\bar{x}1}^2 + ... + w_{km}^2 \sigma_{\bar{x}m}^2 \right)$$

When $x_i, i = 1, ..., m$ have normal distributions, $z_k, k = 1, ..., m$ have normal distributions.

For the weight w_{ki}, there are different similarity indexes available in the of artificial intelligence or computational linguistics such as cosine similarity. In drug discovery and development, a popular similarity index is the *Tanimoto index* defined by

$$w_{ki} = \frac{n_{ki}}{n_k + n_i - n_{ki}} \tag{5.31}$$

where n_k is the number of bits set to 1 in molecule (disease indication in the current case) k, n_i is the number of bits set to 1 in molecule/indication i, and n_{ki} is the number of set bits common to both k and i. The possible value of w_{ki} ranges between 0 (maximal dissimilarity) and 1 (identical bitstrings). For the example of two indications in Table 5.4, the Tanimoto Index is

$$\tau_{ki} = \frac{4}{5 + 6 - 4} = 0.571.$$

5.6 Summary

Biomarkers are becoming increasingly important for streamlining drug discovery and development in the new era of precision medicine. This chapter provided an overview of classical and adaptive designs to consider if biomarkers are to be incorporated into clinical trials. There are a number of issues to consider before designing a trial with a predictive biomarker component (Huang et al 2015). First, we need to evaluate the strength of preclinical evidence for a potential predictive biomarker. If there is compelling preliminary evidence that the experimental therapy does not provide benefit to all the patients, and the benefit is restricted to a subset of patients expressing a molecular or genetic value, an enrichment strategy may be adopted. Otherwise, an unselected or all-comers strategy may be wise to use. W e need to evaluate whether the prevalence of the biomarker positive group is high, moderate or low. If the prevalence is high, population enrichment may not be required, and a traditional design could render the greatest commercial value and market opportunity. Third, as indicated by the FDA, the accuracy of the measurements used to identify the enrichment population and the sensitivity and specificity of the enrichment criterion in distinguishing responders and non-responders are also critical issues. When the assay is not 100% accurate to dichotomize patients to biomarker positive and negative groups, the efficiency of targeted clinical trials will be affected in a negative way.

An accurate, reproducible and adequately validated assay is essential for establishing desired therapeutic activity and clinical validation of the biomarker (usually realized by a companion diagnostic kit from a central lab) in a prospective manner. In addition, the feasibility and timing to obtain a biopsy (de-novo or archived), serum, or other samples at baseline prior to randomization determines whether the biomarker can be prospectively validated.

Baseline classifier biomarkers can be used for population segmentation or enrichment design and optimization of target patient population. Early measured treatment effect of a predictive biomarker can be used to design BIGSD and other biomarker-adaptive designs. A good predictive biomarker may be labeled and considered as a surrogate that can be used to replace the primary endpoint. However, identifying a surrogate marker is extremely difficult. A prognostic marker will predict the outcome irrespective to the treatment. A higher response rate of a prognostic marker in the test group than the placebo does not necessarily lead to a higher response in the primary endpoint as we have discussed in the non-transitivity of "friendships." We also discussed the design methods for biomarker-stratified design, biomarker-adaptive winner design, and biomarker-informed GSD and provided simulations programs.

The umbrella design is a trial design evaluating the safety and/or efficacy of multiple drugs in a single indication. Basket design is a trial design evaluating a h a single drug for multiple indications. When sample size is large, the method discussed in the section of "Basket Design Method with Familywise Error Control" may be considered for both umbrella and basket trials as long as the test statistics for different drugs in the umbrella trial and for different indications in the basket trial are independently distributed. The difference between common dose-finding trial design and basket design is that the former has a common control arm, thus the test statistics for different doses are correlated, but the latter does not have a common control, thus the test statistics for different indications are independent.

The basket design method based on the totality evidence from weighted effect size from different indications is supported by the general similarity principle. By using the principle, subjectivity is inevitable, and it is true to all sciences. We will discuss this more in the chapter about controversies. A practical challenge of using basket design comes from working with different divisions in FDA (and/or working with different agencies across geographic regions) and obtaining agreement on common criteria for approval.

There are other methods for using biomarkers in clinical trial design, monitoring and data analysis. For example, the threshold regression with biomarker and application to treatment switching in oncology trials (Lee, Whitmore, Chang, 2005) will be discussed in Chapter 7, Survival Trial Design.

To select an optimal design among all the trial options considered, the globally optimal model developed in Chapter 3 can be used. To this end, the estimations of the cost, duration, the number of potential competitors, the time-to-market, and the expected sales are necessary to consider for each design. In addition, prior distribution of the drug profile, mainly the efficacy, but also the safety and quality of life,   should also be considered. Readers can follow the example given in Chapter 4 to design a globally optimized trial for precision medicine.

Bibliography

Baker, S.G., Kramer, B.S., Sargent, D.J. & Bonetti, M. (2012). Biomarkers, subgroup evaluation, and clinical trial design. Discovery Medicine 13: 187-192.

Barker, A.D., Sigman, C,C,, Kelloff, G.J., et al. (2009). I-SPY 2: an adaptive breast cancer trial design in the setting of neoadjuvant chemotherapy. Clinical Pharmacology & Therapeutics 2009; 86: 97-100.

Bayer, R, Galea, S. (2015). Public Health in the Precision-Medicine Era. New England Journal of Medicine; 373:499-501.

Beckman, R., Clark, J. and Chen, C. (2011) Integrating predictive biomarkers and classifiers into oncology clinical development programmes. Nature Reviews Drug Discovery 10, 735-748.

Bio et al. (2016). Clinical Development Success Rates 2006-2015. https://www.bio.org/sites/.

Carini, C., Menon, S.M., Chang (Eds). (2014). Clinical and Statistical Considerations in Precision Medicine. CRC

Chakravarty, A. (2005), Regulatory aspects in using surrogate markers in clinical trials. In: The evaluation of surrogate endpoint, Burzykowski, Molenberghs, and Buyse (eds.) 2005. Springer.

Chang, M. (2012). Paradoxes in Scientific Inference. Taylor & Francis Group, LLC. Boca Raton, FL.

Chang, M. (2014). Principles of Scientific Methods. Mark Chang, Taylor & Francis Group, LLC. Boca Raton, FL

Chang, M. (2006). Bayesian Adaptive Design Method with Biomarkers. Biopharmaceutical Report. Volume 14, No. 2.

Chang, M. (2007). Adaptive Design Theory and Implementation Using SAS and R. Chapman & Hall/CRC, Taylor & Francis. Boca Raton, FL.

Chang, M. (2008). Biomarker Development, in Statistics for Translational Medicine. Taylor and Francis, FL.

Chapman, P,B,, Hauschild, A,, Robert, C, et al. (2011). Improved survival with vemurafenib in melanoma with V600E mutation. New England Journal of Medicine 2011; 364; 2507-16.

Chen, C., Li, N., Shentu, Y., Pang, L., Beckman, R. A. (2016). Adaptive Informational Design of Confirmatory Phase III Trials with an Uncertain Biomarker Effect to Improve the Probability of Success, Statistics in Biopharmaceutical Research. Vol. 8 , Iss. 3.

Chen, C. (2017). Two-stage Adaptive Design of a Confirmatory Basket Trial. ENAR Spring Meetings, 3/12-15, 2017, Washington DC.

Collins, F.S., Varmus, H. (2015). A new initiative on precision medicine. New England Journal of Medicine; 372:793-795.

Conley, B.A. and Taube, S.E. (2004). Prognostic and predictive marker in cancer. Disease Markers 20, 35-43.

FDA, Oct 2013. Paving the Way for Personalized Medicine, FDA's Role in a New Era of Medical Product Development

Freidlin, B, Jiang, W., Simon, R. (2010). The cross-validated adaptive signature design. Clinical Cancer Research 16: 691-698.

Freidlin, B. and Simon, R. (2005). Adaptive signature design: an adaptive clinical trial design for generating and prospectively testing a gene expression signature for sensitive patients. Clinical Cancer Research. 2005 Nov 1;11(21):7872-8.

Freidlin, B. and Korn, E.L. (2014). Biomarker enrichment strategies: matching trial design to biomarker credentials. Nature Reviews Clinical Oncology. 11.2 (Feb. 2014) p81.

Graiger, D. (2016). The mutual benefits of rare disease research and precision medicine. The journal of precision medicine.

Hawgood, S, Barnard, I.G., O'Brien, T.C., Yamamoto, K.R. (2015). Precision medicine: Beyond the inflection point. Science Translational Medicine, 7(300): 300-17.

Heinrich, M.C., Joensuu, H., Demetri, G.D., et al. Phase II, open-label study evaluating the activity of imatinib in treating life-threatening malignancies known to be associated with imatinib-sensitive tyrosine kinases. Clinical Cancer Research 2008; 14: 2717-25.

Heinrich, M.C., Joensuu, H,, Demetri, G.D., Corless CL, Apperley J, Fletcher JA, et al. Phase II, open-label study evaluating the activity of imatinib in treating life-threatening malignancies known to be associated with imatinib-sensitive tyrosine kinases. Clinical Cancer Research 2008; 14: 2717-25.

Huang, B., Wang, J., Menon, S. (2015). Population enrichment designs. Chapter 11. Modern approaches to clinical trials using SAS: Classical, adaptive and Bayesian methods, edited by Sandeep Menon and Richard Zink. SAS Press.

Jameson, J.L., Longo, D.L. (2015). Precision Medicine — Personalized, Problematic, and Promising. New England Journal of Medicine; 372:2229-2234.

Jenkins, M., Stone, A., Jennison, C. (2011). An adaptive seamless phase II/III design for oncology trials with subpopulation selection using correlated survival endpoint. Pharmaceutical Statistics 10(4):347-56.

Jiang, W, Freidlin, B., Simon, R. (2007). Biomarker-adaptive threshold design: a procedure for evaluating treatment with possible biomarker-defined subset effect. Journal of the National Cancer Institute 99: 1036-1043.

Kopetz, S. (2013). Right Drug for the Right Patient: Hurdles and the path forward in colorectal cancer. 2013 ASCO educational book http://meetinglibrary.asco.org/content/19-132.

Lacombe, D., Burocka, S., Bogaertsa, J., et al. (2014). The dream and reality of histology agnostic cancer clinical trials. Molecular Oncology 2014; 8:1057-1063.

Lee, M.L.T, Chang, M. and Whitmore, G.A. (2008). A threshold regression mixture model for assessing treatment efficacy in a multiple myeloma clinical trial. Journal of Biopharmaceutical Statistics 2008;18(6):1136-49

Mandrekar, S.J., Sargent, D. (2009). Clinical trial designs for predictive biomarker validation: theoretical considerations and practical challenges. Journal of Clinical Oncology 27: 4027-4034.

Mirnezami, R., Nicholson, J., Darzi, A. (2012). Preparing for Precision Medicine. New England Journal of Medicine 2012; 366:491.

Sargent, D.J., Conley, B.A., Allegra, C., Collete, L. Clinical trial designs for predictive marker validation in cancer treatment trials. Journal of Clinical Oncology 23(9): 2020-2227, 2005.

Simon, R. (2010). Clinical trial designs for evaluating the medical utility of prognostic and predictive biomarkers in oncology. Journal of Personalized Medicine 2010 January 1; 7(1): 33–47.

Simon, R., Maitournam, A. (2004). Evaluating the efficiency of targeted designs for randomized clinical trials. Clinical Cancer Research 10: 6759-6763.

Simon, N., Simon, R. (2013). Adaptive Enrichment Designs for Clinical Trials. Biostatistics. 2013 Sep;14(4):613-25.

Simon, R., Wang, S.J. (2006). Use of genomic signatures in therapeutics development in oncology and other diseases. The Pharmacogenomics Journal 6: 166-173.

Sleijfer, S., Bogaerts, J., Siu, L.L. (2013). Designing transformative clinical trials in the cancer genome era. Journal of Clinical Oncology 2013; 31:1834-41.

Song, X., Pepe, M.S. (2004) Evaluating markers for selecting a patient's treatment. Biometrics 60: 874-883

Song, Y, Chi, G.Y. (2007). A method for testing a prespecified subgroup in clinical trials. Statistics in Medicine, 26(19): 3535-3549.

Wang, J. (2013). Biomarker informed adaptive design. PhD Desertation, Biostatistics, Boston University, Boston, MA.

Wang, J., Chang, M., and Menon, S. (2014). Biomarker-Informed Adaptive Design, in Clinical and Statistical Considerations in Personalized Medicine (eds. Glaudio, Menon, and Chang). Chapman and Hall/CRC. 2014

Wang, J., Chang, M., Menon, S. (2015). Biomarker informed add-arm design for unimodal response. Journal of Biopharmaceutical Statistics 2015 May 26:1-18.

Wang, S.J., O'Neill R T, Hung J. (2007). Approaches to Evaluation of Treatment Effect in Randomised Clinical Trials with Genomic Subset. Pharmaceutical Statistics. 6(3), 227-244.

Wang, S.J., Hung, J., O'Neill, R.T. (2009). Adaptive patient enrichment designs in therapeutic trials. Biometrical Journal 51: 358–374.

Weir, C.J. and Walley, R.J. (2006). Statistical evaluation of biomarkers as surrogate endpoints: a literature review. Statistics in Medicine 2006; 25:183–203.

Zhou. X., Liu. S., Kim. E.S., Herbst. R.S., Lee, J. (2008). Bayesian adaptive design for targeted therapy development in lung cancer—a step toward personalized medicine. Clinical Trials. 5(3): 181-193.

6

Clinical Trial with Survival Endpoint

6.1 Overview of Survival Analysis

6.1.1 Basic Taxonomy

Survival analysis or time-to-event analysis is a branch of statistics dealing with death (failure) or degradation in biological organisms, mechanical or electronic systems, or other areas. The term lifetime distribution function $F(t)$ is defined as the probability of the event (e.g., death) occurring on or before time t, i.e., $F(t) = P(T \le t)$. The survival function $S(t)$ is the probability of an individual surviving longer than t, i.e., $S(t) = 1 - F(t)$. Thus, the event density is $f(t) = dF(t)/dt$. The hazard function or rate $h(t)$, is defined as the event rate at time t, conditional on survival until time t or later,

$$h(t) = \frac{d}{dt} P(T \le t | T > t) = \frac{f(t)}{S(t)} = -\frac{S'(t)}{S(t)}. \tag{6.1}$$

Integrating (6.1) with respect to t, we obtain $-\ln S(t) = \int_0^t h(u)\,du$ or $S(t) = \exp(-H(t))$, where $H(t) = \int_0^t h(u)\,du$ is called the cumulative hazard function. From (6.1), we can obtain

$$f(t) = h(t) S(t) \tag{6.2}$$

In survival analysis, censorings can be considered as a special type of missing data. Survival data can involve different types of censoring: (1) left-censoring if a data point (time value) is equal to or below a certain value but it is unknown by how much (e.g., missing adverse event start date), (2) right-censoring if a data point is above a certain value but it is unknown by how much (e.g., lost to follow up), and (3) interval censoring if a data point is somewhere in an interval between two values. Censoring can occur at a fixed time point (e.g., prescheduled clinical trial termination) or at a random time (e.g., early termination). Censoring can be informative or noninformative with respect to time (treatment/medical intervention). If it is noninformative, the censoring time is statistically independent of the failure time. However, the statistical independence of the failure time is a necessary but not a sufficient condition for noninformative censoring; there must be no common parameters between survival and censoring parameters to ensure the censoring is noninformative.

6.1.2 Nonparametric Approach

Nelson-Aalen Estimator

Let $Y(t)$ be the number of individuals at risk at (or just before) time t and τ_i the occurrence of the ith event. The Nelson-Aalen estimator for the cumulative hazard is given by

$$\hat{H}(t) = \sum_{\tau_i \leq t} \frac{1}{Y(\tau_i)} \qquad (6.5)$$

with variance estimator

$$\hat{\sigma}_\Lambda^2(t) = \sum_{\tau_i \leq t} \frac{1}{Y(\tau_i)^2}. \qquad (6.6)$$

The estimated cumulative hazard $\hat{H}(t)$ approaches to a normal distribution as the sample size approaches infinity. To improve precision, log-transformation can be used.

Kaplan-Meier Estimator

The Kaplan-Meier estimator is given by

$$\hat{S}(t) = \prod_{\tau_k \leq t} S(\tau_k|\tau_{k-1}) = \prod_{\tau_i \leq t} \left\{ 1 - \frac{1}{Y(\tau_i)} \right\} \qquad (6.7)$$

with variance

$$\hat{\sigma}_S^2(t) = \hat{S}(t)^2 \sum_{\tau_i \leq t} \frac{1}{Y(\tau_i)^2}. \qquad (6.8)$$

Alternatively, the variance can be estimated using Greenwood's formulation:

$$\hat{\sigma}_S^2(t) = \hat{S}(t)^2 \sum_{\tau_i \leq t} \frac{1}{Y(\tau_i)^2 - Y(\tau_i)}. \qquad (6.9)$$

For a large sample size, $\hat{S}(t)$ has approximately a normal distribution. To improve precision, log-transformation can be used.

Many software packages, such as SAS, R, and STATA, have the built-in capability of performing survival analyses with various models.

6.1.3 Proportional Hazard Model

Proportional hazard models are widely used in practice. Just as the name suggests, a proportional hazard model assumes the hazard is proportional (i.e., independent of time) between any two different groups with covariates $\boldsymbol{X}' = \boldsymbol{x}'_1$ and $\boldsymbol{X}' = \boldsymbol{x}'_2$,

$$h(t) = h_0(t) \exp\left(\boldsymbol{X}'\boldsymbol{\beta}\right), \tag{6.10}$$

where $\boldsymbol{X}$ is the vector of observed covariates and $\boldsymbol{\beta}$ are the corresponding parameters. If the baseline hazard function is specified (e.g., $h_0(t) = \lambda \rho t^{\rho-1}$), (6.10) represents a parametric proportional hazard model; otherwise, (6.10) is the well-known Cox semiparametric proportional hazard model (Cox, 1972).

6.1.4 Accelerated Failure Time Model

When the proportional hazard assumption does not hold, we may use the accelerated failure time model with a hazard function:

$$h(t) = \exp\left(\boldsymbol{X}'\boldsymbol{\beta}\right) h_0\left(\exp\left(\boldsymbol{X}'\boldsymbol{\beta}\right)t\right). \tag{6.11}$$

Different baseline functions $h_0(\cdot)$ will lead to different parametric models. For the exponential model, $h_0(t) = \lambda$ and $S_0(t) = \exp(-\lambda t)$, where $\lambda > 0$; for the Weibull model, $h_0(t) = \lambda \rho t^{\rho-1}$ and $S_0(t) = \exp(-\lambda t^\rho)$, where $\lambda, \rho > 0$; for the Gompertz model, $h_0(t) = \lambda \exp(\gamma t)$ and $S_0(t) = \exp\left(-\lambda \gamma^{-1}\left(\exp(\gamma t) - 1\right)\right)$, where $\gamma, \lambda > 0$; and for the loglogistic model, $h_0(t) = \frac{\exp(\alpha)kt^{k-1}}{1+\exp(\alpha)t^k}$ and $S_0(t) = \frac{1}{1+\exp(\alpha)t^k}$, where $\alpha \in \mathbb{R}, k > 0$.

6.1.5 Frailty Model

The notion of frailty provides a convenient way to introduce random effects, association and unobserved heterogeneity into models for survival data. In its simplest form, a frailty is an unobserved random factor that modifies the hazard function of an individual or related individuals. The term frailty was coined by Vaupel et al. (1979) in univariate survival models, and the model was substantially promoted for its application to multivariate survival data in a seminal paper by Clayton (1978) on chronic disease incidence in families. The simplest form of frailty model with a (unobserved) scale frailty variable Z can be written as

$$h(t, Z, \boldsymbol{X}) = Z h_0(t) \exp\left(\boldsymbol{X}'\boldsymbol{\beta}\right). \tag{6.12}$$

We will discuss this approach further later.

6.1.6 Maximum Likelihood Method

Modeling survival data can be based on a parametric or nonparametric method. Here we will focus on parametric models. A parametric model can be specified for the hazard rate $h(t) \geq 0$, survival time $S(t)$, or degradation process.

The maximum likelihood estimate (MLE) method is commonly used for parameter estimation in survival modeling, which is similar to the MLE for other models, the only difference being the presence of censoring. Specifically, the likelihood can be written as

$$L(\boldsymbol{\theta}) = \prod_{t_i \in \Omega_U} P(T = t_i | \boldsymbol{\theta}) \prod_{t_j \in \Omega_L} P(T \le t_j | \boldsymbol{\theta}) \prod_{t_k \in \Omega_R} P(T > t_k | \boldsymbol{\theta})$$
$$\cdot \prod_{(a_m, b_m) \in \Omega_I} P(a_m \le T < b_m | \boldsymbol{\theta}), \qquad (6.1)$$

where Ω_U, Ω_L, Ω_R, Ω_I are the sets for uncensored, left-, right-, and interval-censored data, respectively.

The reason to use four different probabilities in (6.3) is to capture as much information, as precisely as possible. For a subject that died exactly at time t_i we use probability $P(T = t_i | \boldsymbol{\theta})$ or probability density $f(t_i | \boldsymbol{\theta})$; for a subject left-censored at time t_j, we know he/she survived up to t_j thus we use probability $1 - S(t_j | \boldsymbol{\theta}) = P(T \le t_j | \boldsymbol{\theta})$ to capture the information. Similarly, for a subject right-censored at time t_k, we know he/she survived at least t_i, we use $P(T > t_i | \boldsymbol{\theta}) = S(t_i | \boldsymbol{\theta})$, and for interval-censored subject, we know he/she died between time a_m and b_m, thus we use probability $P(a_m < T \le b_{mi} | \boldsymbol{\theta}) = S(a_m | \boldsymbol{\theta}) - S(b_m | \boldsymbol{\theta})$.

The MLE is defined as

$$\hat{\boldsymbol{\theta}}_{mle} = \arg\max L(\boldsymbol{\theta}). \qquad (6.4)$$

Under fairly weak conditions (Newey and McFadden, 1994, Theorem 3.3), the MLE has approximately a normal distribution for a larger sample size n,

$$\sqrt{n} \left(\hat{\boldsymbol{\theta}}_{mle} - E(\boldsymbol{\theta}) \right) \xrightarrow{d} N\left(0, I^{-1}\right),$$

where I is the expected Fisher information matrix given by

$$I = E \left[\nabla_{\boldsymbol{\theta}} \ln f(x | E(\boldsymbol{\theta})) \nabla_{\boldsymbol{\theta}} \ln f(x | E(\boldsymbol{\theta}))' \right],$$

where the gradient operator is given by $\nabla_{\boldsymbol{\theta}} = \sum_i \frac{\partial}{\partial \theta_i}$.

6.1.7 Landmark Approach and Time-Dependent Covariate

One of the main goals of the landmark method is to estimate in an unbiased way the time-to-event probabilities in each group conditional on the group membership of patients at a specific, landmark time point (Dafni, 2011). Landmarking was originated from the debate on the effect of response to chemotherapy on survival (Anderson, Cain, Gelber, 1983) involving subgroups such as "responder" and "non-responder." Simply dividing patients into these two groups will lead to biased estimate of survival time due to the association between survival time and probability of response. A patient who survives longer has more opportunities to respond and a potential responder will only belong to the "responder" group if he/she survives until his/her time of response. Individuals in the responder group are surviving until the respective response time which gives them an unfair survival advantage called immortal time bias. "Responder" versus "non-responder" is something that is not known at baseline and using such as postbaseline variable(s) as independent predictors in the related model will cause controversies.

The problem of time-dependent covariates can come in a number of disguises (Hein Putter, 2013): effect of recurrence on survival in cancer, effect of transplant failure on survival in transplant studies, effect of compliance on recurrence, effect of drug-specific adverse events on recurrence, effect of winning an Oscar on survival for US actors. To deal with such a problem, at least two alternatives are available: Landmark and time-dependent covariate approaches

In the Landmark approach, consider response at a fixed point in time (landmark) and remove patients from analysis who experience an event (or are censored) before the landmark. Patients are separated into two response categories according to whether they have responded up to the landmark, thus the landmark method ignores all responses after the landmark time and all deaths before that time. Another way to look at is that in landmarking analysis, landmark (response) variables are "baseline" variables defined before the landmark, whereas common baseline variables are usually defined before a treatment intervention. We can also use multiple landmarkers. When the landmark model used for predictions, the model is called dynamic predictive model.

Landmark analyses were performed to explore the association of extended clopidogrel use and long-term clinical outcomes of patients receiving drug eluting stents (DES) and bare-metal stents (BMS) for treatment of coronary artery disease (Eisenstein, Anstrom, Kong, et al. 2007). In the context of heart transplant data in which the survival of patients receiving heart transplants is compared with that of control subjects, the patients receiving a heart transplant must have at least survived from time of diagnosis to time of treatment, whereas no such requirement is necessary for the control subjects. This "time-to-treatment" bias is identical to the "time-to-response" bias in the comparison of overall survival between responders and nonresponders (Dafni, 2011).

When landmark method is used for time-to-event probability estimation, HR estimation and statistical tests, conditional on the group classification at a fixed time point (landmark time) to reduce bias, it creates a few issues at the same time. The choice of landmark is somewhat arbitrary. Using a landmark as new baseline for the analysis will weaken the randomization. Therefore, the method carries all the caveats of reaching conclusions based on an observational study instead of a controlled experiment. In the case of "responders," response is possibly just a marker that selects the good prognosis patients. When landmark analysis results demonstrate a significant differential effect between groups as defined by the time of landmark, it can only claim "association" and not a "cause-effect" relationship between benefit and group membership. In this context, it is generally close to impossible to disentangle the effect of a "treatment" from the possibly confounding effects of the underlying factors that lead to "treatment allocation" (Dafni, 2011). The ignoring of early time-to-event can also lead a target population shift and the external validity of the trial will become questionable. Such a disadvantage is shared by the time-varying covariate Cox model that will be discussed next.

To retain the early outcome event information, when group membership is defined during follow-up, as an alternative to alndmark approach, a time-varying Cox model could be used to compare time-to-event outcome between the groups. In the time-varying Cox model, group membership changes from "no risk altering event" to "risk altering event" at the time the intervening event occurs, and thus the arbitrary choice of the appropriate landmark time is not of concern anymore (Dafni, 2011).

In time-dependent covariate model, the hazard rate is expressed as

$$h\left(t, \mathbf{X}\left(t\right)\right) = h_0\left(t\right) \exp\left(\mathbf{X}'\left(t\right)\boldsymbol{\beta}\left(t\right)\right). \tag{6.13}$$

If landmarks are chosen to be the timepoint when the covariates have a change, then time-dependent covariate survival model (6.13) becomes a discreate time Markov model and is equivalent to multistage model discussed in next section.

6.2 Multistage Models for Progressive Disease

6.2.1 Introduction

A multistage model consists of several stages across a time axis. At each stage, a time-to-event model is applied. The rationale for using multistage models is that it may not be easy to specify a single model across the entire time course. For example, the natural course of disease may consist of stages and the time-to-event model is relatively easy to specify for each stage separately. However, in principle, the model within each stage can be the proportional hazard model, frailty model, exponential model, or a combination of them. Multistage models are a simple way to deal with time-dependent covariate model (6.13).

Most common multistage models are semi-Markov processes (continuous time, discrete states). The time-independent hazard rate λ_{ij} can be a function of covariates (i.e., $\lambda_{ij} = \lambda_{ij}\left(\mathbf{X}'\boldsymbol{\beta}\right)$). The transitional probability matrix for a semi-Markov chain is given by

$$\boldsymbol{P}\left(t\right) = e^{\boldsymbol{\Lambda}t} = \boldsymbol{I} + \sum_{k=1}^{\infty} \frac{\boldsymbol{\Lambda}t^k}{k!}, \tag{6.14}$$

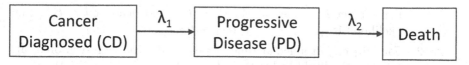

FIGURE 6.1
Progressive Disease Model.

where hazard matrix $\mathbf{\Lambda}$ has elements of of λ_{ij} and $\lambda_{ii} = 1$ $(i, j = 1, K)$.

6.2.2 Progressive Disease Model

We consider the time-dependent Markov progressive model in which the probability of transition is usually dependent on the time relative to the previous state but independent of any earlier states. For example, a individual diagnosed with cancer may have a progressive disease and then die (Figure 6.1). Assume there is no chance for a person with PD to recover and become a healthy person. The possible transition directions are indicated by arrows, with a hazard or event rate λ_1 and λ_2.

Clinically, $\lambda_2 > \lambda_1$ because after PD, the patient gets sicker. If hazard rates λ_1 and λ_2 are assumed only dependent on baseline covariates but independent of time, then the time to PD from CD is $T_1 \sim \lambda_1 \exp(-\lambda_1 T_1)$ and time to death from PD is, $T_2 \sim \lambda_2 \exp(-\lambda_2 T_2)$. Thus, the survival time $T = T_1 + T_2$ has a mixture of exponential distribution. Let $T^* = T/2 = 0.5T_1 + 0.5T_2$, then the density and survival functions are

$$f_{T^*}(t) = \sum_{i=1}^{2} \frac{1}{2} \lambda_i \exp(-\lambda_i t) \text{ and } S_{T^*}(t) = \sum_{i=1}^{2} \frac{1}{2} \exp(-\lambda_i t).$$

Since $T^* = t/2$ implyies $T = t$, we have

$$T \sim f_T(t) = \frac{1}{2} \sum_{i=1}^{2} \lambda_i \exp(-\lambda_i t/2) \tag{6.15}$$

$$F(t) = 1 - \sum_{i=1}^{2} \exp(-\lambda_i t/2)$$

and survival function

$$S(t) = \sum_{i=1}^{2} \exp(-\lambda_i t/2). \tag{6.16}$$

After a multistage model is constructed, we need to formulate the likelihood for the MLE of parameters. The likelihood formulation L (assume the process starting time $t_0 = 0$) can be classified into the following four different cases:

1. For subject i disabled at time $t = t_{11i}$ and dead at $t = t_{12i}$, the likelihood is $l_{1i} = f_1(t_{11i}) f_2(t_{12i} - t_{11i})$.

2. For subject j disabled at time $t = t_{21j}$ and alive (right-censored) at $t = t_{22j}$, the likelihood is $l_{2j} = f_1(t_{21j})(1 - F_2(t_{22j} - t_{21j}))$.

3. For subject k disabled before or at time t_{31k} (left-censored) and dead at $t = t_{32k}$, the likelihood is $l_{3k} = F_1(t_{31k}) f_2(t_{32k} - t_{31k})$.

4. For subject m disabled before or at time t_{41m} (left-censored) and alive (right-censored) at $t = t_{42m}$, the likelihood is $l_{4m} = F_1(t_{41m})(1 - F_2(t_{42m} - t_{41m}))$.

Suppose there are n_1 subjects in category 1 and n_2 subjects in category 2, but no left-censored observations, i.e., $n_3 = n_4 = 0$. The log-likelihood is given by

$$\ln L = (n_1 + n_2) \ln \lambda_1 + n_1 \ln \lambda_2 - \lambda_1 \left(\sum_{i=1}^{n_1} t_{11i} + \sum_{j=n_1+1}^{n_1+n_2} t_{21j} \right) \quad (6.2)$$

$$- \lambda_2 \left(\sum_{i=1}^{n_1} (t_{12i} - t_{11i}) + \sum_{j=n_1+1}^{n_1+n_2} (t_{22j} - t_{21j}) \right).$$

If λ_1 and λ_2 are constants, then their MLEs can be obtained by $\frac{\partial \ln L}{\partial \lambda_i} = 0$. The solutions are

$$\begin{cases} \lambda_1 = \frac{n_1 + n_2}{\sum_{i=1}^{n_1} t_{11i} + \sum_{j=n_1+1}^{n_1+n_2} t_{21j}}, \\ \lambda_2 = \frac{n_1}{\sum_{i=1}^{n_1} (t_{12i} - t_{11i}) + \sum_{j=n_1+1}^{n_1+n_2} (t_{22j} - t_{21j})} \end{cases} \quad (6.18)$$

If $\lambda_i = \lambda_i(\mathbf{X}'\boldsymbol{\beta})$, the partial derivatives should be taken with respect to the parameter vector $\boldsymbol{\beta}$. After MLE of $\boldsymbol{\beta}$ is obtained, the MLE of λ_i can be obtained. Substitute the estimated λ_1 and λ_2 into (6.15) and (6.16), we can determine the density and survival functions.

The mean and median times for the mean model are:

$$T_m = \frac{1}{2} \sum_{i=1}^{2} \int_0^\infty \lambda_i \exp(-\lambda_i t/2) \, t \, dt = 2 \left(\frac{1}{\lambda_1} + \frac{1}{\lambda_2} \right). \quad (6.19)$$

The median time T_M is the solution of the following equation:

$$\sum_{i=1}^{2} \exp(-\lambda_i T_M/2) = 0.5$$

It is interesting to note that when two populations with different distribution $f_1(T)$ and $f_2(T)$ are combined into one single super population for the analysis, the super population has a mixed distribution of $f_1(T)$ and $f_2(T)$.

For example, test statistic based on the blinded (pooled) data of two treatment group with normal primary endpoint will have a mixed normal distribution. If male and female have normal distributions of two different means, then the mixed population has a mixed normal distribution with pdf, $f = p_1\phi_1 + p_2\phi_2$, where p_i and ϕ_i are the proportion and distribution of population i. If a clinical trial involved different patients with different stages of cancers and thus different survival distribution, the combined cancer population has a mixed distribution: $f = w_1f_1 + w_2f_2$, where w_1 and w_2 are the proportions of two patient populations. In contrast, in the CD→PD→death model, the weights $w_1 = w_2 = 1$. From this example we also see that in a cancer study if we assume TTP and OS are exponential distributions, then time from PD to death cannot also be an exponential distribution.

In general, for mixture of K exponential distributions, $T = \sum_{i=1}^{K} w_i T_i$, where $w_i > 0$ and $\sum_{i=1}^{K} w_i = 1$, T has the following pdf, cdf and survival function

$$\begin{cases} f(t) = \sum_{i=1}^{K} w_i \lambda_i \exp\left(-\lambda_i t\right), \\ F(t) = 1 - \sum_{i=1}^{K} w_i \exp\left(-\lambda_i t\right), \quad t > 0. \\ S(t) = \sum_{i=1}^{K} w_i \exp\left(-\lambda_i t\right), \end{cases} \quad (6.20)$$

For the mixed exponential distribution, the failure rate is

$$\lambda(t) = \frac{1}{\sum_{j=1}^{K} w_j \exp\left(-\lambda_j t\right)} \sum_{i=1}^{K} w_i \lambda_i \exp\left(-\lambda_i t\right) \quad (6.21)$$

This is a weighted average of the λ_i's. As t becomes larger, weight moves away from the larger λ_i's and toward the smaller λ_i's, thus decreasing the failure rate. This is often true in clinical trials since sicker patients will die first and the remaining less sick patients will have fewer expected failures (deaths).

6.3 Piecewise Model for Delayed Drug Effect

6.3.1 Introduction

The logrank test has been the "standard" method for survival analysis in clinical trials. It is (asymptotically) optimal under proportional hazards alternatives, with equal censoring patterns in the two groups (Yang and Prentice, 2010). However, the proportional hazard assumption can often be violated in clinical trials such as due to delayed drug effects. When the proportional hazard model does not hold, piecewise or multistage model with a weighted logrank test can be used. The weight, if chosen appropriately, can improve the power (Lagakos, Lim, and Robins, 1990; Zucker, 1992; Prentice, 1978; Fleming and Harrington, 1991, Gastwirth, 1985; Zucker and Lakatos, 1990; Tarone, 1981; Fleming and Harrington, 1991; Breslow et al., 1984).

Assume a minimum treatment period T_d is necessary before the possibility of a drug exerting an effect (T_d is actually different for different patients). As an example, we use piecewise exponential model to evaluate performance of logrank and weighted logrank tests. Conceptually, events occurred before the delayed time T_s do not contribute to the power. Therefore, the total number events should increase when the drug is expected a delayed effect. The sample size can be determined through simulations.

6.3.2   Piecewise Exponential Distribution

Let T_d be the drug's effect-delayed time. At the moment we consider exponential models. Before the drug take effect, the hazard rate is λ_1, after a period of T_d, the hazard rate for the survivors are λ_2. Again, if λ_1 and λ_2 are independent of time, then the survival function $S(T)$ for $T > T_d$ is the product of probability of surviving up to T_d and the probability of surviving from T_d to T, that is $S(T) = \exp(-\lambda_1 T_d)\exp(-\lambda_2(T - T_d))$. Taking the derivative of failure function $F(T) = 1 - S(T)$ with respect to T, we can obtain pdf of failure time T:

$$T \sim \begin{cases} \lambda_1 \exp(-\lambda_1 T), & T \leq T_d \\ \exp(-\lambda_1 T_d)\lambda_2 \exp(-\lambda_2(T - T_d)), & T > T_d \end{cases} \qquad (6.22)$$

Here the term $\exp(-\lambda_1 T_d))$ is the probability survival longer than T_d.

We use inverse CDF method to generate random numbers from the distribution. For $T \leq T_d$, the CDF is $x = 1 - e^{-\lambda_1 T}$. Solving T to get the inverse CDF: $T = -\frac{\ln(1-x)}{\lambda_1}$. For $T > T_d$, the CDF: $x = \left(1 - e^{-\lambda_1 T_d}\right) + e^{-\lambda_1 T_d}\left(1 - e^{-\lambda_2(T-T_d)}\right)$. Solving T to get the inverse CDF:

$$T = T_d - \frac{1}{\lambda_2}\ln\left(\frac{1-x}{e^{-\lambda_1 T_d}}\right)$$

Therefore, we have

$$\begin{cases} T = -\frac{\ln(1-x)}{\lambda_1}, & T \leq T_d \text{ or } x \leq F(T_d) = 1 - e^{-\lambda_1 T_d} \\ T = T_d - \frac{1}{\lambda_2}\ln\left(\frac{1-x}{e^{-\lambda_1 T_d}}\right) & T > T_d \text{ or or } x > F(T_d) = 1 - e^{-\lambda_1 T_d} \end{cases} \qquad (6.23)$$

Note that the hazard rates can be a function of baseline covariates, $\lambda_i = \lambda_i\left(X'\beta\right)$. The parameter vector β can be estimated using MLE method as demonstrated in the previous examples.

6.3.3   Mean and Median Survival Times

When no delay $T_d = 0$ or when $\lambda_1 = \lambda_2$, the model is equal to a standard survival mode. Consider when $T_d \neq 0$ or $\lambda_1 \neq \lambda_2$. Is this distribution function

$f(T)$ continuous at T_d? When $T \to T_{d+}$, $f(T) \to \lambda_2 e^{\lambda_1 T_d} \neq \lambda_1 e^{-\lambda_1 T} = f(T)$. Thus $f(T)$ is not continuous at $T = T_d$ (but the cdf will be continuous). For treatment delay, $\lambda_2 < \lambda_1$, then $\lambda_2 e^{\lambda_1 T_d} < \lambda_1 e^{-\lambda_1 T}$, this means that pdf decreases at $T = T_d$ and pushes survival to longer times.

The median time T_m can be obtained through

$$0.5 = \begin{cases} 1 - e^{-\lambda_1 T_m}, & T_m \leq T_d \\ 1 - e^{-\lambda_1 T_d} + \int_{T_d}^{T_m} e^{-\lambda_1 T_d} \lambda_2 e^{-\lambda_2 (T - T_d)} dT, & T_m > T_d \end{cases}$$

$$T_m = \begin{cases} \frac{\ln 2}{\lambda_1}, & \frac{\ln 2}{\lambda_1} \leq T_d \\ \frac{\ln 2 - \lambda_1 T_d + \lambda_2 T_d}{\lambda_2}, & \text{otherwise} \end{cases} \tag{6.24}$$

The mean time T_a can be obtained using

$$T_a = \int_0^{T_d} T \lambda_1 e^{-\lambda_1 T} dT + \int_{T_d}^{\infty} T e^{-\lambda_1 T_d} \lambda_2 e^{-\lambda_2 (T - T_d)} dT.$$

That is,

$$T_a = \frac{1}{\lambda_1} + \frac{\lambda_1 - \lambda_2}{\lambda_1 \lambda_2} e^{-T_d \lambda_1}. \tag{6.25}$$

A key distinction between the piecewise survival model and multistage model is that the former has a known fixed time interval as when the hazard will change, whereas the later the time interval for changing the hazard is a random variable.

In general, for k-piecewise distribution pdf with the changing rate time point at $t_1, t_2, \cdots, t_k$ where $t_1 = 0$, and the corresponding exponential rates are $\lambda_1, \lambda_2, \cdots, \lambda_k$. The simple exponential pdf is $f(t; \lambda_i) = \lambda_i e^{-\lambda_i t} I(t \geq 0)$ and cdf is $F(t, \lambda_i) = (1 - e^{-\lambda_i t}) I(t \geq 0)$, where $I(t \geq 0)$ is an indicator function.

The pdf of piecewise exponential distribution is:

$f(t; t_1, t_2, ... t_k, \lambda_1, \lambda_2, ..., \lambda_k)$

$$= \begin{cases} f(t; \lambda_1) I(0 \leq t \leq t_1) \\ \Pi_{i=1}^m (1 - F(t_i - t_{i-1}; \lambda_i)) f(t - t_m; \lambda_m) I(t > t_m), 2 \leq m \leq k \end{cases} \tag{6.26}$$

6.3.4 Weighted LogRank Test for Delayed Treatment Effect

The logrank test statistic compares estimates of the hazard functions of the two groups at each observed event time. It is constructed by computing the observed and expected number of events in one of the groups at each observed event time and then adding these to obtain an overall summary across all-time points where there is an event.

Let $j = 1, ..., J$ be the distinct times of observed events in either group. For each time j, let N_{1j} and N_{2j} be the number of subjects "at risk" (have not yet had an event or been censored) at the start of period j in the two groups (often treatment vs. control), respectively. Let $N_j = N_{1j} + N_{2j}$. Let O_{1j} and O_{2j} be the observed number of events (not cumulative) in the groups respectively at time j, and define $O_j = O_{1j} + O_{2j}$.

Given that O_j events happened across both groups at time j, under the null hypothesis (of the two groups having identical survival and hazard functions) O_{1j} has the hypergeometric distribution with parameters N_j, N_{1j}, and O_j. This distribution has expected value $E_{1j} = \frac{O_j}{N_j} N_{1j}$ and variance

$$V_j = \frac{O_j\,(N_{1j}/N_j)\,(1 - N_{1j}/N_j)\,(N_j - O_j)}{N_j - 1}. \tag{6.29}$$

The logrank statistic compares each O_{1j} to its expectation E_{1j} under the null hypothesis and is defined as

$$Z = \frac{\sum_{j=1}^{J} w_j\,(O_{1j} - E_{1j})}{\sqrt{\sum_{j=1}^{J} w_j^2 V_j}}, \tag{6.30}$$

where $w_j > 0$ is weight. For standard logrank test, $w_j \equiv 1$. We implemented the weight system in SAS: If observed survival time $t_j < t_{Lap}$, weight $w_j = 1$; otherwise weight $= 2$.

If the two groups have the same survival function, the logrank statistic is approximately standard normal. A one-sided level α test will reject the null hypothesis if $Z > z_{1-\alpha}$. If the hazard ratio is θ, there are n total subjects, d is the probability a subject in either group will eventually have an event (so that $D = nd$ is the expected number of events at the time of the analysis), then under exponential model, the logrank statistic is approximately normal

$$Z \sim N\left(\log\theta\sqrt{f_1 f_2 D}, 1\right), \tag{6.31}$$

where f_1 and f_2 are the sample size fractions for the two groups (Schoenfeld, 1981).

Suppose in a group sequential design, Z_1 and Z_2 are the logrank statistics at stage 1 and stage 2. Z_1 and Z_2 are approximately bivariate normal with means $\log\theta\sqrt{f_1 f_2 D_1}$ and $\log\theta\sqrt{f_1 f_2 D_2}$, and correlation $\sqrt{\frac{D_1}{D_2}}$, where D_1 and D_2 are the numbers of deaths at the stages 1 and 2, respectively.

Example 6.1: Before the delayed time T_d, $\lambda_1 = \lambda_2 = 0.87(1/\text{year})$. After T_d, $\lambda_1 = 0.87$ (1/year), $\lambda_2 = 0.65$ (1/year). For exponential distribution with $\lambda = 0.87$ (1/year), mean time $= 1.1494$ year and median $= 0.7967$ year. For exponential distribution with $\lambda = 0.65$, mean time $= 1.5385$ and median $= 1.0663$. Total number of deaths $= 700$. The comparison of power performed among ordinal logrank test and the weighted LogRank: weight $= 1$ if before the estimated delayed-time $\hat{T}_d = 0.3$ and weight $= 2$ after $\hat{T}_d = 0.3$. From table 1, we can see (1) a small delay can cause a huge drop in power and (2) the weighted logrank tests generally perform better than logrank test.

The SAS code to invoke the macro:

%PWExp(n1=700, n2=700, lambdaPRE1=0.87, lambdaLAG1=0.87, lag1=0.1, lambdaPRE2=0.87, lambdaLAG2=0.65, lag2=0.1, DeathsNeed=700, estLag=0.3);

TABLE 6.1
Delayed Treatment Effect on Simulated Power (%).

	\multicolumn{10}{c}{True Delay Time, Td (year)}
	0	0.1	0.2	0.3	0.4	0.5	0.6	0.7	0.8	0.9
LogRank	97.1	88.9	74.9	54.7	34.6	19.9	10.9	5.2	2.6	2.5
wLogRank	95.8	90.5	83.1	72.0	48.4	28.3	14.5	6.0	2.7	2.5

Note: wLogRank=weighted logRank Test. One-sided $\alpha = 0.025$

6.4 Oncology Trial with Treatment Switching

6.4.1 Descriptions of the Switching Problem

To evaluate the efficacy and safety of a test treatment for progressive diseases, such as cancers and HIV, a parallel-group, active-control, randomized clinical trial is often conducted. In this type of trial, qualified patients are randomly assigned to receive either an active control (a standard therapy or a treatment currently available in the marketplace) or a test treatment under investigation. Due to ethical considerations, patients are allowed to switch from one treatment to another if there is evidence of lack of efficacy or disease progression. In practice, it is not uncommon that up to 80% of patients may switch from one treatment to another. Sommer and Zeger (1991) referred to the treatment effect among patients who complied with treatment as "biological efficacy." Robins and Finkelstein (2000) developed the inverse probability of censoring weighted logrank test and Jiménez-Moro and Gómez (2014) implemented the method in SAS. Branson and Whitehead (2002) widened the concept of biological efficacy to encompass the treatment effect as if all patients adhered to their original randomized treatments in clinical studies allowing treatment switching using Inverse-Probability Censoring Weight (IPCW). Despite allowing a switch in treatment, many clinical studies are designed to compare the test treatment with the active control agent as if no patients had ever been switched. This certainly has an impact on the evaluation of the efficacy of the test treatment, because the response-informative switching causes the treatment effect to be confounded. The power for the methods without considering the switching is often lost dramatically because many patients from two groups eventually took the same drugs (Shao, Chang, and Chow, 2005). Currently, more approaches have been proposed, including a mixture of the

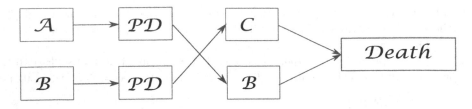

FIGURE 6.2
Effect of Treatment Switching In a Clinical Trial.

Wiener processes (Lee, Chang, and Whitmore, 2008). Latimer et al. (2014, 2016) conducted simulation studies and conclude that randomization-based adjustment methods, such as the Rank Preserving Structural Failure Time Model (RPSFTM, Robins and Tsiatis, 1991) and the iterative parameter estimation (IPE) algorithm, usually produced low bias. For the IPCW, data must be available on all prognostic factors for mortality that independently predict informative censoring and models for switching and survival must be correctly specified. IPCW is not applicable if there are any covariates which ensure (i.e. the probability equals 1) that treatment switching will occur (Robins, 1994, 1999; Yamaguchi and Ohashi, 2004). However, the common treatment effect assumption associated with the RPSFTM and IPE methods may result in the survival times of switchers being over-adjusted (Ray, et al. 2013). Patterns in the direction of bias were not observed for the IPCW and two-stage adjustment methods.

6.4.2   Treatment Switching

In Example 2, a progressive disease (PD) is an indication of treatment failure and the patient usually has to switch from the initial treatment to an alternative. Thus, treatment for a patient is a time-dependent variable: before PD with one treatment, after PD with another treatment (Figure 6.2).

Example 2: Multistage Model for Clinical Trial Treatment Switch

Suppose patients in a two-group oncology clinical trial are randomized to receive either treatment A or B. If progressive disease is observed, meaning the patient has developed a resistance to the drug to (or never responded to), then the patient will switch the treatment from A to B or B to C (the best treatment option available). The hazard rates are denoted by β_{11} for treatment A before PD, β_{21} for treatment A after PD, β_{12} for treatment B before PD, and β_{22} for treatment C after PD.

For simplicity we assume PD is always observed immediately (i.e., no censoring on PD). Thus, a typical patient i initially treated with drug A will have the following two possible likelihood functions:

1. PD at time $t = t_{11i}$ and death at $t = t_{12i}$, $l_i = \beta_{11}e^{-\beta_{11}t_{11i}}\beta_{21}e^{-\beta_{21}(t_{12i}-t_{11i})}$, where $i = 1, ..., n_1$.

2. PD at time $t = t_{21i}$ and alive (right-censored) at $t = t_{22i}$, $l_i = \beta_{11}e^{-\beta_{11}t_{21i}}e^{-\beta_{21}(t_{22i}-t_{21i})}$, where $i = n_1 + 1, ..., n_1 + n_2$.

Similarly, a typical patient i initially treated with drug B will have the following two possible likelihood functions:

1. PD at time $t = t_{31i}$ and death at $t = t_{32i}$, $l_i = \beta_{12}e^{-\beta_{12}t_{31i}}\beta_{22}e^{-\beta_{22}(t_{32i}-t_{31i})}$, where $i = n_1+n_2+1, ..., n_1+n_2+n_3$.

2. PD at time $t = t_{41i}$ and alive (right-censored) at $t = t_{42i}$, $l_i = \beta_{12}e^{-\beta_{12}t_{41i}}e^{-\beta_{22}(t_{42i}-t_{41i})}$, where $i = n_1 + n_2 + n_3 + 1, ..., n_1 + n_2 + n_3 + n_4$.

The likelihood function based on the total $n_1 + n_2 + n_3 + n_4$ observations is the same as (3). The log-likelihood function can be given explicitly by

$$
\begin{aligned}
\ln L = {} & (n_1 + n_2)\ln\beta_{11} + (n_3 + n_4)\ln\beta_{12} + n_1 \ln\beta_{21} + n_3 \ln\beta_{22} \\
& -\beta_{11}\left(\sum_{i=1}^{n_1} t_{11i} + \sum_{i=n_1+1}^{n_1+n_2} t_{21i}\right) \\
& -\beta_{21}\left(\sum_{i=1}^{n_1} (t_{12i} - t_{11i}) + \sum_{i=n_1+1}^{n_1+n_2} (t_{22i} - t_{21i})\right) \\
& -\beta_{12}\left(\sum_{i=n_1+n_2+1}^{n_1+n_2+n_3} t_{31i} + \sum_{i=n_1+n_2+n_3+1}^{n_1+n_2+n_3+n_4} t_{41i}\right) \\
& -\beta_{22}\left(\sum_{i=n_1+n_2+1}^{n_1+n_2+n_3} (t_{32i} - t_{31i}) + \sum_{i=n_1+n_2+n_3+1}^{n_1+n_2+n_3+n_4} (t_{42i} - t_{41i})\right)
\end{aligned}
$$

Letting $\frac{\partial \ln L}{\partial \beta_{jk}} = 0$, we can obtain

$$
\begin{cases}
\beta_{11} = \frac{n_1+n_2}{\sum_{i=1}^{n_1} t_{11i}+\sum_{i=n_1+1}^{n_1+n_2} t_{21i}}, \\
\beta_{12} = \frac{n_3+n_4}{\sum_{i=1}^{n_1} (t_{12i}-t_{11i})+\sum_{i=n_1+1}^{n_1+n_2} (t_{22i}-t_{21i})}, \\
\beta_{21} = \frac{n_1}{\sum_{i=n_1+n_2+1}^{n_1+n_2+n_3} t_{31i}+\sum_{i=n_1+n_2+n_3+1}^{n_1+n_2+n_3+n_4} t_{41i}}, \\
\beta_{22} = \frac{n_3}{\sum_{i=n_1+n_2+1}^{n_1+n_2+n_3} (t_{32i}-t_{31i})+\sum_{i=n_1+n_2+n_3+1}^{n_1+n_2+n_3+n_4} (t_{42i}-t_{41i})}.
\end{cases}
$$

The relative treatment efficacy between the treatment groups can be measured by the hazard ratio:

$$
\begin{cases}
HR_1 = \frac{\beta_{11}}{\beta_{12}}, \text{ before PD,} \\
HR_2 = \frac{\beta_{21}}{\beta_{22}}, \text{ after PD.}
\end{cases}
$$

The median survival time for group i if treatment switching is not allowed can be expressed

$$T_{mi} = \frac{\ln 2}{\beta_{1i}} + \frac{\ln 2}{\beta_{2i}}$$

The median survival time for group i if treatment switching is allowed can be expressed

$$\begin{cases} T_{m1} = \frac{\ln 2}{\beta_{11}} + \frac{\ln 2}{\beta_{22}} \\ T_{m2} = \frac{\ln 2}{\beta_{12}} + \frac{\ln 2}{\beta_{21}} \end{cases}$$

In practice, cancer drugs are categorized by the number of PDs: newly diagnosed patients usually use first-line drugs, after one PD they use second-line drugs, and so on. Therefore, treatment benefit after PD is the benefit treating the next line patients.

6.4.3   Inverse Probability of Censoring Weighted LogRank Test

The Inverse Probability of Censoring Weighting (IPCW) developed by Robins et al (1994, 1999), attempts to reduce the bias caused by treatment change recreating a scenario where any patient switched to the alternative treatment arm. The weights estimated to reduce the bias are usually based on a logistic regression model, where the response variable tells whether the patient switched to the other treatment or not. The key idea in the IPCW method is the determination of weights in the Cox regression model so that the bias introduced by treatment change is minimized.

For patients that switch from treatment A to treatment B, we need to compensate for the impact of switching. Therefore, the basic idea is that, in treatment A, we try to find patients with similar characteristics to those patients that switched treatment and give the patient that remained on treatment A, a higher weight and attribute a zero weight to the patients moving to treatment B from the time of crossover onwards. That way, the patients that remained on treatment A are weighted in a way that compensates for the switch of patient to the other arm. However, as pointed out by an evaluation of pazopanib for renal cancer (Bukowski, et al. 2010), IPCW is subject to the assumption of no unmeasured confounders and randomization is not preserved.

To obtain these weights, the likelihood of remaining uncensored is going to be estimated. This procedure can be easily done by means of a logistic regression. Specifically, we need to perform two logistic regression models, one using only baseline covariates and other using both baseline and time dependent covariates. The coefficient between these two estimated probabilities of switching is going to give us the assigned weights. Subsequently, patients that switched will have a lower weight that patients that did not, and patients in

TABLE 6.2

Dummy Trial Dataset (dIPCW)with Treatment Switch for IPCW.

ID	trt	TTS	switch	OS	regions	age	sensor	ps	aes	OS2	censor2
1	A	8.2	1	9	2	40	0	0	2	8.2	1
1	A	8.2	1	9	5	40	0	1	1	8.2	1
2	B	9.5	0	12	1	38	1	1	3	12	0
2	B	9.5	0	12	2	38	1	0	4	12	0

treatment arm A will have a weight equal to 1 since there is no need to compensate for switching. More formally, this procedure follows the next formula.

$$
w_{ij} = \frac{\prod_{k=0}^{j} P\left(C\left(k\right)_i = 0 | C(k-1)_i = 0, X_i\right)}{\prod_{k=0}^{j} P\left(C\left(k\right)_i = 0 | C\left(k-1\right)_i = 0, X_i, Z\left(k\right)_i\right)} \tag{6.32}
$$

We follow the procedure outlined by Luis, Moro and Gómez (2014). The dummy dataset (dIPCW) used to illustrate the procedure includes patient ID (ID), treatment group (trt), time-to-switch (TTS) or PFS, overall survival (OS), age (age), number of regions (regions) affected at baseline, performance status (PS) and the number of grade 3 adverse events (AEs) at the end of cycle 2. PS and AEs are the two time-dependent covariates. Switch (switch) is indication variable (1=treatment switch, 0=no switch), censor=1 if OS is censored; otherwise censor=0. These variables are sufficient for IPCW analysis. However, if we want to compare the IPCW results with the classical method that considered switch as a censor for the OS, then we can create another censor variable, censor2=1 if censor=1 or Switch=1; otherwise censor2= 0. And the modified survival time, OS2=min(OS, TTS) if Switch=1 and OS2=OS if Switch=0. See the dataset structure in table 6.2.

We first can use the PROC LOGISTIC with only baseline variables and specifying which is the event we are modeling. In this case 0 means uncensored as specified in the formula, so we need to specify it. Note that the dataset "**dIPCW**" has two observations per patient as shown in Table 6.2. Since we are no using the time dependent covariates, we should remove the duplicated observations to avoid possible problems.

/*Logistic model with baseline variables*/
proc logistic descending data=dIPCW;
    model switch(censor='0')=age regions;
    output out=out1 prob=tn;
    run;

Next, we need to estimate again the probability of remaining uncensored but using both baseline and time dependent covariates. We use PROC GENMOD because it allows us to model longitudinal data in a logistic regression model. Since the event of interest is not specified we need to sort the data in a way that the procedure models the probability of switch = 0. This is achieved by the next SAS commands:

```
proc sort data=dIPCW; by descending crossover; run;
/*Logistic model with baseline and time dependent variables*/
proc genmod data=dIPCW descending order=data;
    class switch id;
    model switch= regions ps aes / d=bin link=logit;
    repeated subject=id; estimate "ps" ps 1 -1 / exp;
    estimate "aes" aes 1 -1 / exp;
    output out=out2 prob=td;
    run;
```

Now we only need to merge the obtained probabilities and obtain the weights which are in the dataset "wIPCW" in the variable "w".

```
proc sort data=out1;by id;run; proc sort data=out2;by id;run;
data Com; merge out1 out2; by id; run;
data wIPCW(drop= tn td); set Com; by id; w=tn/td; run;
```

To estimate the Hazard Ratio of the IPCW method, we need to implement a weighted Cox regression model using the option "freq" in SAS to weight the data and there is where we have introduce the estimated weights. It's also important to use the option "notruncate" to avoid truncation problems with the weights.

```
/*Hazard Ratios with treatment switch using IPCW */
proc phreg data=wIPCW; model OS*censor(0) = trt; freq w/notruncate; run;
```

If we want to compare the IPCW results with the results from classical censoring analysis (switch is considered a censor), we can use the following SAS code to obtain the latter.

```
/*Hazard Ratios with treatment switch using Censoring Analysis*/
proc phreg data=wIPCW; model OS2*sensor2(0) = trt; run;
```

However, keep in mind that the weights used in the Cox regression model introduce variability in the model and hence the 95% CI of the IPCW method are unadjusted. This problem can be fixed using bootstrapping (Barker, 2005). A more controversial issue in time-dependent variable in the model as discussed in Chapter 5 Designing Trial for Precision Medicine.

6.4.4 Removing Treatment Switch Issue by Design

The carryover effect is difficult to handle when a patient switches treatment in a cancer trial. Suppose that if progressive disease (PD) is observed for a patient (from either group), the patient will switch to the best alternative treatment C available on the market. This way, the control group represents the situation without the test drug, and the test group represents the situation with the test drug. The difference between these two is the benefit (or risk) that patients may experience by adding the test drug to the market.

The efficacy should be compared in terms of increases in survival time between the two conditions with and without the new drug B. (1) Without drug B, the patients would be treated with A initially and then treated with physician's best choice C (not include B) after PD. (2) With drug B, the patients will be initially treatment B and then treated with C after PD. The

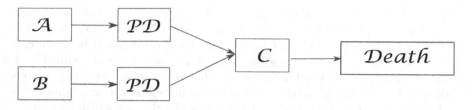

FIGURE 6.3
A New Oncology Trial Design.

difference between the two groups should then measure the survival benefit (Figure 6.3).

6.5 Competing Risks

6.5.1 Competing Risks as Bivariate Random Variable

A competing risks situation arises when an individual can experience more than one type of event and the occurrence of one type of event hinders or interferences the occurrence of other types of events. For instance, in a trial for heart disease, patients are followed in order to observe a myocardial infarction (MI). By the end of the study patients were either observed to have MI, die from other causes, or to be alive and well (censored). This is a competing risks situation because death from other causes prohibits the occurrence of MI. MI is considered the event of interest, while death from other causes is considered a competing risk. As a second example, death is often the event of interest in a cancer trial. A patient may or may not have progressive disease (PD) before death. If PD did occur, it indicated that the patient got sicker; consequently, his hazard rate of death should increase. In this case the competing event is PD that interferes with but does not prevent the main event, death.

When competing risks are present, Kaplan–Meier estimates (denoted by KM) cannot be interpreted as probabilities. Their complement (1-KM) can be interpreted as the probability of an event of interest in an ideal world where the other types of events do not exist. The logrank test and Cox regression are well established methods of analysis in the survival literature. These methods ignore the competing risks and test the 'pure' effect, which may be useful. In contrast, the more recent techniques developed by Pepe and Mori (1993), Gray (1988) and Fine and Gray (1999) take into account the competing risks (Pintilie, 2006).

In the absence of competing risks, survival data are usually presented as a bivariate random variable or pair (T, C). The censoring variable, C, is 1 if the event of interest was observed, and is 0 if the observation was censored. When

$C = 1$ the first member of the pair, T, is the time at which the event occurred and when $C = 0$, T is the time at which the observation was censored. When there are $K \geq 2$ types of competing risks, the data can still be represented as a pair (T, C) , and the censoring indicator C will again be defined as 0 if the observation is censored. In the event that the observation is not censored, though, C will take on the value i, where i is the type of the first failure/event observed $(i = 1, 2..., K)$. If $C = i$ then T is the time at which the event of type i occurred; otherwise it is the time of censoring (Kalbfleisch and Prentice, 1980).

The cumulative incidence function (CIF) or subdistribution for an event of type i, $i = 1, 2, ..., K$, is defined as the (joint) probability that an event of type i occurs at or before time t.

$$F_i(t) = \Pr(T \leq t, C = i). \tag{6.35}$$

The overall distribution function is the probability that an event of any type occurs at or before time t. That is,

$$F(t) = \Pr(T \leq t) = \sum_{i=1}^{p} \Pr(T \leq t, C = i). \tag{6.36}$$

If define $S_i(t) = \Pr(T > t, C = i)$, then $F_i(t) + S_i(t) = \Pr(C = i) = F_i(\infty)$. The subdensity function and the subhazard for events of type i is defined as $f_i(t) = \frac{\partial F_i(t)}{\partial t}$ and $h_i(t) = \frac{\partial F_i(\tau|\tau>t)}{\partial \tau} = \frac{f_i(t)}{S(t)}$, respectively. The overall hazard of an event of any type is $h(t) = \sum_{i=1}^{K} h_i(t)$. The cumulative subhazard function is defined as $H_i(t) = \int_0^t h_i(\tau) \, d\tau$. The hazard function of subdistribution (Gray, 1988) is defined as $\gamma_i(t) = \frac{\partial F_i(\tau|\tau>t \text{ or } (\tau \leq t \cap C \neq i))}{\partial \tau} = \frac{f_i(t)}{1-F_i(t)}$.

In many practical situations, we may only be interested in one type of time-to-event, and all the competing risks can combined into to one competing risk.

6.5.2   Solution to Competing Risks Model

Denote the failure function for cause-specific without competing risks by $F_{0i}(t)$ and density function by $f_{0i}(t)$ (Figure 6.4). In this case, the CIF for cause i is

$$
\begin{aligned}
F_i(t) &= \Pr(T \leq t, C = i) = \Pr(T \leq t|C = i)\Pr(C = i) \tag{6.3}\\
&= \Pr(T_i \leq t)\prod_{j \neq i}\Pr(T_j \geq T_i)\\
&= F_{0i}(t)\int_0^\infty f_{0i}(t_i)\prod_{j \neq i}S_{0j}(t_i)\,dt_i
\end{aligned}
$$

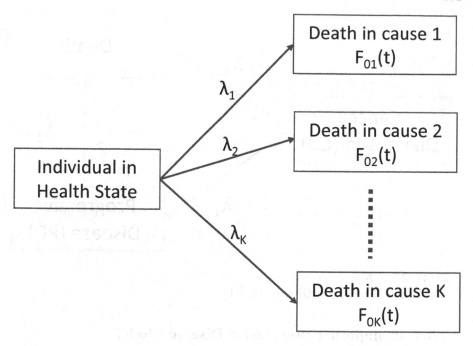

FIGURE 6.4
Competing Risks.

For exponential distributions with or without covariates, $T_i \sim f_{0i}(t) = \lambda_i \exp(-\lambda_i t)$ and $S_{0j}(t) = \exp(-\lambda_i t)$, the integration can be carried out:

$$F_i(t) = \frac{\lambda_i}{\sum_{j=1}^{K} \lambda_j} F_{0i}(t) \qquad (6.38)$$

(6.38) is a very intuitive result: The CIF F_i is proportional to λ_i and the "pure" failure function F_{0i} without competing risks. Here λ_i can be a function of baseline covariates but independent time. Given the death at time t, the probability of death due to cause i is $\frac{\lambda_i}{\sum_{j=1}^{K} \lambda_j}$, but when the person will in cause i is determined by F_{0i}.

The overall death function is

$$F(t) = \frac{1}{\sum_{j=1}^{K} \lambda_j} \sum_{i=1}^{K} \lambda_i F_{0i}(t) \qquad (6.39)$$

Note censoring will not affect CIF or overall death function, but it will affect the MLEs of of the parameters in the models. This is the key difference between competing risk and censoring.

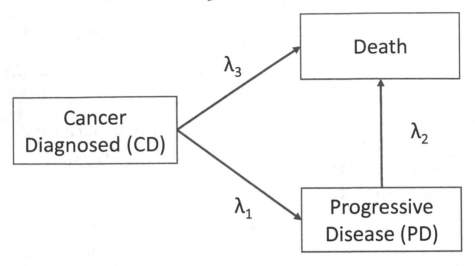

FIGURE 6.5
Competing Progressive Disease Model.

6.5.3   Competing Progressive Disease Model

Death and PD are not independent. In fact, a PD will change the hazard/death rate and death before PD will prevent PD from occurring. For this reason, the competing progressive disease model is not necessarily a Markov chain.

There are two paths of death, direct and indirect through PD (Figure 6.5). The probability of direct death is $\frac{\lambda_3}{\lambda_1+\lambda_3}$ and the probability of indirect death is $\frac{\lambda_1}{\lambda_1+\lambda_3}$. The direct death function $F_{03}(t)$ and death function with PD is $\int_0^t f_1(t_1) F_{02}(t-t_1)\,dt_1$. Therefore, the total death function is

$$F(t) = \frac{\lambda_3}{\lambda_1+\lambda_3} F_{03}(t) + \frac{\lambda_1}{\lambda_1+\lambda_3}\int_0^t f_1(t_1) F_{02}(t-t_1)\,dt_1 \qquad (6.40)$$

For exponential distributions, $F_{03}(t) = \left(1 - e^{-\lambda_3 t}\right)$, $f_1(t_1) = \lambda_1 e^{-\lambda_1 t_1}$, and $F_{02}(t-t_1) = 1 - e^{-\lambda_2(t-t_1)}$

$$F(t) = 1 - \frac{\lambda_1}{\lambda_1+\lambda_3}\frac{\lambda_2}{\lambda_2-\lambda_1}e^{-\lambda_1 t} - \frac{\lambda_1}{\lambda_1+\lambda_3}\frac{\lambda_1}{\lambda_1-\lambda_2}e^{-\lambda_2 t} - \frac{\lambda_3}{\lambda_1+\lambda_3}e^{-\lambda_3 t} \qquad (6.41)$$

$$f(t) = \frac{\lambda_1}{\lambda_1+\lambda_3}\frac{\lambda_1\lambda_2}{\lambda_2-\lambda_1}e^{-\lambda_1 t} + \frac{\lambda_1}{\lambda_1+\lambda_3}\frac{\lambda_1\lambda_2}{\lambda_1-\lambda_2}e^{-\lambda_2 t} + \frac{\lambda_3^2}{\lambda_1+\lambda_3}e^{-\lambda_3 t}, \qquad (6.42)$$

where $\lambda_2 > \lambda_1$ because patient will get sicker after PD and the starting time for λ_2 is different from λ_1.

With the pdf $F(t)$ and cdf $f(t)$, we can have MLS technology discussed in Section 1 and will be further elaborated the next section. For hypothesis test, the logrank test can be used for testing the treatment and covariate effects.

If we consider the drug effect delayed time T_d, a random variable with exponential distribution rather than a constant, we can change "time to PD" to "time-to-drug's effect" in the model in Figure 6.2 and (6.28) becomes a model for delayed drug effect. If the drug is very effective, $\lambda_2 < \lambda_1$; if the drug has a little effect, $\lambda_2 > \lambda_1$, when $\lambda_1 = \lambda_2$, (6.26) will lead to the following model:

$$F(t) = 1 - \frac{\lambda_1(1+t)}{\lambda_1 + \lambda_3} e^{-\lambda_1 t} - e^{-\lambda_3 t}. \tag{6.43}$$

$$f(t) = \frac{\lambda_1}{\lambda_1 + \lambda_3}(\lambda_1 t - 1)e^{-\lambda_1 t} - \lambda_3 e^{-\lambda_3 t}. \tag{6.44}$$

Software packages are available in SAS Proc Phreg and R.

6.5.4 Hypothesis Test Method

Gray's method

Without loss of generality, only two types of events are considered: the event of interest and the competing risk event. The test introduced by Gray (1988) compares the weighted averages of the hazard of the subdistribution functions for the event of interest. The score for treatment group i is

$$z_i = \int_0^\tau W_i(t)\{h_i(t) - h_0(t)\} dt,$$

where τ is the maximum time observed in both groups, $W_i(t)$ is a weight function, $h_i(t)$ is the hazard of the subdistribution for group i defined in (5.1) and $h_0(t)$ is the hazard of the subdistribution for all groups together.

Pepe-Mori's method

Pepe-Mori's method (1993) compares the cumulative incidence curves directly. The test is essentially the weighted area between the two CIFs. It was proven by Pepe (1991) that under the null hypothesis of no treatment effect

$$s = \sqrt{\frac{N_1 N_2}{N_1 + N_2}} \int_0^\tau W(t)\{F_1(t) - F_2(t)\} dt$$

is asymptotically normal with mean 0 and standard deviation σ. In this formula $F_i(t)$ represents the cumulative incidence function for the event of interest for group i, N_i is the total number of subjects in group i and $W(t)$ is a weight function.

Some challenges in analyses of treatment switch are, the delayed or carryover effect from primary therapy to the secondary therapy after PD or switch. The question arises as to how to deal with a treatment that may decrease the hazard rate for cancer but increase the death rate for CV diseases or other unspecified reasons. For this reason, the overall survival, not CIF, should be the primary endpoint for a clinical trial with competing risks.

6.6 Threshold Regression with First-Hitting-Time Model

Biomarker or clinical responses and survival time, can be modeled using stochastic processes $X(t)$. When the stochastic process reaches a certain level (i.e., $X(t) = ß$) for the first time, it is called first hitting time (FHT). FHT usually indicates a critical state such as a biological inhibition, degradation, or death. The critical value ß, called the boundary or threshold, can be a constant or function of time t. Threshold regression (TR) refers to the first-hitting-time models with regression structures that accommodate covariate data (Lee and Whitmore, 2006).

A stochastic process $\{X(t), t \geq 0\}$ is said to be a Brownian motion (Wiener Process) with a drift μ if (1) $X(0) = 0$; (2) $\{X(t), t \geq 0\}$ has stationary and independent increments; and (3) for every $t > 0$, $X(t)$ is normally distributed with mean μt and variance $\sigma^2 t$,

$$X(t) \sim \frac{1}{\sqrt{2\pi\sigma^2 t}} \exp\left(-\frac{(x - \mu t)^2}{2\sigma^2 t}\right). \tag{6.45}$$

For any given timepoint $t = t_c$, $X(t = t_c)$ has a normal distribution. The covariance of the Brownian motion is $\text{cov}[X(t), X(s)] = \sigma^2 \min\{s, t\}$. The standard Brownian motion $B(t)$ is the Brownian motion with drift $\mu = 0$ and diffusion $\sigma^2 = 1$. The relationship between the standard Brownian motion and Brownian motion with drift μ and diffusion parameter σ^2 can be expressed as

$$X(t) = \mu t + \sigma B(t). \tag{6.46}$$

The cdf. is given by

$$\Pr\{X(t) \leq y | X(0) = x\} = \Phi\left(\frac{y - x - \mu t}{\sigma\sqrt{t}}\right), \tag{6.47}$$

where $\Phi(\cdot)$ is the cdf. of the standard normal distribution.

The first hitting time T is a random variable when $X(t)$ starts from the initial position $X(0) = 0 \in \Omega \backslash ß$ (inside the space not at boundary)but and reaches a given constant boundary $ß = b$ of the domain Ω (non-negative values). The FHT for Brownian motion is the inverse normal distribution:

$$T \sim f(t|\mu, \sigma^2, b) = \frac{b}{\sqrt{2\pi\sigma^2 t^3}} e^{-\frac{(b+\mu t)^2}{2\sigma^2 t}}. \tag{6.48}$$

The cdf. corresponding to (6.48) is given by

$$F(t|\mu, \sigma^2, b) = \Phi\left[-\frac{(\mu t + b)}{\sqrt{\sigma^2 t}}\right] + e^{-\frac{2b\mu}{\sigma^2}} \Phi\left[\frac{\mu t - b}{\sqrt{\sigma^2 t}}\right]. \tag{6.49}$$

Note that if $\mu > 0$, then the FHT is not certain to occur and the pdf. is improper. Specifically, in this case, $P(t = \infty) = 1 - \exp(-2b\mu/\sigma^2)$.

In general, an FHT model $< X(t), ß>$ has two essential components: (1) a parent stochastic process $\{X(t),\ t \in T\ ,\ x \in \mathbb{R}\}$ with initial value $X(0) = 0$, where T is the time space and $\mathbb{R}$ is the state space of the process, and (2) a boundary set or threshold $ß$, where $ß \subset \mathbb{R}$. Note that $ß$ can be a constant or function vector of time t or a stochastic process.

In an FHT model, both the parent process $\{X(t)\}$ and boundary $ß$ can have parameters that depend on covariates. As a simple sample, the Wiener process has mean parameter μ and variance parameter σ^2. The boundary $ß$ has parameter x_0, the initial position. In FHT regression models, these parameters will be connected to linear combinations of covariates using a suitable regression link function,

$$g\left(\boldsymbol{\theta}\right) = \boldsymbol{Z}\boldsymbol{\beta}', \tag{6.50}$$

where $g\left(\cdot\right)$ is the link function that has the inverse function $g^{-1}\left(\cdot\right)$, $\boldsymbol{\theta}$ is the parameter vector in the FHT model, $\boldsymbol{Z} = (1, Z_1, ..., Z_k)$ is the covariate vector (with a leading unit to include an intercept term), and $\beta = (\beta_0, \beta_1, ..., \beta_k)$ is the associated vector of regression coefficients. The commonly used link functions include the identity and logistic functions.

There are two different covariates: time-independent (e.g., DNA markers) and time-dependent covariates (e.g., RNA markers).

We can solve (6.50) for $\boldsymbol{\theta}$:

$$\boldsymbol{\theta} = g^{-1}\left(\boldsymbol{Z}\boldsymbol{\beta}'\right). \tag{6.51}$$

The parameter estimations for FHT models have been dominated by the maximum likelihood method. Consider a latent health status process characterized by a Wiener diffusion process. The FHT for such a process follows an inverse Gaussian distribution. The inverse Gaussian distribution depends on the mean and variance parameters of the underlying Wiener process (μ and σ^2) and the initial health status level (x_0), i.e., $\boldsymbol{\theta} = (\mu, \sigma, x_0)$. Let $f(t|\boldsymbol{\theta})$ and $F(t|\boldsymbol{\theta})$ be the pdf. and cdf. of the FHT distribution, respectively. Using (6.51), we can obtain

$$\begin{cases} f(t|\boldsymbol{\theta}) = f(t|g^{-1}\left(\boldsymbol{Z}\boldsymbol{\beta}'\right)), \\ F(t|\boldsymbol{\theta}) = F(t|g^{-1}\left(\boldsymbol{Z}\boldsymbol{\beta}'\right)). \end{cases} \tag{6.52}$$

To form a likelihood function, denote by $\boldsymbol{Z}_i$ $(i = 1, ...n_e)$ the realization of covariate vector $\boldsymbol{Z}$ on the ith subject who had an event at time t_i, and by $\boldsymbol{Z}_j$ $(j = n_e + 1, ...n_e + n_s)$ the realization of covariate vector $\boldsymbol{Z}$ on the jth subject, who is right-censored at time t_j. Then the likelihood function is given by

$$L\left(\beta\right) = \prod_{i=1}^{n_e} f\left(t_i|g^{-1}\left(\boldsymbol{Z}_i\boldsymbol{\beta}'\right)\right) \prod_{j=n_e+1}^{n_e+n_s} S(t_j|g^{-1}\left(\boldsymbol{Z}_j\boldsymbol{\beta}'\right)). \tag{6.53}$$

To estimate parameters β, the likelihood or the log-likelihood function can be used. Numerical gradient methods can be used to find the maximum likelihood estimates for β. Then the parameter vector $\boldsymbol{\theta}$ can be found using

(6.51), and the distribution function $f(t|\boldsymbol{\theta})$ and $F(t|\boldsymbol{\theta})$ can be obtained from (6.52).

In randomized oncology trials, a patient's treatment may be switched in the middle of the study because of a progressive disease (PD), which indicates a failure of the initial treatment regimen. In such cases, the total survival time is the sum of two event times: randomization to switching and switching to death. If the test drug is more effective than the control, then the majority of patients in the control group will switch to the test drug and the survival difference between the two treatment groups will be significantly reduced in comparison with the case without treatment switching.

Since the actual or censored survival time can be composed of two intervals, representing the time on the primary therapy and the time on the alternative therapy, the disease may progress at different rates in these two intervals (irrespective of the treatment). Instead of using two different hazards at different stages. we transform survival times from calendar time to the so-called running time, which has the form

$$r = a_1\tau_1 + \tau_2, \tag{6.54}$$

where τ_1 and τ_2 correspond to time to progression and progression to death, respectively, and a_1 is a scale parameter to be estimated.

Threshold regression has been used for assessing treatment efficacy of VEL-CADE in a multiple myeloma clinical trial with treatment switch (Lee, Chang, and Whitmore, 2006). VELCADE (bortezomib) is indicated for the treatment of patients with multiple myeloma. The pivotal study was a multi-center, international, randomized, open-label study designed to determine whether treatment with VELCADE prolongs time-to-progression (TTP) relative to treatment with high-dose Dexamethasone in patients with multiple myeloma. Patients were assigned to receive VELCADE or high-dose Dexamethasone by random allocation at a 1:1 ratio. Randomization was stratified based on the number of treatment regimens the patient previously received (one previous treatment regimen versus more than one previous treatment regimen) and stem cell transplant history (history of transplant versus no history of transplant). Patients who developed confirmed PD after treatment were allowed to switch treatment.

Figure 6.6 illustrate some possible paths for the trial with the threshold regression. The first region describes health status after randomization until the patient experiences PD. The second region describes health status between PD and death. The setup assumes that PD always precedes death. Patient records in this study are subject to censoring for both PD and death. The figure shows four illustrative sample paths for a multiple myeloma patient participating in the study. Path 1 illustrates a patient who experiences PD under the assigned primary therapy and then dies before the end of follow-up. The dashed sample path indicates that the patient is assigned to the alternate therapy at PD. Time of PD and time of death are both known in this case. Path 2 illustrates a patient who is switched to the alternate therapy prior

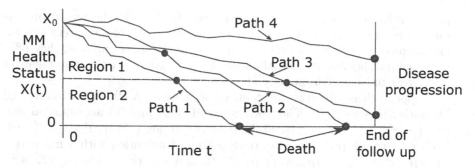

FIGURE 6.6
FTH model: Health Status vs Time to PD and Death.

to PD and happens to die before the end of follow-up. The time of PD is not observed in this case, but the time of death is known. Path 3 illustrates a patient who experiences PD on the primary therapy, is switched to the alternate therapy, and then is living at the end of follow-up. The time of PD is known in this case, but survival time is censored. Path 4 is a patient who does not experience PD under the primary therapy. This patient is censored for both times of PD and death. In all cases, we note that the time on the primary therapy and the time on the alternate therapy are both measured, with the time measurement ending at death or end of follow up as the case may be. There are other possible paths too that are not shown in the Figure 6.6.

The covariates used in the threshold regression (TR) analysis are as follows. (1) treatment primary treatment before PD, (2) PD, (3) treatment by PD Interaction term, (4) the number of previous treatments, (5) baseline level of beta-2 microglobulin, and (6) age. The analyses show that although the Cox regression results agree broadly with TR results in this trial, TR provides more subtle insights into the source and nature of the comparative benefits of VELCADE than offered by the Cox methodology.

Regression analysis can be performed using threg package in R (Xiao et al., 2015).

6.7 Multivariate Model with Biomarkers

In Chapter 5, Designing for Precision Medicine, we discussed the utilization of biomarkers in clinical trials. In this section, we will further discuss this topic from different perspectives and also will discuss how to use the biomarker process to assist in tracking the progress of the parent process if the parent process is latent or only infrequently observed. In this way, the marker process forms a basis for a predictive inference about the status of the parent process and its progress toward an FHT. As markers of the parent process, they offer potential insights into the causal forces that are generating the movements of the parent process (Whitmore et al., 1998).

Suppose there are the parent survival process, $X(t)$, and a correlated biomarker process, $Y(t)$. They form a two-dimensional Wiener diffusion process $\{X(r), Y(r)\}$ for $r \geq 0$ and the initial condition $\{X(0), Y(0)\} = \{0, 0\}$. Vector $\{X(r), Y(r)\}$ has a bivariate normal distribution with a mean vector $r\boldsymbol{\mu}$, where $\boldsymbol{\mu} = (\mu_x, \mu_y)'$, $\mu_x \geq 0$, and covariance matrix $r\boldsymbol{\Sigma}$ with $\boldsymbol{\Sigma} = \begin{pmatrix} \sigma_{xx} & \sigma_{xy} \\ \sigma_{yx} & \sigma_{yy} \end{pmatrix}$. The correlation coefficient is $\rho = \sigma_{xy}/\sqrt{\sigma_{xx}\sigma_{yy}}$.

The key is to formulate the probability or pdf. for the survival and failing subjects. For a survivor at time t, an observed value $Y(t) = y(t)$ for the biomarker constitutes a censored observation of failure time because we know $S > t$. The pdf. for survival subjects is given by

$$p_s(y) = \Phi(c_1)\phi(c_2) - e^{\frac{2\mu_x}{\sigma_{xx}}} \Phi\left(c_1 - 2\sqrt{\frac{(1-\rho^2)}{\sigma_{xx}t}}\right)\phi\left(c_2 - \frac{2\sigma_{xy}}{\sigma_{xx}\sqrt{\sigma_{yy}t}}\right),$$

(6.56)

where ϕ and Φ are, respectively, the standard normal pdf. and cdf., and

$$\begin{cases} c_1 = \frac{1-\mu_x t - \sigma_{xy}(y-\mu_y t)}{\sigma_{yy}\sqrt{\sigma_{xx}(1-\rho^2)t}}, \\ c_2 = \frac{y-\mu_y t}{\sqrt{\sigma_{yy}t}}. \end{cases}$$

(6.57)

For a subject that died at time $S = s$ with an observed value $Y(S) = y(s)$ for the biomarker, the joint pdf. is

$$p_f(y, s) = \frac{\exp\left(-\frac{1}{2}W^T\Sigma^{-1}W\right)}{2\pi\sqrt{|\Sigma|}s^2},$$

(6.58)

where

$$W^T = \left(\frac{y-\mu_y s}{\sqrt{s}}, \frac{1-\mu_x s}{\sqrt{s}}\right).$$

(6.59)

The probability of surviving longer than time t is

$$P(S > t) = \int_{-\infty}^{\infty} p_s(y)\, dy.$$

(6.60)

Numerical methods can be used to calculate $P(S > t)$.

To carry out MLE of the parameters, we denote the independent sample observations on failing items by $(\hat{y}_i, \hat{s}_i)$, $i = 1, ..., \nu$, and those on surviving items by $\hat{y}_i$, $i = \nu + 1, ..., n$. The log-likelihood can then be written as

$$\ln L (\mu, \Sigma) = \sum_{i=1}^{\nu} \ln p_f (\hat{y}_i, \hat{s}_i) + \sum_{i=\nu+1}^{n} \ln p_s (\hat{y}_i). \qquad (6.61)$$

The MLEs of the parameters μ and Σ can be found based on (6.61).

From (6.56) through (6.61), we have assumed the threshold for failure is $x = 1$. If failure is defined as $x = a$, then the estimates $\hat{\mu}_x$, $\hat{\sigma}_{xx}$, and $\hat{\sigma}_{xy}$ from (6.61) should be multiplied by a constant a. Other estimates and probabilities are independent of a. Thus, no changes are needed.

So far, we have considered a single-marker case. In practice, there is usually more than one relevant marker, while each marker will have a certain degree of correlation with the underlying parent process. We wish to find that the linear combination of the available markers will have the largest possible correlation with the degradation component. Whitmore et al. (1998) extended their method to include a composite marker or a combination of several markers.

Suppose there are k candidate markers available, denoted by $Z(t) = (Z_1(t), ..., Z_k(t))$, with the initial condition $Z(0) = 0$. Assume that vector $Z(t)$, together with the degradation component $X(t)$, forms a $k+1$−dimension Wiener process. We define the composite marker denoted by $Y(t)$ as

$$Y(t) = Z(t) \beta' = \sum_{j=1}^{k} Z_j(t) \beta_j, \qquad (6.62)$$

where $\beta = (1, \beta_2, ..., \beta_k)$ is a $k \times 1$ vector of coefficients that we wish to estimate. The linear structure of (6.25) assures that the joint process for $Y(t)$ and $X(t)$ retains its bivariate Wiener form. The parameterization is defined by

$$\mu_y = \mu_Z \beta', \; \sigma_{yy} = \beta \Sigma_{ZZ} \beta', \; \sigma_{yy} = \Sigma_{XZ} \beta', \qquad (6.63)$$

where μ_Z and Σ_{ZZ} denote the $k \times 1$ mean vector and $k \times k$ covariance matrix of markers $Z(t)$ and Σ_{XZ} denotes the $1 \times k$ covariate vector of $X(t)$ with $Z(t)$.

The MLEs presented earlier for a single marker can be extended to estimate the optimal composite marker in (6.25). This extension requires rewriting the likelihood function in (6.24) in terms of the new parameterization in (6.26).

6.8 Summary

Survival data are characterized by incompleteness of data (or censoring) and competing risks. Issues of censoring or competing risks are different but related. A censored event is expected to happen sooner or later, but has not been observed during the time interval concerned. Competing risks are different, as an example, death related to cancer and death related to CV disease can be competing risks: the occurrence of one would prevent the occurrence of another. We often separate event of interest from competing risk. In this example we would call death due to cancer the event of interest and death due to cardiovascular (CV) a competing risk if it is a cancer trial. If it is a CV trial, we would call death related to CV the event of interest and death related to cancer a competing risk. We used a generalized definition of competing risk: a competing risk is an event whose occurrence will prevent the main event from occurring . An example for the latter is disease progression, which will change the hazard rate of survival in a cancer trial. There are three different practical situations: (1) events occur in sequence: cancer diagnosed → Disease progression → die, (2) events coexisting or occurring in parallel: one event of interest, and the others are considered as censoring , (3) conventional competing risks: simultaneous process but the occurrence of one event will predispose to other events occurring.

Survival data can be analyzed using nonparametric Kaplan-Meier and Nelson-Aalen methods, or parametric model such as proportional hazard model, accelerated failure time model, and frailty model. MLE is widely used because its simplicity and has asymptotically normal distribution. Landmark analysis is a simple way to deal with potential bias in the conventional responder analysis. Because people who survive longer have more chance of getting tumor responses, landmark approach using a fixed time point to define the responders may be utilized to avoid bias. The second method to deal with responder analysis is to adopt a time-dependent hazard model. The multistage model is to model the event process using semi-Markov model (discrete in stage and continuous in time), the hazard between two states are usually assumed a constant as seen in the Progressive Disease Model (Figure 6.1). Similar to the multistage semi-Markov model, the piecewise (exponential) model has been used to study the drug-delayed effect. In the model both the state and time are discrete, that is, the piecewise exponential model is a Markov chain. The SAS simulation program for trial design with a delayed drug effect can be found in the Appendix. It is interesting to know that if we consider the delayed time is not fixed but randomly varies from patient to patient, then it can be modeled using a semi-Markov process.

Treatment switch or crossover in cancer trials is a challenging issue since the crossover diminishes the treatment different between the two treatment groups if the majority of patients from the control group switch to the test group. After we use a simple multistage model to illustrate the analysis, the IPCW logrank test is discussed and the SAS program is provided. Treatment switch problem will be even more challenging when there is potential carryover of the drug effect. We propose a new trial design to avoid the problem at the design stage.

We derived CIF for the general competing risks and discussed the competing progressive disease model. The commonly used methods for hypothesis testing of CIF difference are Gray's method and Pape-Mori's Method. However, a drug can reduce the death of interest but increase the death due to other causes. In clinical trials we argue the most appropriate method is to compare the overall survival rather than cause-specific death using a logrank test for example. The software packages for completing risk analysis are available in SAS Proc Phreg and the R Package CFC.

Threshold regression (TR) is a powerful model for time-to-event analysis. It can deal the time-dependent covariates using running time without any difficulties. A trial application with treatment switch is discussed. The software package for TR is available in R package threg.

Bibliography

Anderson, J.R., Cain, K.C., Gelber, R.D. (1983). Analysis of survival by tumor response. Journal of Clinical Oncology 1983;1:710 –719.

Bukowski, R.M., Yasothan, M., and Kirkpatrick. P. (2010). Pazopanib. Nature Reviews Drug Discovery 9.1 (2010): 17-18.

Breslow, N., Elder, L., Berger, L. (1984). A two sample censored-data rank test for acceleration. Biometrics. 1984; 40:1042–1069.

Branson, M, Whitehead, W. (2002). Estimating a treatment e ect in survival studies in which patients switch treatment. Statistics in Medicine 2002; 21:2449 –2463.

Clayton, D.G. (1978) A model for association in bivariate life tables and its application in epidemiological studies of familial tendency in chronic disease incidence. Biometrika 65, 141-151

Cox, D.R. (1972). Regression models and life-tables (with Discussion). J. R. Statist. Soc. B. 1972; 34:187–220.

Cox, D.R., Oakes, D. (1984). Analysis of Survival Data. Monographs on Statistics and Applied Probability. Chapman & Hall: London, 1984.

Dafni, U. (2011). Landmark Analysis at the 25-Year Landmark Point. Circ Cardiovasc Qual Outcomes. 2011;4:363-371

Eisenstein, E.L., Anstrom, K.J., Kong, D.F., et al. (2007). Clopidogrel use and long-term clinical outcomes after drug-eluting stent implantation. JAMA. 2007;297: 159–168.

Fine, J. and Gray, R. (1999). A proportional hazards model for the subdistribution of a competing risk. Journal of the American Statistical Association, 94(446):496–509.

Fleming, T.R., Harrington, D.P. (1991) Counting processes and survival analysis. John Wiley and Sons, New York.

Gastwirth, J.L. (1985). The use of maximum efficiency robust tests in combining contingency tables and survival analysis. Journal of the American Statistical Association. 1985; 80:380–384.

Gray, R.J. (1988). A Class of K-Sample Tests for Comparing the Cumulative Incidence of a Competing Risk. Annals of Statistics Volume 16, Number 3 (1988), 1141-1154.

Jiménez-Moro, J.L. and García, J.G. (2014). Inverse Probability of Censoring Weighting for Selective Crossover in Oncology Clinical Trials. PhUSE Annual Conference, 12th-15th Oct 2014, London, UK

Kalbfeisch, J.D., Prentice, R.T. (1980). The Statistical Analysis of Failure Time Data. Wiley: New York, 1980.

Lagakos, S.W., Lim, L.L.-Y. (1990). Robins JM. Adjusting for early treatment termination in comparative clinical trials. Statistics in Medicine. 1990; 9:1417–1424.

Latimer, N. R., Abrams, K., Lambert, P., et al. (2014). Adjusting for Treatment Switching in Randomised Controlled Trials - A Simulation Study and a Simplified Two-Stage Method. Statistical Methods in Medical Research, 2014. I

Latimer, N. R. , Henshall, C., Siebert, U. and Bell, H. (2016). Treatment switching: Statistical and decisionmaking challenges and approaches. International journal of technology assessment in health care, 32(3): 160–166, 2016.

Lee, M.-L. T., Whitmore, G. A. (2006). Threshold regression for survival analysis: modeling event times by a stochastic process. Statistical Science 21:501–513.

Lee, M.L.T., Chang, M. and Whitmore, G.A. (2008). A Threshold regression mixture model for assessing treatment efficacy in Multiple Myeloma Clinical Trial. Journal of Biopharmaceutical Statistics 2008;18(6):1136-49

Lee, M.-L.T., DeGruttola, V. and Schoenfeld, D. (2000). A model for markers and latent health status, Journal of the Royal Statistical Society, Series B, 62, 747-762.

Lee, M.-L. T. and Whitmore G. A. (2004). First hitting time models for lifetime data. In: Handbook of Statistics: Volume 23, Advances in Survival Analysis, C. R. Rao, N. Balakrishnan, editors, 537-543.

Newey, W.K., McFadden, D. (1994). Large sample estimation and hypothesis testing. Handbook of econometrics, vol.IV, Ch.36. Elsevier Science. pp. 2111–2245.

Pepe, M.S., Mori, M. (1993). Kaplan-Meier marginal or conditional probability curves in summarizing competing risks failure time data? Statistics in Medicine. 1993; 12:737–751.

Pepe, M. S. and Fleming, T. R. (1991). Weighted Kaplan-Meier statistics: large sample and optimality considerations. Journal of the Royal Statistical Society B 53, 341-352.

Pintilie, M. (2006). Competing Risks: A Practical Perspective. John Wiley & Sons Ltd, The Atrium, Southern Gate, Chichester, West Sussex PO19 8SQ, England

Prentice, R.L. (1978). Linear rank tests with right censored data. Biometrika. 1978; 65:167–179.

Putter, H. (2013). The Landmark Approach: An Introduction and Application to Dynamic Prediction in Competing Risks. Dynamic prediction workshop, Bordeaux. October 10, 2013

Robins, J. M. and Tsiatis, A. A. (1991). Correcting for non-compliance in randomized trials using rank preserving structural failure time models. Communications in Statistics Theory and Methods, 20: 2609–2631, 1991

Robins, J.M. (1994). Correcting for non-compliance in randomized trials using structural nested mean models. Communications in Statistics 1994; 23:2379–2412.

Robins, J.M. (1999). Marginal structural models versus structural nested models as tools for causal inference, in Statistical Models in Epidemiology, the Environment, and Clinical Trials, Halloran ME, Berry D (eds). Springer: New York, 1999; 95–133.

Robins, J.M., Finkelstein DM. Correcting for non-compliance and dependent censoring in an AIDS Clinical Trial with inverse probability of censoring weighted (IPCW) log-rank tests. Biometrics 2000; 56:779-788.

Shao, J., Chang, M., Chow, S. C. (2005). Statistical inference for cancer trials with treatment switching. Statistics in Medicine 24:1783–1790.

Schoenfeld, D. (1981). The asymptotic properties of nonparametric tests for comparing survival distributions. Biometrika 68: 316–319.

Sommer, A., Zeger, S.L. (1991). On estimating e cacy from clinical trials. Statistics in Medicine 1991; 10:45–52.

Tarone, R.E. (1981). On the distribution of the maximum of the logrank statistic and the modified Wilcoxon statistic. Biometrics. 1981; 37:79–85.

Vaupel, J.W., Manton, K.G., Stallard, E. (1979). The Impact of Heterogeneity in Individual Frailty on the Dynamics of Mortality. Demography 16, 439 - 454.

Whitmore, G. A., M. J. Crowder and J. F. Lawless (1998). Failure inference from a marker process based on a bivariate Wiener model, Lifetime Data Analysis, 4, 229-251.

Wu, J. (2014). A New One-Sample Log-Rank Test. J Biomet Biostat 5: 210.

Xiao, T., Whitmore, G.A., He, X., and Lee, ML. T. (2015). The R Package threg to Implement Threshold Regression Models. Journal of Statistical Software August 2015, Volume 66, Issue 8.

Yamaguchi, T. and Ohashi, Y. (2004). Adjusting for differential proportions of second-line treatment in cancer clinical trials. Part I: structural nested models and marginal structural models to test and estimate treatment arm effects. Stat Med. 2004 Jul 15;23(13):1991-2003.

Yang, S. & Prentice, R.L. (2010). Improved Logrank-Type Tests for Survival Data Using Adaptive Weights, Biometrics. 2010 March; 66(1): 30–38.

Zucker, D.M. (1992). The efficiency of a weighted log-rank test under a percent error misspecification model for the log hazard ratio. Biometrics. 1992; 48:893–899.

Zucker, D.M., Lakatos, E. (1990). Weighted log rank type statistics for comparing survival curves when there is a time lag in the effectiveness of treatment. Biometrika. 1990; 77:853–864.

7

Practical Multiple Testing Methods in Clinical Trials

7.1 Multiple-Testing Problems

7.1.1 Sources of Multiplicity

It is well known that multiple-hypothesis testing (multiple-testing) can inflate the type-I error dramatically without proper adjustments for the p-values or significance level. This is referred to as a multiplicity issue. The multiplicity can come from different sources, for example, in clinical trials, it can come from (1) multiple-treatment comparisons, (2) multiple tests performed at different times, (3) multiple tests for several endpoints, (4) multiple tests conducted for multiple populations using the same treatment within a single experiment, and (5) a combination of some or all of the sources above.

Multiple-treatment comparisons are often conducted in dose-finding studies. Multiple time-point analyses are often conducted in longitudinal studies with repeated measures, or in trials with group sequential or adaptive designs.

Why are multiple-endpoint analyses required? Moyé (2003, p. 76) points out three primary reasons why we conduct a multiple-endpoint study: (1) a disease has an unknown aetiology or no clinical consensus on the single most important clinical efficacy endpoint exists; (2) a disease manifests itself in multidimensional ways; and (3) a therapeutic area for which the prevailing methods for assessment of treatment efficacy dictate a multifaceted approach both for selection of the efficacy endpoints and for their evaluation.

The statistical analyses of multiple-endpoint problems can be categorized as (1) a single primary efficacy endpoint with one or more secondary endpoints, (2) coprimary endpoints (more than one primary endpoint) with secondary endpoints, (3) composite primary efficacy endpoints with interest in each individual endpoint, or (4) a surrogate primary endpoint with supportive secondary endpoints. A surrogate endpoint is a biological or clinical marker that can replace a gold standard endpoint such as survival.

In the case of diseases of unknown etiology, where no clinical consensus has been reached on the single most important clinical efficacy endpoint, coprimary endpoints may be used. When diseases manifest in multidimensional ways, drug effectiveness is often characterized by the use of composite endpoints, global disease scores, or the disease activity index (DAI). When a composite primary efficacy endpoint is used, we are often interested in the particular aspect or endpoint where the drug has demonstrated benefits. An ICH guideline (European Medicines Agency, 1998) suggests: "If a single primary variable cannot be selected from multiple measurements associated with the primary objective, another useful strategy is to integrate or combine the multiple measurements into a single or 'composite' variable, using a predefined algorithm... This approach addresses the multiplicity problem without requiring adjustment to the type-I error." For some indications, such as oncology, it is difficult to use a gold standard endpoint, such as survival, as the primary endpoint because it requires a longer follow-up time and patients switch treatments after disease progression. Instead, a surrogate endpoint, such as time-to-progression, might be chosen as the primary endpoint with other supporting efficacy evidence, such as infection rate. Huque and Röhmel (2010) provide an excellent overview of multiplicity problems in clinical trials from the regulatory perspective. Following are some illustrative examples.

(1) A trial compares two doses of a new treatment to a control with respect to the primary efficacy endpoint . (2) In a clinical trial, there are two endpoints; at least one needs to be statistically significant or all need to be statistically significant . (3) Given three specified primary endpoints E1, E2 and E3, either E1 needs to be statistically significant or both E2, and E3 need to be statistically significant. (4) One of the two specified endpoints must be statistically significant and the other one needs to show noninferiority. (5) A trial tests for treatment effects for multiple primary and secondary endpoints at low, medium and high doses of a new treatment compared with a placebo with the restriction that tests for the secondary endpoints for a specific dose can be carried out only when certain primary endpoints show meaningful treatment efficacy for that dose. (6) A clinical trial uses a surrogate endpoint S for an accelerated approval and a clinically important endpoint T for a full approval. (7) In a multiple-group oncology trial, each treatment group represents a single drug or combination of drugs. The goal is to identify the most effective drug or combination of drugs, if any. (9) In pharmacovigilance or sequential drug safety monitoring in postmarketing, how can false signals be effectively controlled? (9) In adaptive sequential design, multiple tests are performed at different time points. How can the type-I error rate be controlled?

7.1.2 Multiple-Testing Taxonomy

Let H_i $(i = 1, ..., K)$ be the null hypotheses of interest in an experiment. There are at least three different types of global multiple-hypothesis testing that can be performed.

(1) **Union-Intersection Testing**

$$H_o : \cap_{i=1}^{K} H_i \text{ versus } H_a : \bar{H}_o. \tag{7.1}$$

In this setting, if any H_{0i} is rejected, the global null hypothesis H_o is rejected. For union-intersection testing, if the global testing has a size of α, then this has to be adjusted to a smaller value for testing each individual H_{oi}, called the local significance level.

In a typical dose-finding trial, patients are randomly assigned to one of several (K) parallel dose levels or a placebo. The goal is to find out if there is a drug effect and which dose(s) has the effect. In such a trial, H_i will represent the null hypothesis that the ith dose level has no effect in comparison with the placebo. The goal of the dose-finding trial can be formulated in terms of hypothesis testing (7.1). Union-intersection testing is the focus of this chapter.

(2) Intersection-Union Testing

$$H_o : \cup_{i=1}^{K} H_i \text{ versus } H_a : \bar{H}_o. \tag{7.2}$$

In this setting, if and only if all H_i $(i = 1, ..., K)$ are rejected is the global null hypothesis H_o rejected. For intersection-union testing, the global α will apply to each individual H_i testing.

As an example, Alzheimer's trials in mild to moderate disease generally include ADAS Cog and CIBIC (clinician's interview based impression of change) endpoints as coprimaries. The ADAS Cog endpoint measures patients' cognitive functions, while the CIBIC endpoint measures patients' deficits in activities of daily living. For proving a claim of a clinically meaningful treatment benefit for this disease, it is generally required to demonstrate statistically significant treatment benefit on each of these two primary endpoints (called coprimary endpoints). If we denote H_1 as the null hypothesis of no effect in terms of the ADAS Cog and H_2 as the null hypothesis of no effect in terms of CIBIC, then the hypothesis testing for the efficacy claim in the clinical trial can be expressed as (7.2). Intersection-union testing (IUT) will be discussed in the context of coprimary endpoints.

Of course, there can be a mixture of UIT and IUT. For instance, as a combination of Example 1.1 and Example 1.2, suppose this dose-finding trial has $K = 2$ dose levels and a placebo. For each dose level, the efficacy claim is based on the coprimary endpoints, ADAS Cog and CIBIC.

Familywise Error Rate

Familywise Error Rate (FWER) is the maximum (sup) probability of falsely rejecting H_o under all possible null hypothesis configurations:

$$FWER = \sup_{H_o} P\left(\text{rejecting } H_o\right). \tag{7.3}$$

In intersection-union testing, a null hypothesis configuration can be just a combination of some H_i $(i = 1, ..., K)$.

TABLE 7.1

Error Inflation Due to Correlations between Endpoints.

Level α_A	Level α_B	Correlation R_{AB}	FWER
		0	0.098
		0.25	0.097
0.05	0.05	0.50	0.093
		0.75	0.083
		1.00	0.050

Note: $\alpha_A = \alpha$ for endpoint A, $\alpha_A = \alpha$ for endpoint B.

The strong FWER control requires that

$$FWER = \sup_{H_o} P\,(\text{rejecting } H_o) \le \alpha. \qquad (7.4)$$

That is, strong FWER control requires that the supremum of the error rate under all possible null configurations is no more than α, the size of the test or significance level. On the other hand, the weak FWER control requires only α control under the global null hypothesis. The test procedure with strong FWER control is the focus of this chapter.

Local alpha: A local alpha is the type-I error rate allowed (often called the size of a local test) for individual H_i testing. In most hypothesis test procedures, the local α is numerically different from (smaller than) the global (familywise) α to avoid FWER inflation. Without the adjusted local α, FWER inflation usually increases as the number of tests in the family increases.

Suppose we have two primary endpoints in a two-arm, active-control, randomized trial. The efficacy of the drug will be claimed as long as one of the endpoints is statistically significant at level α. In such a scenario, the FWER will be inflated. The level of inflation is dependent on the correlation between the two test statistics (Table 7.1). The maximum error rate inflation occurs when the endpoints are independent. If the two endpoints are perfectly correlated, there is no alpha inflation. For a correlation as high as 0.75, the inflation is still larger than 0.08 for a level 0.05 test. Hence, to control the overall α, an alpha adjustment is required for each test. Similarly, to study how alpha inflation is related to the number of analyses, simulations are conducted for the two independent endpoints, A and B. The results are presented in Table 7.2. We can see that alpha is inflated from 0.05 to 0.226 with five analyses and to 0.401 with ten analyses.

Closed family: A closed family is one for which any subset intersection hypothesis involving members of the testing family is also a member of the family. For example, a closed family of three hypotheses H_1, H_2, H_3 has a total of seven members, listed as follows: H_1, H_2, H_3, $H_1 \cap H_2$, $H_2 \cap H_3$, $H_1 \cap H_3$, $H_1 \cap H_2 \cap H_3$.

Closure principle: This was developed by Marcus, et al. (1976). This principle asserts that one can ensure strong control of FWER and coherence (see

TABLE 7.2

Error Inflation Due to Different Numbers of
Endpoints.

Level α_A	Level α_B	Number of analyses	FWER
		1	0.050
		2	0.098
0.05	0.05	3	0.143
		5	0.226
		10	0.401

below) at the same time by conducting the following procedure. Test every member of the closed family using a local α-level test (here, α refers to the comparison-wise error rate, not the FWER). A hypothesis can be rejected provided (1) its corresponding test was significant at the α-level, and (2) every other hypothesis in the family that implies it has also been rejected by its corresponding α-level test.

Closed testing procedure: A test procedure is said to be closed if and only if the rejection of a particular univariate null hypothesis at an α-level of significance implies the rejection of all higher-level (multivariate) null hypotheses containing the univariate null hypothesis at the same α-level. The procedure can be described as follows (Bretz, et al., 2006):

1. Define a set of elementary hypotheses, $H_1; ...; H_K$, of interest.

2. Construct all possible $m > K$ intersection hypotheses, $H_I = \cap H_i$, $I \subseteq \{1, ..., K\}$.

3. For each of the m hypotheses find a suitable local α-level test.

4. Reject H_i at FWER α if all hypotheses H_I with $i \in I$ are rejected, each at the (local) α-level.

This procedure is not often used directly in practice. However, the closure principle has been used to derive many useful test procedures, such as those of Holm (1979), Hochberg (1988), Hommel (1988), and gatekeeping procedures.

α-exhaustive procedure: If $P (\text{Reject } H_I) = \alpha$ for every intersection hypothesis $H_I, I \subseteq \{1, ..., K\}$, the test procedure is α-exhaustive.

Partition principle: This is similar to the closed testing procedure with strong control over the familywise α-level for the null hypotheses. The partition principle allows for test procedures that are formed by partitioning the parameter space into disjointed partitions with some logical ordering. Tests of the hypotheses are carried out sequentially at different partition steps. The process of testing stops upon failure to reject a given null hypothesis for predetermined partition steps (Hsu, 1996; Dmitrienko, et al., 2010, p. 45—46). We will discuss this more later in this chapter.

Coherence and *consonance* are two interesting concepts in closed testing procedures. *Coherence* means that If hypothesis H implies H^*, then whenever

H is retained, so must be H^*. *Consonance* means whenever H is rejected, at least one of its components is rejected, too. Coherence is a necessary property of closed test procedures; consonance is desirable but not necessary. A procedure can be coherent but not consonant because of asymmetry in the hypothesis testing paradigm. When H is rejected we conclude that it is false. However, when H is retained, we do not conclude that it is true; rather, we say that there is not sufficient evidence to reject it. Multiple comparison procedures that satisfy the closure principle are always coherent but not necessarily consonant (Westfall, et al., 1999).

7.2   Union-Intersection Testing

7.2.1   Single-Step Procedure

Definition of a single-step procedure: the rejection or non-rejection of a single hypothesis does not depend on the decision on any other hypothesis. The p-values or test statistics for each individual or elementary hypotheses are statistically correlated, but that does not mean that the test procedure is not a single test procedure (See SPPM method).

Weighted Bonferroni Method
     The alpha doesn't have to be split equally among all tests. When we suspect there are different effect sizes among the different endpoints and doses, we can use the so-called weighted Bonferroni tests, for which the adjusted α and p-value are given by

$$\alpha_k = w_k \alpha. \tag{7.5}$$

If $p_k \leq \alpha_k$, reject H_{ok}.

Simes Global Testing Method
     The Simes method is a global test in which the type-I error rate is controlled for the global null hypothesis (7.1). We reject the null hypothesis H_o if

$$p_{(k)} \leq \frac{k\alpha}{K} \text{ for at least one } i = 1, ..., K, \tag{7.6}$$

where $p_{(1)} < ... < p_{(K)}$ are the ordered p-values. Therefore, the Simes method does not control FWER strongly.

Dunnett's Method
     Dunnett's method can be used for multiple comparisons of active groups against a common control group, which is often done in clinical trials with multiple parallel groups. Let n_0 and n_i $(i = 1, ..., K)$ be the sample sizes for

the control and the ith dose group; the test statistic (one-sided) is given by (Westfall, et al., 1999, p. 77)

$$T = \max_i \frac{\bar{y}_i - \bar{y}_0}{\sigma\sqrt{1/n_i + 1/n_0}}, \tag{7.7}$$

The multivariate t-distribution of T in (7.7) is called one-sided Dunnett distribution with $v = \sum_{i=1}^{K+1}(n_i - 1)$ degrees of freedom. For a balanced design, the correlation between the pairwise statistics of pairwise comparisons is $\rho = 0.5$. For larger sample size, the critical values can be calculated using the following R code for the two active groups?

```
library(mvtnorm)
alpha=0.025; rho=0.5; s=matrix(c(1,rho, rho, 1), 2,2)
qmvnorm(1-alpha, mean=rep(0,2), sigma = s, tail = "lower")
```

Examples of critical values for a large trial with a balanced design are given in Table 7.3.

TABLE 7.3
Critical Value for Dunnett's Test with Equal Size.

Number of Active Groups, K						
1	2	3	4	5	6	7
1.960	2.212	2.349	2.442	2.512	2.567	2.613

Note: one-sided $\alpha = 0.025$ with a large sample assumption.

Fisher-Combination Test

To test the global null hypothesis $H_o = \cap_{i=1}^{K} H_{oi}$, the Fisher combination statistic can be used:

$$\chi^2 = -2\sum_{i=1}^{K} \ln(p_i), \tag{7.8}$$

where p_i is the p-value for testing H_{oi}. When H_{oi} is true, p_i is uniformly distributed over $[0,1]$. Furthermore, if the p_i ($i = 1, ..., K$) are independent, the test statistic χ^2 is distributed as a chi-square statistic with $2K$ degrees of freedom. Thus H_o is rejected if $\chi^2 \geq \chi^2_{2K,1-\alpha}$. Note that if the p_i are not independent or H_o is not true (e.g., one of the H_{oi} is not true), then χ^2 is not necessarily a chi-square distribution. The test procedure does not control FWER.

7.2.2 Stepwise Procedures

Stepwise procedures are different from single-step procedures in the sense that a stepwise procedure must follow a specific order to test each hypothesis. There are four categories of stepwise procedures which are dependent on how the stepwise tests proceed: fixed-sequence, stepup, stepdown, and fallback procedures.

Stepdown Procedure

A stepdown procedure starts with the most significant p-value and ends with the least significant. In this procedure, the p-values are arranged in ascending order,

$$p_{(1)} \leq p_{(2)} \leq \cdots \leq p_{(K)}, \tag{7.9}$$

with the corresponding hypotheses

$$H_{(1)}, H_{(2)}, ..., H_{(K)}.$$

The test proceeds from $H_{(1)}$ to $H_{(K)}$. If $p_{(k)} > C_k \alpha$ $(k = 1, ..., K)$, retain all $H_{(i)}$ $(i \geq k)$; otherwise, reject $H_{(k)}$ and continue to test $H_{(k+1)}$. The critical values C_k are different for different procedures.

Stepup Procedure

A stepup procedure starts with the least significant p-value and ends with the most significant p-value. The procedure proceeds from $H_{(K)}$ to $H_{(1)}$. If, $P_{(k)} \leq C_k \alpha$ $(k = 1, ..., K)$, reject all $H_{(i)}$ $(i \leq k)$; otherwise, retain $H_{(k)}$ and continue to test $H_{(k-1)}$.

Hochberg stepup

The critical values C_k for the *Hochberg stepup procedure* are $C_k = K - k + 1$ $(k = 1, .., K)$. The procedure controls FWER when the test statistic is non-negatively correlated, but it is a little conservative when p-values are independent (Westfall et al., 1999, p. 33).

Fixed-Sequence Test

This is a stepdown procedure using a predetermined order of hypotheses:

$$H_1, H_2, ..., H_K.$$

The test proceeds from H_1 to H_K. If $p_k > \alpha$ $(k = 1, ..., K)$, retain all H_i $(i \geq k)$. Otherwise, reject H_k and continue to test H_{k+1}.

Holm Stepdown Procedure

Suppose there are K hypothesis tests H_i $(i = 1, ..., K)$. The Holm stepdown procedure (Holm 1979, Dmitrienko et al., 2010) can be outlined as follows:

Step 1. If $p_{(1)} \leq \alpha/K$, reject $H_{(1)}$ and go to the next step; otherwise retain all hypotheses and stop.

Step i $(i = 2, ..., K - 1)$. If $p_{(i)} \leq \alpha/(K - i + 1)$, reject $H_{(i)}$ and go to the next step; otherwise retain $H_{(i)}, ..., H_{(K)}$ and stop.

Step K. If $p_{(K)} \leq \alpha$, reject $H_{(K)}$; otherwise retain $H_{(K)}$.

Hommel (Stepup) Procedure

Step 1: If $p_{(m)} > \alpha$, accept $H_{(m)}$ and go to Step 2; otherwise reject all null hypotheses and stop.

Step $i = 2, ..., m - 1$: If $p_{(m-i+j)} > j\alpha/i$ for all $j = 1, ..., i$, accept $H_{(m-i+j)}$ and go to Step $i + 1$; otherwise reject all remaining null hypotheses $H_{(j)}$ with $p_{(j)} \leq \alpha/(i - 1)$ and stop.

Step m: If $p_{(j)} > j\alpha/m$ for all $j = 1, ..., m$, accept $H_{(1)}$; otherwise reject $H_{(1)}$ if $p_{(1)} \leq \alpha/(m - 1)$.

Three-Hypothesis Testing

The procedure is simplified as follows:

Step 1: If $p_{(3)} > \alpha$, accept $H_{(3)}$ and go to Step 2; otherwise reject all null hypotheses and stop.

Step 2: If $p_{(2)} > \alpha/2$, accept $H_{(2)}$ and go to Step 3; otherwise reject all remaining null hypotheses and stop.

Step 3: If (1) $\alpha/2 < p_{(2)} \leq 2\alpha/3$ and $p_{(1)} \leq \alpha/2$ or (2) $p_{(1)} \leq \alpha/3$, reject $H_{(1)}$; otherwise, accept $H_{(1)}$.

Hochberg's procedure is uniformly more powerful than Holm's procedure and Hommel's procedure is uniformly more powerful than Hochberg's procedure (Dmitrienko, Tamhane, Bretz, 2010, p.67). Stepup Dunnett procedure is uniformly more powerful than Hochberg and single-step Dunnett procedure. Stepup Dunnett procedure is not always more powerful than stepdown Dunnett procedure follow standard cite method: (Dmitrienko, 2013).

Fallback Procedure

The Holm procedure is based on a data-driven order of testing, while the fixed-sequence procedure is based on a prefixed order of testing. A compromise between them is the fallback procedure introduced by Wiens (2003) and further studied by Wiens and Dmitrienko (2005) and Hommel and Bretz (2008). The test procedure can be outlined as follows:

Suppose hypotheses H_i $(i = 1, ..., K)$ are ordered according to (7.10). We allocate the overall error rate α among the hypotheses according to their weights w_i, where $w_i \geq 0$ and $\sum_i w_i = 1$. For fixed-sequence test, $w_1 = 1$ and $w_2 = ... = w_K = 0$.

(1) Test H_1 at $\alpha_1 = \alpha w_1$. If $p_1 \leq \alpha_1$, reject this hypothesis; otherwise retain it. Go to the next step.

(2) Test H_i at $\alpha_i = \alpha_{i-1} + \alpha w_i$ $(i = 2, ..., K - 1)$ if H_{i-1} is rejected and at $\alpha_i = \alpha w_i$ if H_{i-1} is retained. If $p_i \leq \alpha_i$, reject H_i; otherwise retain it. Go to the next step.

(3) Test H_K at $\alpha_K = \alpha_{K-1} + \alpha w_K$ if H_{K-1} is rejected and at $\alpha_K = \alpha w_K$ if H_{K-1} is retained. If $p_K \leq \alpha_K$, reject H_K; otherwise retain it.

7.2.3   Single-Step Progressive Parametric Procedure

Single-step progressive parametric multiple (SPPM) testing is a special single-step but powerful test method for multiple testing problems with normal endpoint, proposed by Chang, Deng, Balser (2017) and Deng and Chang (2018). Their methods are based on the idea that to construct a powerful multiple testing procedure, three issues need to be considered: (1) α-exhaustive status; (2) synergized strength of data for local hypothesis or marginal p-values, and (3) ability to use correlations between local test statistics or local p-values.

The test procedure is described as follows, but the derivations will be presented later.

For a two-hypothesis union-intersection test (UIT):

$$H_o : H_1 \cap H_2 \text{ versus } H_a : \bar{H}_1 \cup \bar{H}_2$$

where $\bar{H}_i$ is the negation of H_i. The decision rules are as follows:

$$\begin{cases} \text{If } p_1 p_2 \leq \alpha_1 \text{ and } p_1 \leq \alpha_0, \text{ reject } H_1, \text{ otherwise retain } H_1. \\ \text{If } p_1 p_2 \leq \alpha_2 \text{ and } p_2 \leq \alpha_0, \text{ reject } H_2, \text{ otherwise retain } H_2. \\ \text{If only if } H_1 \text{ or } H_2 \text{ is rejected, } H_o \text{ will be rejected.} \end{cases} \quad (7.10)$$

p_k is the univariate local p-value for H_k, and the critical values α_1 and α_2 can be determined through the exhaustion of the FWER.

The idea is that the totality of the evidence against H_o should be considered in rejecting any of the hypotheses H_i. If the evidences against H_1 and H_2 are consistent (e.g., pointed two the same directions), then any of the H_i should should have less chance to be rejected. If the evidences against H_1 and H_2 are conflicting (e.g., pointed two different directions), then any of the H_i should be less chance to be rejected.

According to the closure principle, a hypothesis is rejected if all intersection hypotheses containing this hypothesis are rejected, and testing each intersection hypothesis using a local α-level can strongly control the FWER.

$$\begin{cases} \Pr(\text{reject } H_1 | H_1) = \Pr\left(p_1 p_2 \leq \alpha_1 \cap p_1 \leq \alpha_0 | H_1\right) = \alpha \\ \Pr(\text{reject } H_2 | H_2) = \Pr\left(p_1 p_2 \leq \alpha_2 \cap p_2 \leq \alpha_0 | H_1\right) = \alpha \\ \Pr(\text{reject } H_1 \text{ or } H_2 | H_0) = \Pr(p_1 p_2 \leq \min(\alpha_1, \alpha_2) \cap \\ \max(p_1, p_2) \leq \alpha_0 | H_0) = \alpha \end{cases} \quad (7.11)$$

For independent and uniform p under H_0, (7.11) leads to $\alpha_0 = \alpha$ and

$$\alpha_1 + \alpha_1 \ln \frac{\alpha}{\alpha_1} + \alpha_2 + \alpha_2 \ln \frac{\alpha}{\alpha_2} - \alpha^2 = \alpha, \ \alpha^2 \leq \min(\alpha_1, \alpha_2) \leq \alpha \quad (7.12)$$

By choosing $\alpha_1 = \alpha_2$, (7.12) can be simplified as

$$2\left(\alpha_1 + \alpha_1 \ln \frac{\alpha}{\alpha_1}\right) - \alpha^2 = \alpha. \quad (7.13)$$

The critical values α_1 and α_2 for a given α can be determined using (7.12): (1) choose α_1 so that $\alpha^2 \leq \alpha_1 \leq \alpha$, (2) solve (7.12) for α_2. When p_i, $(i = 1, 2, ...K)$ are correlated numerical integration or simulations have to be used to determine the critical values (Deng and Chang, 2018). Table 7.4

TABLE 7.4

Critical Values α_1 (α_2) for One-sided Two-Hypothesis Testing.

ρ	$\alpha = 0.025$	$\alpha = 0.05$	ρ	$\alpha = 0.025$	$\alpha = 0.05$
0	0.004855	0.01010	0.45	0.002035	0.00546
0.05	0.004465	0.00947	0.50	0.001825	0.00508
0.10	0.004085	0.00888	0.55	0.001635	0.00472
0.15	0.003735	0.00831	0.60	0.001465	0.00439
0.20	0.003395	0.00776	0.65	0.001305	0.00408
0.25	0.003085	0.00725	0.70	0.001175	0.00380
0.30	0.002785	0.00676	0.75	0.001055	0.00353
0.35	0.002515	0.00630	0.80	0.000945	0.00329
0.40	0.002265	0.00587	0.85	0.000845	0.00306

Note: $\alpha_0 = \alpha$. e.g., for $\alpha = 0.025$ and $\rho = 0.05$, $\alpha_1 = \alpha_2 = 0.004465$.

gives examples of critical values for the two-hypothesis UIT with $\alpha_1 = \alpha_2$ and ρ is the correlation between the two normal test statistics.

For three-hypothesis UIT, the SPPM's procedure is defined as:

$$\begin{cases} p_1 p_2 p_3 \leq \alpha_4 \cap p_1 p_2 \leq \alpha_1 \cap p_1 p_3 \leq \alpha_1 \cap p_1 \leq \alpha, \text{ reject } H_1 \\ p_1 p_2 p_3 \leq \alpha_4 \cap p_2 p_3 \leq \alpha_2 \cap p_2 p_1 \leq \alpha_2 \cap p_2 \leq \alpha, \text{ reject } H_2 \\ p_1 p_2 p_3 \leq \alpha_4 \cap p_3 p_1 \leq \alpha_3 \cap p_3 p_3 \leq \alpha_3 \cap p_3 \leq \alpha, \text{ reject } H_3 \\ \text{If only if } H_1, H_2 \text{ or } H_3 \text{ is rejected, } H_o \text{ will be rejected.} \end{cases}$$

To determine the critical values α_1, α_2, α_3, and α_4, the α–exhaustive condition is applied to all null hypothesis configurations. The solution can be obtained through numerical integrations or simulations (Deng and Chang, 2018). Table 7.5 lists examples of critical values.

Table 7.5 gives examples of critical values for the two-hypothesis UIT with $\alpha_1 = 3\alpha_2$, $\alpha_1 = 5\alpha_2$, and $\alpha_1 = 10\alpha_2$.

Note that data-dependent critical values can be converted to non-data-dependent critical values because $T < c$ is equivalent to $T^* = T/c\alpha < \alpha$.

If p_1, p_2, and p_3 are mutually independent and uniformly over $[0, 1]$ under H_0 such as in a basket design and $\alpha_1 = \alpha_2 = \alpha_3$, then

$$\begin{cases} 2\alpha_1 \left(1 - \ln \frac{\alpha}{\alpha_1}\right) = \alpha + \alpha^2 \\ \alpha_4 \left(\left(1 + \ln \frac{\alpha_1}{\alpha_4}\right)^2 + 1\right) - \alpha_1 (2\alpha - \alpha_1) - \frac{\alpha_1^2}{\alpha} = \frac{\alpha}{3}(1 - \alpha^2) \end{cases} \quad (7.14)$$

From Eq (7.14) α_1 and α_4 can be solved sequentially for a given α.

R-Code for numerical integrations is provided in Appendix 12.5 for calculations of the critical values beyond those in Tables 7.4 through 7.6. When the correlations between the test statistics are unknown, the observed correlation can be used without any meaningful inflation of α as long as the sample size is larger than 30.

TABLE 7.5
Critical Values for Two-Hypothesis Testing with Unequal α_i.

ρ	α_1 $(3\alpha_2)$	α_1 $(5\alpha_2)$	α_1 $(10\alpha_2)$	ρ	α_1 $(3\alpha_2)$	α_1 $(5\alpha_2)$	α_1 $(10\alpha_2)$
0	.00795	.00965	.01200	0.45	.00344	.00434	.00582
0.05	.00733	.00891	.01120	0.50	.00310	.00393	.00534
0.10	.00675	.00823	.01044	0.55	.00280	.00355	.00491
0.15	.00617	.00760	.00967	0.60	.00252	.00323	.00442
0.20	.00562	.00695	.00897	0.65	.00227	.00292	.00402
0.25	.00513	.00636	.00830	0.70	.00205	.00264	.00363
0.30	.00466	.00580	.00763	0.75	.00184	.00238	.00326
0.35	.00422	.00525	.00698	0.80	.00166	.00216	.00295
0.40	.00382	.00479	.00639	0.85	.00151	.00193	.00264

Note: one-sided $\alpha = 0.025$. 100,000,000 simulations per scenario.

TABLE 7.6
Critical Values of Three Hypothesis Testing.

ρ	α_1	α_4	ρ	α_1	α_4
0	0.004855	0.0026778	0.45	0.002035	0.0004686
0.05	0.004465	0.0023174	0.50	0.001825	0.0003642
0.10	0.004085	0.0020055	0.55	0.001635	1.0000000
0.15	0.003735	0.0016730	0.60	0.001465	1.0000000
0.20	0.003395	0.0014100	0.65	0.001305	1.0000000
0.25	0.003085	0.0011417	0.70	0.001175	1.0000000
0.30	0.002785	0.0009502	0.75	0.001055	1.0000000
0.35	0.002515	0.0007560	0.80	0.000945	1.0000000
0.40	0.002265	0.0005972	0.85	0.000845	1.0000000

Note: one-sided $\alpha = 0.025, \alpha_1 = \alpha_2 = \alpha_3$.

The SPPM testing procedure takes into account the correlation among test statistics to control the FWER. For a multiple-arm trial with a common control, the correlation coefficient $\rho = \sqrt{\frac{n}{N}}$. However, in general, correlation is unknown, but can also be estimated with the sample data. The question is will the FWER be inflated? Deng and Xuan (2018) show that the impact on the FWER is negligible Table 7.7).

7.2.4   Power Comparison of Multiple Testing Methods

Power comparisons of various testing procedures for two-hypothesis test- ing are summarized in Table 7.8 and three-hypothesis testing in Table 7.9.

Tables 7.8 and 7.6 demonstrate that equal [Greek alpha symbol] SPPM is more powerful when the effects corresponding to different hypotheses are consistently pointing to the same positive directions, reflecting a larger totality of evidences. Parameter values that indicate different directions for alternative hypotheses mean that a smaller totality a smaller totality of evidence against

TABLE 7.7
FWER of SPPM Using Estimated Correlation.

Correlation	N=30	N=90	N=180
0.00	0.024	0.024	0.025
0.25	0.025	0.025	0.024
0.50	0.024	0.024	0.025
0.75	0.024	0.024	0.026

H_0, SPPM will be less powerful. When the parameters in the alternative hypotheses (e.g., effects of the different endpoints) are very different, we should use different α_1, α_2, and α_3 such that their trend is opposite to the trend of parameters in the alternative hypotheses. In most of the situations presented in Tables 7.8 and 7.9, SPPM clearly provides a power advantage. In SPPM rejection a hypothesis is based on the totality of evidence, that is, the rejection will depend on the evidences (p-values) against all hypotheses. Therefore, the combination of evidences must be clinically meaningful, such as when the tests are for multiple endpoints for same disease, the multiple doses for same drug, or the same drug with the same mechanism of action for different indications (e.g., cancers). In the stepwise procedure, the rejections of hypotheses in the downstream of the testing procedure will depend on the evidences against previous hypotheses. Therefore, the same clinical meaningfulness is required.

7.2.5 Application to Armodafinil Trial

Armodafinil is a small molecule with a 273.35 molecular weight. It is a white to off-white, crystalline powder that is slightly soluble in water, sparingly soluble in acetone, and soluble in methanol. Armodafinil was developed as a wakefulness-promoting agent for oral administration, though the mechanism of action is not clear.

This randomized, placebo-controlled study was conducted to compare the overnight efficacy and plasma concentration-time profiles of armodafinil (250, 200, and 150 mg) in patients with chronic shift work sleep disorder (SWSD). The primary endpoint was the change in multiple sleep latency test (MSLT) from the baseline to the last visit. MSLT is an objective assessment of sleepiness that measures the likelihood of falling asleep. The details of this trial can be found at https://clinicaltrials.gov. The three individual hypotheses might be of interest:

$$H_i : \mu_i - \mu_c = 0 \ vs : \bar{H}_i : \mu_i - \mu_c > 0, \qquad (7.15)$$

where i ($i = 1, 2, 3$) and μ_c are the true means of the change in MSLT from baseline in 250, 200, 150 mg, and the placebo groups, respectively. The procedure dealing with the multiple testing is required and parametric testing procedure could be potentially more powerful by utilizing the correlation among the test statistics. The measurements of change in MSLT from baseline and

TABLE 7.8
Power Comparisons for Two-Hypothesis Testing.

ρ	Method	μ_1/μ_2 0.0/0.3	0.15/0.3	0.2/0.3	0.3/0.3
0.0	Bonferroni		0.784	0.829	0.927
	Fallback		0.784	0.829	0.927
	Hommel		0.792	0.838	0.934
	Dunnett Stepup		0.792	0.838	0.934
	SPPM^E		0.844	**0.891**	**0.963**
	SPPM^U		**0.853**	0.887	0.953
0.25	Bonferroni		0.762	0.798	0.898
	Fallback		0.762	0.798	0.898
	Hommel		0.769	0.807	0.906
	Dunnett Stepup		0.769	0.808	0.906
	SPPM^E		0.795	0.847	**0.938**
	SPPM^U		**0.825**	**0.855**	0.923
0.5	Bonferroni		0.744	0.769	0.866
	Fallback		0.744	0.769	0.866
	Hommel		0.749	0.778	0.875
	Dunnett Stepup		0.754	0.782	0.877
	SPPM^E		0.737	0.795	**0.903**
	SPPM^U		**0.794**	**0.821**	0.885
0.75	Bonferroni		0.732	0.742	0.824
	Fallback		0.732	0.742	0.824
	Hommel		0.735	0.749	0.838
	Dunnett Stepup		0.751	0.763	0.847
	SPPM^E		0.672	0.737	**0.861**
	SPPM^U		**0.787**	**0.809**	0.858

Notes: one-sided $\alpha = 0.025$, $\sigma = 1$, $N = 90$.
SPPM^E with $\alpha_1 = \alpha_2$, SPPM^U with $10\alpha_1 = \alpha_2$.

one-sided p-values for the comparisons between treatment and placebo groups are in Table 7.10. The pooled estimate for variance as 19 was used (p-value from the Bartlett's test is 0.559). The correlation matrix of the test statistics is determined by sample size and is:

$$\sum = \begin{bmatrix} 1 & 0.499 & 0.499 \\ 0.499 & 1 & 0.479 \\ 0.499 & 0.479 & 1 \end{bmatrix}$$

Therefore, the equal pairwise correlation as 0.48 is assumed in this case for the simplicity. The critical values using the SPPM procedure are: $\alpha_1 = \alpha_2 = \alpha_3 = 0.00191$ and $\alpha_4 = 0.000406$ for one-sided test significance level as 0.025.

Using the SPPM procedure, we can reject H_1 because $p_1 p_2 p_3 = 3.1610^{-5} < \alpha_4$, $p_1 p_2 = 0.00031 < \alpha_1$, $p_1 p_3 = 0.00162 < \alpha_1$, and $p_1 < \alpha$; we cannot reject H_2 because $p_2 p_3 = 0.00199 > 2$; and we cannot reject H_3 because $p_3 > \alpha$.

TABLE 7.9

Power Comparisons for Three-Hypothesis Testing.

ρ	Method	μ_1/μ_2 0.03/0.3	0.2/0.3	0.1/0.2	0.1/0.1	0.3/0.3
0.0	Hommel	0.733	0.787	0.608	0.531	0.869
	Dunnett Stepup	0.728	0.781	0.602	0.528	0.862
	SPPM^E	0.774	0.883	0.696	0.595	0.941
	SPPM^U	0.786	0.865	0.721	0.657	0.917
0.25	Hommel	0.689	0.729	0.565	0.505	0.808
	Dunnett Stepup	0.689	0.726	0.567	0.510	0.805
	SPPM^E	0.666	0.798	0.593	0.511	0.876
	SPPM^U	0.700	0.794	0.659	0.609	0.850
0.5	Hommel	0.646	0.671	0.528	0.485	0.743
	Dunnett Stepup	0.658	0.680	0.544	0.502	0.750
	SPPM^E	0.551	0.706	0.504	0.431	0.798
	SPPM^U	0.609	0.722	0.599	0.561	0.778
0.75	Hommel	0.601	0.612	0.495	0.472	0.671
	Dunnett Stepup	0.634	0.642	0.534	0.516	0.698
	SPPM^E	0.445	0.619	0.439	0.392	0.716
	SPPM^U	0.514	0.657	0.545	0.516	0.700

Notes: SPPM^E with $\alpha_1 = \alpha_2 = \alpha_3$, SPPM^U with $\alpha_1 = \alpha_2 = 10\alpha_3$; one-sided $\alpha = 0.025$, $\mu_3 = 0.3$, $\sigma = 1$. $N = 60$.

We now study the results when 8 different test procedures are applied to the data.

(1) Weighted Bonferroni Procedure

Suppose we suspect the high dose may be more toxic than the low dose. Unless the high dose is more efficacious than the low dose, we will choose the low dose as the target dose. For this reason, we want to spend more alpha in the low-dose comparison than in the high-dose comparison. Specifically, we choose one-sided significance levels $\alpha_1 = 0.01$, $\alpha_2 = 0.008$, and $\alpha_3 = 0.007$ ($\alpha_1 + \alpha_2 + \alpha_3 = \alpha$), which will be used to compare p_1, p_2, and p_3, respectively, for rejecting or accepting the corresponding hypotheses. Since $p_1 = 0.016 >$

TABLE 7.10

Multiple Latency Test Change from Baseline in Five Groups.

	Armodafinil 250 mg/Day	200 mg/Day	150 mg/Day	Placebo
Number of Subjects	27	23	23	25
MSLT: Mean (SD)	3.7 (4.33)	3.7 (5.07)	2.7 (4.24)	1.1 (3.76)
p-value	0.016	0.020	0.102	-

Note: p-values for comparisons between armodafinil and placebo.

α_1, $p_2 = 0.020 > \alpha_2$, and $p_3 = 0.102 > \alpha_3$, we cannot reject any of the hypotheses. If we unweighted Bonferroni test with $\alpha_1 = \alpha_2 = \alpha_3 = \alpha/3 = 0.025/3 = 0.00833$, the conclusion will be the same.

(2) Dunnett's Procedure

It is approximately a balanced design, the critical value 3+1 arm design is $c_\alpha = 2.349$ (Table 7.3) or $\alpha_D = 0.0094$ on p-scale. Since p_1, p_2, and $p_3 > \alpha_D$, we cannot reject any of the hypotheses.

(3) Fisher's Combination Method

This method usually requires independent p-values; otherwise, the test may be on the conservative or liberal side. However, for illustrating the calculation procedure, let's pretend the p-values are independent. From (7.8), we can calculate the χ-square value: $\chi^2 = -2\ln((0.016)(0.020)(0.102)) = 20.660$ with 6 degrees of freedom. The corresponding p-value is $0.0021 < \alpha$. Thus, the global null hypothesis is rejected and conclude at least one hypothesis is not true, but we don't know which one.

(4) Hochberg's Stepup Procedure

Since $p_{(3)} = 0.102 > \alpha = 0.025$, H_3 cannot be rejected; $p_{(2)} = 0.020 > \alpha/2 = 0.0125$, H_2 cannot be rejected either; $p_{(1)} = 0.016 > \alpha/3 = 0.00833$, H_3 cannot be rejected either.

(5) Fixed-Sequence Procedure

Since a higher dose usually has a high efficacy response, we may fix test sequence as H_1, H_2, H_3 before we see the data. Since $p_{(1)} = 0.016 < \alpha$, we reject H_1. Similarly, $p_{(2)} = 0.02 < \alpha$, H_2 is also rejected. However, since $p_{(3)} = 0.102 > \alpha$, H_3 cannot be rejected.

(6) Holm's Stepup Procedure

In this example, , the procedure and conclusion are identical Hochberg's stepup procedure.

(7) Hommel's Stepup Procedure

H_1 and H_2 cannot be rejected since the rejection criteria are the same as Holm procedure. For H_3, we need to check the condition if $\alpha/2 < p_2 < 2\alpha/3$ and $p_1 \leq \alpha/2$. The condition does not meet the criterion because $p_2 = 0.02 > \frac{2}{3}\alpha = 0.0167$. Thus, none of the hypotheses can be rejected.

(8) Fallback Procedure

Choose equal weights $w_i = 1/K = 1/3$. $\alpha_1 = \alpha/3 = 0.00833$, $\alpha_2 = \alpha_1 + \alpha/3 = 0.0167$, and $\alpha_3 = \alpha_2 + \alpha/3 = \alpha = 0.025$. Since $p_1 = 0.016 > \alpha_1$, $p_2 = 0.020 > \alpha_2$, and $p_3 = 0.102 > \alpha_3$, none of the three hypotheses can be rejected.

7.3   Intersection-Union Testing

7.3.1   Need for Coprimary Endpoints

Multiple endpoints are often used as co-primary endpoints in clinical trials for the purpose of assessing different aspects of a treatment to gain a comprehensive picture of the treatment effect for an indication. For example, when assessing treatment effect in patients with osteoarthritis of the knee and hip, usually three endpoints – patient global assessment of disease status, pain, and functionality, are used. In order to support the treatment claim, all the endpoints should be able to provide evidence of efficacy. Therefore, it is not appropriate to base a claim on one endpoint that could show statistical significance at a stringent level after certain multiplicity adjustments (Li, 2009; Li and Huque, 2003). The requirement of coprimary endpoints is carried from (1) lack of a consensus on a single most important efficacy endpoint, and (2) diseases with no clear aetiology. The combined chance of missing the efficacy criteria on individual endpoints, under the IUT approach could lead to a lower success probability even if the new treatment is indeed effective on all the co-primary endpoints (Chuang-Stein et al, 2007).

7.3.2   Conventional Approach

Because coprimary endpoints issues are IUT, to control FWER, the decision rules are: reject H_0 if the p-vlaue p_i for every individual hypothesis is less than or equal to α, the significance level; otherwise retain H_o. That is,

$$\text{If } p_i \leq \alpha \text{ for } i = 1, 2, ..., K, \text{ then reject } H_0. \tag{7.16}$$

IUT is also called reverse multiplicity problem. The regulatory position on the reverse multiplicity problem is that there is no need to adjust the individual significance levels downwards, neither is upward adjustment accepted (Chuang-Stein, et al, 2007).

The requirement to show statistical significance on all the coprimary endpoints results in low power, especially as the number of coprimary endpoints increases. It is inefficient to make up for the reduction in the study power by increasing the sample size. The reduction of power gets worse for IUT as the number of tests, K, increases and/as the number of tests, K, and/or the correlation p between statistics increases (Table 7.11). A solution to the reverse multiplicity problem is to reduce the multiple coprimary endpoints to a single primary endpoint. This includes creating a composite measure or declaring one endpoint to be the single primary endpoint. For diseases where the dimensions of the coprimary endpoints cannot be reduced, statistical solutions are needed to address the needed balance between type I error rate and study power.

TABLE 7.11

Power of K Coprimary Endpoints.

ρ	K						
	1	2	3	4	5	8	10
0.0	0.900	0.810	0.729	0.656	0.590	0.430	0.349
0.2	0.900	0.820	0.747	0.688	0.636	0.516	0.456
0.5	0.900	0.835	0.782	0.741	0.708	0.633	0.597
0.7	0.900	0.849	0.810	0.783	0.761	0.712	0.689
0.9	0.900	0.871	0.850	0.837	0.827	0.794	0.795

Note: From numerical integration using mvtnorm in R.

The typical R-code of numerical integrations for generating the powers in Table 7.11 is presented below:

```
library(mvtnorm)
N=131; u=0.4005*sqrt(N/2); rho=0.2
s=matrix(c(1,rho, rho, 1), 2,2)
Power= pmvnorm(lower=rep(1.96, 2), upper=rep(Inf, 2), mean=rep(u, 2),
sigma=s)
```

7.3.3 Average Error Method

Chuang-Stein, et al (2007) proposed an approach to control the average type I error rate over all possible null configurations.

Denote by δ_1 and δ_2 the effect sizes for the two coprimary normal endpoints; the three type-I error rates, corresponding critical value α^*, under the three null configurations are:

$$\begin{cases} \sup_{-\infty < \delta_2 < \infty} \Pr(p_1 \leq \alpha^* | \delta_1 = 0, \delta_2) = \Pr(p_1 \leq \alpha^* | 0, \infty) \\ \sup_{-\infty < \delta_1 < \infty} \Pr(p_1 \leq \alpha^* | \delta_1 = 0, \delta_2) = \Pr(p_1 \leq \alpha^* | \infty, 0) \\ \sup_{\delta_1 \leq 0, \delta_2 \leq 0} \Pr(p_1 \leq \alpha^* | \delta_1 = 0, \delta_2) = \Pr(p_1 \leq \alpha^*, p_2 \leq \alpha^* | 0, 0) \end{cases} \quad (7.17)$$

Therefore, the critical value α^* for two coprimary endpoints can be obtained by solving the following equation:

$$\frac{1}{3}(\Pr(p_1 \leq \alpha^* | 0, \infty) + \Pr(p_1 \leq \alpha^* | \infty, 0) + \Pr(p_1 \leq \alpha^*, p_2 \leq \alpha^* | 0, 0)) = \alpha \quad (7.18)$$

That is,

$$\frac{1}{3}(2\Pr(p_1 \leq \alpha^* | 0, \infty) + \Pr(p_1 \leq \alpha^*, p_2 \leq \alpha^* | 0, 0)) = \alpha \quad (7.19)$$

Similarly, for three coprimary endpoints there are 7 null configurations.

TABLE 7.12

Critical Values for Average Error Method.

Correlation	Number of Coprimary Endpoints			
ρ	2	3	4	5
0	0.036	0.055	0.082	0.121
0.2	0.036	0.052	0.075	0.106
0.4	0.035	0.048	0.066	0.089
0.6	0.032	0.043	0.055	0.070
0.8	0.030	0.037	0.044	0.052

Note: One-sided $\alpha = 0.025$.

Thus, the critical value α^* can be obtained by solving the following equation:

$$\frac{1}{7}(3\Pr(p_1 \leq \alpha^*|0,\infty,\infty) + 3\Pr(p_1 \leq \alpha^*|0,0,\infty)$$
$$+ \Pr(p_1 \leq \alpha^*, p_2 \leq \alpha^*|0,0,0)) = \alpha \qquad (7.1)$$

The power is, for given δ_1 and δ_2,

$$Power = \Pr(p_1 \leq \alpha^*, p_2 \leq \alpha^*|\delta_1, \delta_2). \qquad (7.21)$$

7.3.4 Li's and Huque's Method

Li-Huque's method used to derive the decision rules for coprimary endpoint evaluation is similar to the one developed by Li (2009) and Li and Huque (2003) for the purpose of evaluating multiple independently conducted studies. Here the method is extended to the evaluation of multiple dependent (correlated) coprimary endpoints as described as described in Table 7.12.

Ordering the p-values for the K individual hypotheses, we obtain $p_{(1)} \leq p_{(2)} \leq \cdots \leq p_{(K)}$. An overall null H_0 is rejected if

$$p_{(1)} \leq \gamma_1, \; p_{(2)} \leq \gamma_2, ..., p_{(K)} \leq \gamma_K \qquad (7.22)$$

where the constant vector $(\gamma_1, \gamma_2, ..., \gamma_K)$ is called a decision rule (or p-value cutpoints) with the order of $\gamma_1 \leq \gamma_2 \leq ... \leq \gamma_K \leq 1$. The decision rule should satisfy the following probability inequality:

$$FWER = \Pr\left(p_{(1)} \leq \gamma_1, \; p_{(2)} \leq \gamma_2, ..., p_{(K)} \leq \gamma_K\right) \leq \alpha. \qquad (7.23)$$

In determining the decision rule, Li and Huque propose to control the error rate under the global null (i.e., all hypothesis H_i ($i = 1, 2, ..., H_K$) are true) at α level. However, they argue that the impact of making a false rejection will be different in different situations (null configurations). For example, For example, if we claim drug efficacy when a drug has no effect on any of the endpoints, the impact of such false claim is larger than the impact of a false positive claim when drug has effects on all endpoints except one. Therefore, we should control the impact of the errors and give a larger α when the drug is effective on some of the endpoints. Li and Huque suggested one-sided $\alpha = 0.025$ when the global null $H^{1/K}$ is true and 0.07 when the drug has no effect only on one endpoint, $H^{K/K}$.

The decision rules can be derived using simulations: generate the p-values for the individual endpoints based on the standardized multivariate normal distribution . By moving the correlation parameters from -1 to 1 in small increments, the simulation covers all possible correlation matrices which are positive-defined (see Table 1 in Li and Huque, 2003).

TABLE 7.13
Critical Values for Li-Huque Method.

Number of Primary Endpoints K	γ_1	γ_2	γ_3	γ_4
2	0.016	0.065		
	0.023	0.030		
	0.025	0.025		
3	0.023	0.025	0.070	
	0.024	0.025	0.030	
	0.025	0.025	0.025	
4	0.023	0.023	0.070	0.070
	0.024	0.024	0.045	0.045
	0.025	0.025	0.025	0.025

Note: Error rate ≤ 0.025 and 0.07 under $H_0^{1/K}$ and $H_0^{K/K}$.

Fallback Procedure

When efficacy of a treatment is measured by co-primary endpoints, efficacy is claimed only if for each endpoint an individual statistical test is significant at level α. While such a strategy controls the FWER, it is often strictly conservative and allows for no inference if not all null hypotheses can be rejected. Hierarchical testing allows for inference if the main objective is not met. This is sometimes desirable because, for example, when the main hypothesis for co-primary is not rejected, rejecting subset of a subset of hypotheses is valuable for publications of the research results. This approach, however, has the limitation that the co-primary endpoints need to be tested sequentially according to a pre-defined ordering. Ristl et al. (2016) proposed, for the case of two and three co-primary endpoints, fallback tests that have the same conjunctive power as the classical test for co-primary endpoints, but have a higher disjunctive power.

According to Ristl and others (2016), the Hommel test is a fallback test for coprimary endpoints because both are shortcuts of a closed test where the intersection hypotheses are tested based on the Simes inequality: An intersection of n hypotheses is rejected if $p_{(k)} \leq k\alpha/K$ for some $k = 1, \dots K$, where $p_{(k)}$ are the ordered elementary p-values. However, for multivariate normal and t-distributed test statistics, the Simes and consequently the Hommel test (which is equivalent to the Simes test in the case of two endpoints) has only been shown to be conservative for non-negative correlations but does not control the level for arbitrary correlation structures. To construct a fallback test for two coprimary endpoints that controls the type I error rate for arbitrary correlations, Ristl et al. (2016) proposed a modification of the classical Simes test. Diagonally trimmed Simes test steps for two hypotheses two hypotheses with normal test statistics with unit standard deviation, Z_1 for H_1 and Z_2 for H_2 are:

1. If $\min(Z_1, Z_2) \geq z_{1-\alpha}$, reject both H_1 and H_2.
2. If $Z_1 \geq z_{1-\alpha/2}$ and $Z_1 + Z_2 \geq 0$, reject H_1.
3. If $Z_2 \geq z_{1-\alpha/2}$ and $Z_1 + Z_2 \geq 0$, reject H_2.

For three-hypothesis testing, A 2 out of 3 fallback tests for three co-primary endpoints ($\alpha \leq 0.5$). A fallback test for three endpoints is defined by the following procedure:

1. If $\min(Z_1, Z_2, Z_3) \geq z_{1-\alpha}$, reject all elementary hypotheses H_1, H_2, H_3 and stop the procedure.
2. If there exist i, $j \in \{1, 2, 3\}$, $i \neq j$ such that $\min(Z_i, Z_j) \geq z_{1-\alpha}$, reject the intersection hypothesis $H_i \cap H_j$.
3. If $Z_i \geq z_{1-\alpha/2}$ and there exists a $j \in \{1, 2, 3\}$, $i \neq j$ such that $\min(Z_i, Z_j) \geq z_{1-\alpha}$ and $\min(Z_1, Z_2, Z_3) + Z_i \geq 0$, reject H_i.

The power to reject all null hypotheses simultaneously is called conjunctive power and the power to reject at least one elementary null hypothesis is called disjunctive power (Bretz, 2016). Fallback tests can improve the disjunctive power but not the conjunctive power over classical tests for the coprimary endpoints.

7.3.5 Application to Glaucoma Trial

This is a phase III, multi-center, randomized, double-masked study involving binocular topical application of trabodenoson ophthalmic formulation 3.0% or 6.0% once-daily (QD) or 4.5% twice-daily (BID), placebo BID, or timolol 0.5% BID for 12 weeks in adult subjects with OHT or POAG. Note, the data are simplified to provide a brief example.

All subjects who meet the study's enrollment criteria following screening will undergo washout of all prohibited medications, including their routine glaucoma medications. During the placebo run-In period, placebo (vehicle control matched to trabodenoson) is administered twice daily to both eyes in all subjects. During the treatment period, study drug is applied to both eyes for a total of 12 weeks followed by an observation period of approximately 7 days wherein no study eye drops are instilled.

Efficacy Requirement: Time-matched IOP profiling will be performed, using the 8AM, 10AM, 12PM and 4PM IOP measurement taken on the following days: baseline (Day -1), Day 14, Day 28, Day 42. The change from Baseline will be calculated for 12 posttreatment timepoints (4 timepoints on three days). Statistical significance values for all 12 timepoints were required by the regulatory agency.

The regulatory requirement to achieve significance represents an unreasonable burden. Chance alone may likely yield false negatives even when the treatment is highly effective. Given the moderate correlations of IOP between different time points and 90% power for each time point, the probability of achieving statistical significance at all time points will be approximately 53%. Therefore, the probability of observing a false negative is as high as 47%.

We must first step back to better understand the scientific question to be addressed:

1. The drug must be demonstrated to be efficacious over a sufficiently long period (significance up to 84 days).

2. The drug must be demonstrated to be efficacious during an entire day, peak and trough (significance on 8AM, 10AM, 12PM, and 4PM).

Therefore, the scientific question can be addressed in two stages:

1. To prove the first point, the mean daily IOP must be statistically significant against the control group at Day 14, Day 28, and Day 42 (demonstrating overall IOP lowering effect vs the placebo group).

2. To prove the second point mean IOP values at 8AM, 10AM, 12 noon, and 4PM should be statistically better than placebo values.

3. In addition, each individual IOP time point must demonstrate numerical separation from placebo in the right direction (directionality).

To prove Point 1, there are three hypothesis tests with a one-sided FWER of 2.5%. To prove Point 2, there are four hypothesis tests with a one-sided FWER of $\alpha = 2.5\%$. This stepwise method method exhibits more power than 12 simultaneous tests at a one-sided FWER of $\alpha = 2.5\%$.

The p-values from ranked mixed-effects models for the tests on the 3 days were $p_1 = 0.001$, $p_2 = 0.001$, $p3 = 0.001$. The p-values for the tests on the 4 timepoints are $p_4 = 0.06$, $p_5 = 0.01$, $p_6 = 0.003$, and $p_7 = 0.008$. Each individual IOP time point has demonstrated numerical separation from placebo.

Considering the classical Chuang-Stein and Li-Huque methods, it is obvious that the significance is achieved for the 3 days for all three methods. For the 4 timepoints, there are some differences. If the classical method is used, which applies $\alpha = 0.025$ to all p-values, we cannot conclude the efficacy of the drug because, $p_4 = 0.06$ for 8AM IOP was not significant. If Stein's method (considering moderate correlation $\rho = 0.6$) with $\alpha^* = 0.055$, efficacy can also not be concluded in this instance. However, if Li-Huque's method is employed with critical values for the 4 timepoints: $\gamma_1 = \gamma_2 = 0.023$, $\gamma_3 = \gamma_4 = 0.07$, the efficacy can be concluded since $p_{(1)} = p_6 = 0.003 < \gamma_1 = 0.023$, $p_{(2)} = p_7 = 0.008 < \gamma_2$, $p_{(3)} = p_5 = 0.01 < \gamma_3 = 0.07$, and $p_{(4)} = p_4 = 0.06 < \gamma_4 = 0.07$.

SAS software includes three macros useful for trial designs and power studies.

7.4 Priority Winner Test for Multiple Endpoints

Multiple endpoints are often necessary in clinical trials. For example, in a trial of treatments for HIV, therapies are compared on the basis of mortality. However, changes in the CD4 lymphocyte count can be used to measure the effect of treatment, as falling CD4 counts are highly correlated with the declining course of the disease.

For trials of therapies to prevent opportunistic infections, the primary measure of efficacy is the occurrence of infections, though HIV infected patients die of many often-undetermined causes. Ethical issues also permeate the choice of endpoints. Pediatric AIDS is a disease of long duration leading to progressive declines in growth and neurologic development gradually leading to death. The usual solution is to compare treatments on the basis of an event which is defined by a complicated combined measure of failure of therapy which includes death, the occurrence of an opportunistic infection, achieving a specified profound degree of neurologic impairment and failure to thrive. A change of therapy may be warranted for a patient who experiences such complications.

Another example in cardiovascular disease (CVD) trials is a major adverse cardiovascular (CV) event, which is the time to the first of either CV death, non-fatal stroke (stroke) or non-fatal myocardial infarction (MI). Clearly, CV death is more important than stroke. Without taking this into account, an intervention with a strong effect on stroke but no effect on CV death may appear to be preferable over an intervention with a moderate effect on both CV death and stroke (Pocock, 2012).

A composite endpoint consists of multiple endpoints combined in one outcome. Such an unweighted composite endpoint is often criticized for the equal treatment of all endpoints that are in fact of different importance. With respect to weighted multiple endpoints, Bakal et al (2015) surveyed a panel of clinical investigators to score the relative importance of components. The weights are determined, 1.0 for death, 0.5 for stroke, 0.3 for congestive heart failure, and 0.2 for recurrent myocardial infarction. Tong et al. (2012) reanalyzed the Synergy between Percutaneous Coronary Intervention with Taxus and Cardiac Surgery (SYNTAX) trial with the composite endpoint of major adverse cardiac and cerebrovascular events (death, stroke, myocardial infarction, or revascularization), based on 224 respondents on a survey. The relative weights are 0.23 for death, 0.18 for stroke, 0.14 for myocardial infarction, and 0.11 for revascularization.

Recently Finkelstein and Schoenfeld (1999) proposed a winner test and Pocock et al. (2012) introduced the win ratio test to overcome the criticism of conventional composite-endpoint method. The win-ratio method can be applied to the matched pair, unmatched pair, and the mixture case. On the estimation aspect, Oakes (2016) studied the special case of bivariate Lehmann models and showed that the win ratio does not depend on the time horizon or follow-up time. Bebu and Lachin (2016) derive a asymptotic formulation for the confidence intervals win ratio and win difference in proportions. Wang and Pocock (2016) suggested a bootstrap method for constructing the confidence interval for win ratio. Luo et al. (2015) developed a close-form variance estimator of the win ratio for the unmatched pair approach, based on a composite endpoint with two components and a specific algorithm determining winners, losers and ties. Dong et al. (2016) extend the unmatched pair approach to provide a generalized analytical solution to both hypothesis testing and confidence interval construction for the win ratio, based on its logarithmic asymptotic distribution. This asymptotic distribution is derived via U-statistics following Wei and Johnson (1985).

7.4.1   Finkelstein-Schoenfeld Method

Suppose in a two-group parallel trial with multiple endpoints, A, B, and C, there are N_T and N_C patients in treatment (T) and placebo (P) groups, respectively. The endpoint A is more important than B and B is more important than C.

The hypothesis test is defined as $H_0 : T$ does not provide a better benefit in terms of the endpoints than P versus H_a: T provides a better benefit than C.

The method starts with the construction of winning score W_{ij} between a typical subject i and a typical subject j $(i, j = 1, ..., N = N_T + N_P)$ defined by the following algorithm:

1. If subject i has a better outcome in A than subject j, then $W_{ij} = 1$;

2. If subject i has a worse outcome in A than subject j, then $W_{ij} = -1$;

3. If subject i has the same outcome in A than subject j, then further compare in endpoint B :

   (a) If subject i has a better outcome in B than subject j, then $W_{ij} = 1$;

   (b) If subject i has a worse outcome in B than subject j, then $W_{ij} = -1$;

   (c) If subject i has the same outcome in B than subject j, then further compare in endpoint C :

      i. If subject i has a better outcome in C than subject j, then $W_{ij} = 1$;

ii. If subject i has a worse outcome in C than subject j, then $W_{ij} = -1$;

iii. If subject i has the same outcome in C than subject j, then $W_{ij} = 0$;

The algorithm remains the same even if fewer or more categories are used. Only the last category with the lowest priority can have a tie with score $W_{ij} = 0$.

The sum of the winning scores for the ith subject is

$$U_i = \sum_{j=1}^{N} W_{ij} \qquad (7.24)$$

Note $W_{ii} = 0$. We sum up the total winning scores for all subjects in the test group:

$$\varsigma = \sum_{i=1}^{N} D_i U_i, \qquad (7.25)$$

where D_i is a treatment group indicator function defined as $D_i = 1$ if $i = T$ and 0 if $i = P$. The variance of T is (Finkelstein and Schoenfeld, 1999) is

$$V_\varsigma = \frac{N_T N_P}{N(N-1)} \sum_{i=1}^{N} U_i^2 \qquad (7.26)$$

The test statistic is defined as

$$Z = \frac{\varsigma}{\sqrt{V}} \sim N(\theta, 1). \qquad (7.27)$$

The test statistic Z has asymptotically a normal distribution with mean θ and standard deviation of 1. Under H_0, i.e., T and C have the same effect on all endpoints, $\theta = 0$, from which the p-value can be calculated for an observed Z value.

Patients who are heterogeneous can be grouped into different strata A_k, $(k = 1, ..., K)$ and the winning scores U_i are calculated within each stratum. Then ς statistic is calculated as

$$\varsigma = \sum_{k=1}^{K} \sum_{i \in A_k} D_i U_i, \qquad (7.28)$$

and the variance of T is

$$V_\varsigma = \sum_{k=1}^{K} \frac{n_{kT} n_{kP}}{n_k (n_k - 1)} \sum_{i \in}^{N} U_i^2, \qquad (7.29)$$

where n_{kT} and n_{kC} are the sample sizes for the groups T and P, respectively. The test statistic is the same as defined by (7.27).

When stratum A_k has only two patients, one for each group, for all $k = 1, ..., K$, the trial becomes a paired patient design. In general, (7.29) and (7.29) can be applied to mixture of paired and unpaired data. Note that the effect of ties is considered in the V_ς.

Finkelstein and Schoenfeld (1999) applied the method to ACTG 98 phase III trial that compared uconazole versus clotrimazole troches for prevention of invasive fungal infections in patients with HIV. See the original paper for details.

7.4.2 Win-Ratio Test

Pocock proposed the win-Ratio test that is based on the ratio between the total wins and total losses. The total wins for in group T is defined as

$$W = \sum_{k=1}^{K} \sum_{i \in A_k} \sum_{j=1}^{N} D_i I(W_{ij} > 0), \tag{7.30}$$

and the total losses are defined as

$$L = \sum_{k=1}^{K} \sum_{i \in A_k} \sum_{j=1}^{N} D_i I(W_{ij} < 0), \tag{7.31}$$

where I is an indication function. (7.30) and (7.31) are applicable to paired, unpaired, and mixture data.

Define win-ratio as:

$$R_w = \frac{W}{W + L} \tag{7.32}$$

Without proof, Pocock and others (Pocock et al, 2012) assume R_w follows a normal distribution and has a confidence interval:

$$R_w \pm Z_{1-\alpha/2} \left(\frac{R_w (1 - R_w)}{W + L} \right)^{1/2} \tag{7.33}$$

It follows that under H_0 and the larger sample assumption, the test statistic

$$z = \frac{R_w - 0.5}{\sqrt{\frac{R_w(1-R_w)}{W+L}}} \sim N(0,1), \tag{7.34}$$

where the value 0.5 is for the continuity correction. The p-value can be calculated as

$$p = 1 - \Phi(z). \tag{7.35}$$

We can see that the ties in W_{ij} has no effect on the test z. Recently, Dong and others (2016) modified the win ratio slightly $R_w = \frac{W}{L}$ and in log scale, $\ln R_w$ and calculated the variance $\sigma^2_{\ln R_w}$ differently to factor in the effect of ties on the variance using delta method (another approximation).

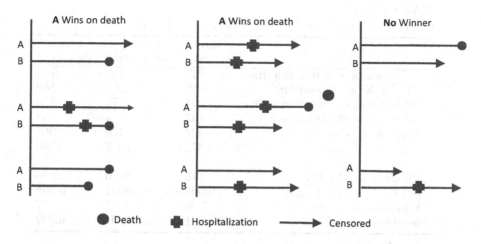

FIGURE 7.1
A diagram Illustration of scenarios for determining winner.

Win score calculation with survival data:

For survival endpoint, the determination of a winner is a little more involved (Figure 7.1).

The method has also some disadvantages: (1) it does not consider the magnitude difference, (2) it does not consider the fact that a later censoring implies a larger probability of surviving longer, and (3) an intervention can lead to a total win when in reality the win constitutes a less clinically relevant variable such as a non-fatal stroke and a loss on CV death results.

7.4.3 Application to CHARM Trial

The Child Health Advanced Records Management (CHARM) program compared candesartan with placebo in chronic heart failure,12 the three patient types being, the following (Pocock et al 2012): CHARM Added for ejection fraction, 40% and on ACE-inhibitor, CHARM Alternative for ejection fraction, 40% and intolerant to ACE-inhibitor, and CHARM Preserved for ejection fraction $\geq 40\%$.

For the composite primary endpoint, CV death, or HF hosp, the published hazard ratios (HR) with covariate adjustment are in Table 7.14. The added and alternative treatment differences are highly significant; the preserved group showed a one-sided p-value of 0.025. Win-ratio analyses were also performed. Overall, the win ratio approach made greater use of CV death data than the conventional approach. The win-ratio method made p-values smaller for the Added group and larger for the Preserved group.

Because there were three p-values for the three different patient populations, we can use SPPM for the multiplicity adjustment. The decision rules

TABLE 7.14
CHARM Trial Hazard Ratio and Win-Ratio Results.

	Charm Added	Charm Alternative	Charm Preserved
CV death on candesartan first	220	148	136
CV death on placebo first	289	202	150
HF hosp on candesartan first	104	74	115
HF hosp on placebo first	132	114	144
None of the above	527	475	964
Total no. of pairs	1272	1013	1509
Classic hazard ratio	0.85	0.70	0.86
p-value for hazard ratio	0.005	<0.0001	0.025
Win ratio for composite	1.30	1.42	1.17
p-value for win-ratio	<0.0001	<0.0001	0.032

Note: One-sided p-values

are:

$$\begin{cases} p_1 p_2 p_3 \leq \alpha_4 \cap p_1 p_2 \leq \alpha_1 \cap p_1 p_3 \leq \alpha_1 \cap p_1 \leq 0.025, \text{ reject } H_1 \\ p_1 p_2 p_3 \leq \alpha_4 \cap p_2 p_3 \leq \alpha_1 \cap p_2 p_1 \leq \alpha_1 \cap p_2 \leq 0.025, \text{ reject } H_2 \\ p_1 p_2 p_3 \leq \alpha_4 \cap p_3 p_1 \leq \alpha_1 \cap p_2 p_3 \leq \alpha_1 \cap p_3 \leq 0.025, \text{ reject } H_3 \end{cases}$$

where $\alpha_1 = 0.004855$ and $\alpha_4 = 0.0026778$ for $\rho = 0$. In terms of HR, $p_1 = 0.0001$, $p_2 = 0.005$, and $p_3 = 0.025$: thus, all three hypotheses are rejected and treatment effects for all three patient populations are concluded. In terms of Win Ratio, $p_1 = 0.0001$, $p_2 = 0.0001$, and $p_3 = 0.032$, thus, the drug was shown to be effective for the Added and Alternative groups but not for the Preserved group.

7.5 Summary

Union-intersection testing (UIT) and intersection-union testing (IUT) are two common multiplicity problems in clinical trials. Familywise error rate, coherence, and consonance are three important concepts in discussing different testing procedures. Testing procedures include single, stepwise, gatekeeping, and tree-structured procedures. A single step procedure is the rejection or non-rejection of a single hypothesis and does not depend on the decision on any other hypothesis. The closure and partitioning principles are very useful in deriving different stepwise test procedures.

With respect to UIT, Hochberg's procedure is uniformly more powerful than Holm's procedure and Hommel's procedure is uniformly more powerful than Hochberg's procedure. Dunnett's stepup procedure procedure is uniformly more powerful than Hochberg's and Dunnett's single-step procedure. Furthermore, Dunnett's stepup procedure is not always more powerful than his stepdown procedure. Stepup Dunnett procedure is not always more powerful than stepdown Dunnett procedure.

Single-step progressive procedure incorporates the totality of evidence by combining evidence from multiple sources (different endpoints, different doses, different populations). Evidence from different sources that points to the same positive differences provides strong evidence against the corresponding null hypothesis. On the other hand, if the evidences from some sources point to a negative direction, they will weaken the evidence against the hypothesis concerned. As a result, when test statistics for different hypothesis tests are mutually independent or positively correlated, the power will increase; if largely negatively correlated if largely correlated, the the statistics will reduce the power.

A powerful test procedure should be α-exhaustive, synergize strengths, and be capable of using correlations between local test statistics or local p-values. The Chang-Deng-Balser method has achieved the three aspects for two-hypothesis and three-hypothesis UIT. The method also ensures coherence and consonance. SPPM is statistically powerful and stresses the importance of clinical and practical meanings to be derived from data. The method also provides consistency of total evidence gleaned from different endpoints, doses, and populations. The test procedure is simple and performs well in broad situations. When the true standardized effect size (value of the parameter) is very different for different hypothesis, the critical values don't have to the same for rejecting all the hypotheses. Instead, the critical values can be different and optimized based on the prior information on effect size or considering the clinical importance of different endpoints.

For IUT, the classsical test methods requiring p-values for all local tests are less than equal to α will control FWER. All other methods that attempt to improve power involve trade-offs of α-inflation. Chuang Stein's method control the average type-I error rate. Li's method relaxes the criterion by increasing α or the null confutation when a few null hypotheses are true.

In dealing with multiple-endpoint problems, priority-based winner methods include the Finkelstein-Schoenfeld method and Pocock's win-ratio system. Alternatively, SPPM can also be used to increase the power.

Bibliography

Bakal, JA, Westerhout, CM, Armstrong, PW (2015). Impact of weighted composite compared to traditional composite endpoints for the design of randomized controlled trials. Statistical Methods. in Medical Research 2015; 24(6):980–988

Bebu, I. and Lachin, JM. (2016). Large sample inference for a win ratio analysis of a composite outcome based on prioritized components. Biostatistics (2016), 17, 1, pp. 178–187.

Bretz, F. et al. (2006). Confirmatory seamless phase II/III clinical trials with hypotheses selection at interim: General concepts. Biometrical Journal 48:4.

Chang, M., Deng, X., and Balser, J. (2016). American Journal of Biostatistics. 2016, 6 (2): 30.41.

CHMP (2002). Points to consider on multiplicity issues in clinical trials, 2002.

Chuang-Stein, C., Stryszak, P., Dmitrienko, A, and Offen, W. (2007). Challenge of multiple co-primary endpoints: A new approach. Statistics in Medicine 2007; 26:1181–1192

Deng, X. and Chang, M. (2018). Single-Step Progressive Parametric method. SBR, submitted.

Dmitrienko, A, Tamhane, AC, Bretz, F. (2010), Multiple Testing Problems in Pharmaceutical Statistics. p.67. CRC. FL

Dmitrienko, A. (2013). Multiple Testing Procedures in Clinical Trials. IBS workshop, Berlin, Sep 19-20, 2013.

Dong, G, Li, D., Ballerstedt, S., and Vandemeulebroecke, M. (2016). A generalized analytic solution to the win ratio to analyze a composite endpoint considering the clinical importance order among components. Pharmaceutical Statistics 2016, 15 430–437

European Medicines Agency (1998). ICH Topic E 9 Statistical Principles for Clinical Trials, Step 5. http://www.ema.europa.eu

Finkelstein, DM, Schoenfeld, DA. (1999). Combining mortality and longitudinal measures in clinical trials. Statistics in Medicine 1999; 18(11):1341–1354.

Hochberg, Y. (1988). A sharper Bonferroni procedure for multiple tests of significance. Biometrika 1988; 75(4):800–802.

Holm, S. (1979). A simple sequentially rejective multiple test procedure. Scandinavian Journal of Statistics 1979; 6:65–70.

Hommel, G. (1988). A stagewise rejective multiple test procedure based on a modified Bonferroni test. Biometrika 1988; 75(2): 383–386.

Homme,l G, Bretz, F. (2008). Aesthetics and power considerations in multiple testing–a contradiction? Biometrical Journal 2008; 50(5):657–666

Huque, M. and Röhmel, J. (2010). Multiplicity problems in clinical trials: a regulatory perspective, in Dmitrienko, A., Tamhane, A.C., and Bretz, F. (2010).

Li, Q.H. (2009). Evaluating Co-primary Endpoints Collectively in Clinical Trials. Biometrical Journal 51 (2009) 1, 137–145.

Li, Q. H. and Huque M. F. (2003). A decision rule for evaluating several independent clinical trials collectively. Journal of Biopharmaceutical Statistics 13, 621–628.

Luo, X. L., Tian, H., Mohanty, S. & Tsai, W. Y. (2015). An alternative approach to confidence interval estimation for the win ratio statistic. Biometrics 71, 139–45.

Marcus, R, Eric, P, Gabriel, KR (1976). On closed testing procedures with special reference to ordered analysis of variance. Biometrika 1976; 63(3):655–660.

Moyé, LA. (2003). Multiple Analyses in Clinical Trials: Fundamentals for Investigators (Statistics for Biology and Health). Springer; NY, NY.

Oakes, D. (2016). On the win-ratio statistic in clinical trials with multiple types. Biometrika (2016), 103, 3, pp. 742–745.

Pocock, S. J., Ariti, C. A., Collier, T. J. & Wang, D. (2012). The win ratio: A new approach to the analysis of composite endpoints in clinical trials based on clinical priorities. European Heart Journal 13, 176–82.

Tong, BC, Huber, JC, et al. (2012). Weighting composite endpoints in clinical trials: essential evidence for the heart team. Annals of Thoracic Surgery 2012; 94(6):1908–1913.

Wang, D. and Pocock, S. (2016). A win ratio approach to comparing continuous non-normal outcomes in clinical trials. Pharmaceutical Statistics 2016, 15 238–245.

Wei, LJ, Johnson, WE (1985). Combining dependent tests with incomplete repeated measurements. Biometrika 1985; 27:359–364.

Westfall, P.H. Tobias, R.D., Rom, D., Wolfinger, R.D., Hochberg, Y. (1999). Multiple comparisons and multiple tests using SAS system. SAS Institute. SAS Institute, Cary, NC.

Wiens, B.L. (2003). A fixed-sequence Bonferroni procedure for testing multiple endpoints. Pharmaceutical Statistics 2003; 2:211–215.

Wiens, B.L. Dmitrienko, A. (2005). The fallback procedure for evaluating a single family of hypotheses. Journal of Biopharmaceutical Statistics 2005; 15(6):929–942.

8

Missing Data Handling in Clinical Trials

8.1 Missing Data Problems

8.1.1 Missing Data Issue and Its Impact

Missing data are common in scientific research and our daily life. In a survey, "no response" constitutes missing data. In clinical trials, missing data can be caused by many different variables, including but not limited to patient refusal to continue in the study, treatment failures, data entry errors, adverse events, or patient relocations.

Missing data will complicate the data analysis. In many medical settings missing data can cause difficulties in estimation, precision and inference. In clinical trials, missing data can undermine randomization (Little, et al. 2010) as well as the interpretation and validity of study results. The European Union's Committee for Medicinal Products for Human Use (CHMP, 2009) provides advice on how the presence of missing data in a confirmatory clinical trial should be addressed in a regulatory submission. It is stated that the pattern of missing data (including reasons for and timing of the missing data) observed in previous related clinical trials should be taken into account when planning a confirmatory clinical trial.

An analysis that ignores subjects with missing data is termed a completer analysis. On one hand, a completer analysis can reduce the power of hypothesis testing due to a reduction in sample size; on the other hand, non-completers might be more likely to have extreme values (e.g., treatment failure leading to dropout, extremely good response leading to loss of follow-up). Therefore, the loss of these non-completers could lead to an underestimate of variability, hence artificially narrowing the confidence interval for the treatment effect, and artificially increasing the power of the study. Therefore, the overall effect of missing data depends on the situation.

A completer analysis can potentially cause bias if missing data are not random, i.e., missingness relates to observed or unobserved or both measurements. Generally missing data will not be expected to lead to bias in the completer analysis if they are not related to the observed or unobserved measurements (e.g. poor outcomes are no more likely to be missing than good outcomes). However, it is virtually impossible to elucidate whether the relationship between missing values and the unobserved outcome variable is completely absent. Therefore, unbiasedness cannot be firmly asserted in reality.

If subjects with missing data are excluded from the analysis in a clinical trial, the exclusion may affect the comparability of the treatment groups and the representativeness of the study sample in relation to the target population (external validity) is questionable.

8.1.2 Missing Mechanism

Let Y_{ij} denote the random variable measured at the jth time point on the ith subject, where $i = 1, ..., n$ and $j = 1, ..., n_i$. We use vector $\boldsymbol{Y}_i = (Y_{i1}, ..., Y_{in_i})'$ to denote the measurements on subject i, where the apostrophe $(\prime)$ represents for the matrix transport. We use an upper case letter to denote a random variable and the lower case letter for a corresponding observation. We use superscripts or subscripts "obs" and "mis" to indicate observed and missing quantities, respectively. Therefore, y_{ij} consists of y_{ij}^{obs} and y_{ij}^{mis}. The indicator $R_{ij} = 1$ if the value of Y_{ij} is observed; otherwise $R_{ij} = 0$. Let $\boldsymbol{R}_i = (R_{i1}, ..., R_{in_i})'$. The mechanism of missingness will be denoted by ϖ_i and the matrix of covariates for the ith subject is denoted by $X_i = (X_{i1}...X_{in_i})$.

According to Rubin (Rubin, 1976; Little and Rubin, 2002), the missing value process can be characterized into three different categories in terms of its marginal probability distribution.

(1) If the probability of missing an observation does not depend on observed or unobserved measurements then the observation is classified as missing completely at random (MCAR). The marginal density for the missing is given by

$$f\left(\boldsymbol{r}_i | \boldsymbol{y}_i, \varpi_i, \boldsymbol{\psi}\right) = f\left(\boldsymbol{r}_i | \varpi_i, \boldsymbol{\psi}\right), \qquad (8.1)$$

where $\boldsymbol{\psi}$ is the parameters characterizing the mechanism of missingness.

MCAR is difficult to find in reality. One may consider a patient moving to another city for non-health reasons is MCAR. However, we can reason that if this patient was responding well to a new oncology drug that was only available in certain cities, the patient may be unlikely to move out of the city. A car accident may be considered as MCAR, but it can also be related to a patient's health condition.

(2) If the probability of missing an observation depends only on observed measurements then the observation is classified as missing at random (MAR). This assumption implies that the behavior (i.e., distribution) of the post dropout observations can be predicted from the observed values, and therefore that response can be estimated without bias using exclusively the observed data. Mathematically, the density of MAR is given by

$$f\left(\boldsymbol{r}_i | \boldsymbol{y}_i, \varpi_i, \boldsymbol{\psi}\right) = f\left(\boldsymbol{r}_i | \boldsymbol{y}_i^{obs}, \varpi_i, \boldsymbol{\psi}\right). \qquad (8.2)$$

(3) When observations are neither MCAR nor MAR, they are classified as missing not at random (MNAR), i.e. the probability of a missing observation depends on both observed and unobserved measurements. The density of missingness, $f(r_i|y_i, \varpi_i, \psi)$, can not be simplified.

Mathematically, there is no way to know whether a missing component is MACR, MAR, or MNAR. However, we often believe MCAR and MAR can be good approximations in certain situations.

Monotonic missingness is a common and simple pattern. If the missing data pattern is monotone, then all observations after time point t are missing, where t is the time point when the first missing observation occurs.

Another property of missingness is ignorability which ensures that ignoring the unobserved data in the analysis will not lead to biased results. Sufficient conditions for ignorability are the following two requirements.

(1) The joint prior distribution for θ and ψ can factor into independent priors

$$P(\theta, \psi) = P(\theta)P(\psi), \qquad (8.3)$$

i.e., the joint distribution is distinct. In this case, the change in one parameter will not cause a change in the other parameter.

(2) MAR holds. In other words, the missingness distribution depends only on the observed data, and all the missingness information is contained in the observed part of the data. Mathematically, it is characterized as

$$P(R_{ij}|Y, \psi) = P(R_{ij}|Y_{obs}, \psi). \qquad (8.4)$$

A commonly used parametric model for missingness calculates the continuatio probability for subject i, at time j, using

$$p_{ij}(\psi) = P(R_{ij} = 1|Y_{i1}, ..., Y_{ij}, \psi) = \frac{exp(\psi_0 + \psi_1 Y_{i1} + \cdots + \psi_j Y_{ij})}{1 + exp(\psi_0 + \psi_1 Y_{i1} + \cdots + \psi_j Y_{ij})}. \qquad (8.5)$$

For MCAR, $\psi_1 = \cdots = \psi_j = 0$, and for MAR $\psi_j = 0$.

8.2 Implementation of Analysis Methods

8.2.1 Trial Data Simulation

It is important to be able to generate simulation data with a specified missing mechanism, MCAR, MAR, or MNAR. Using these simulated data, we can apply different missing data analysis methods to conduct simulation studies so that we can choose the most appropriate methods for the trial under consideration. One crucial step in studying missing data is to generate correlated data with a certain covariance structure. We have developed an SAS Macro based on Proc SimNormal for generating simulated data. Proc SimNormal is included in the SAS base package, and does not require additional packages such as PROC IML.

First, we generate multivariate normal random numbers for a simulated trial. The continuous variable can be transferred into categorical or binary variables as needed. We can add more variables, and set specific mechanics for performing different analyses for missing data. In what follows, we will illustrate the easy steps to create the data we need.

Suppose we are interested in creating 4-variate normal random variables, y1, y2, y3, y4. We first create SAS dataset scov containing a 4×4 correlation coefficient matrix. Note the values for means are zero.

Title "Correlation matrix for Proc Simnorm - group 1"; Run;
data scov(type=COV); * Cov{i,j}=Coef{i,j}*s{i}*s{j}, MEAN always =0 here;
input _TYPE_ $ 1-4 _NAME_ $ 5-10 y1 y2 y3 y4;
datalines ;
COV   y1   1.0 0.4 0.3 0.2
COV   y2   0.4 1.0 0.4 0.3
COV   y3   0.3 0.4 1.0 0.4
COV   y4   0.2 0.3 0.4 1.0
MEAN   0.0 0.0 0.0 0.0
run;

Then, create dataset MusSigmas containing means and standard deviations for the variables.

Data MusSigmas;
* if data in scov is covariance, then mu and sigma should be 0 and sigma=1;
Array mus{4}(0, 0.1, 0.1, 0.1);
Array sigmas{4}(1, 1, 1, 1);
Run;

We now invoke SAS Macro MVNvars to generate 200 observations with 4 multivariate normal variables and their changes for treatment group 1..

%MVNvars(group=1, nVars=4, nObs=200);

The macro creates ActualY and Trial1 datasets as shown in the snapshots in Tables 8.1 and 8.2. ActualY contains the multivariate variables, $y1, y2, y3$, and $y4$, and patient identification (pID). The Trial dataset contains variable of interest Y and we use the Visit variable to construct vertically, that is, $y2$ is y when Visit = 2, $y2 = y$ when Visit 3, and $y3 = y$ when Visit = 4. The dataset also contains the based baseline values ($basey = y1$) and changes, $chgy$, from baseline at each visit ($y2 - y1, y3 - y1$, and $y4 - y1$).

Similarly, we create random variables for group 2. For simplicity, we assume the two groups have the same correlation coefficient matrix. We only

TABLE 8.1
Snapshot of ActualY Dataset.

Obs	y1	y2	y3	y4	Pid
1	-1.39239	-0.79735	-1.96058	0.86978	1
2	1.54022	1.78284	0.90399	0.06687	2
3	-0.37097	1.47915	2.48977	0.67036	3

TABLE 8.2
Snapshot of Trial1 Dataset.

Obs	Pid	y	Chgy	visit	group	basey
1	1	-0.99735	0.39504	2	1	-1.39239
2	1	-2.16058	-0.76819	3	1	-1.39239
3	1	0.66978	2.06217	4	1	-1.39239
4	2	1.58284	0.04262	2	1	1.54022

need to create datasets for means and standard deviations before invoking the MVNvars macro.

```
Data MusSigmas;
 Array mus{4}(0, 0.15, 0.25, 0.35);
 Array sigmas{4}(1, 1, 1, 1);
 Run;
%MVNvars(group=2, nVars=4, nObs=200);
```

We merge the datesets for the two groups:

```
Data Trial; set Trials1 Trials2; run;
```

We can add more independent variables. For example, we want to create a sex variable with 55% males. We can use the following simple code.

```
Data Trial; set Trial; drop pMale;
    pMale=0.55; * pMale= proportion of males;
    sex="female"; if Rand("UNIFORM")<=0.55 Then sex="male";
Run;
```

We may want to convert the continuous variable chgy to binary endpoint using a threshold (e.g., 0.15) or to ordinal endpoint using cutpoints (e.g., 0.1, 0.2, 0.3). Here is corresponding SAS code:

```
Data Trial; set Trial;
        If .<chgy <0.15 Then Do; yBin=0; baseyBin=0; End;
        If chgy>=0.15 Then Do; yBin=1; baseyBin=1; End;
        If .<chgy<=0.1 Then Do; yCat=1; baseyCat=1; End;
        If 0.1<chgy<=0.2 Then Do; yCat=2; baseyCat=2; End;
        If 0.2<chgy<=0.3 Then Do; yCat=3; baseyCat=3; End;
        If 0.3<chgy Then Do; yCat=4; baseyCat=4; End;
Run;
```

We now discuss how to create missing data with different missing mechanisms, MCAR, MAR, and MNAR. The key is to create probability of missing that is either

(1) independent of observed and unobserved data (MCAR), 50% missing in the following example, or

(2) dependent on observed data only (MAR), a logistic function of baseline value and group, as an example, or

(3) dependent on observed and unobserved data (MNAR), a logistic function of treatment group and visit for period at end.

```
Data TrialMCAR; set Trial; drop pMis;
pMis=0.3; * pMis= assumed proportion of missings;
If Rand("UNIFORM")<=pMis Then Do; y=.; chgy=.; End;
Run;
```

```
Data TrialMAR; set Trial;
* pMis= prob. of missings;
pMis=1/(1+exp(-0.2*Basey+0.1*group));
if Rand("UNIFORM")<=pMis Then Do; y=.; chgy=.;  End;
Run;
```

```
Data TrialMNAR; set Trial;
Tox=0.2*group-0.3*Visit*Rand("UNIFORM"); * Tox=unobserved toxicity;
pMis=1/(1+exp(-Tox));
If Rand("UNIFORM")<=pMis Then Do; y=.; chgy=.; End;
Run;
```

We also want to create monotonic missing patterns of yCat and yBin for later use in the generalized estimating equation (GEE) and weighted GEE (WGEE).

```
Data TrialMCARcat; Set Trial;
```

```
    pMis=0.3;        * probability of missing at Visit 4;
    If Rand("UNIFORM")<pMis And visit=4 Then Do;
         yCat=.; yBin=.;
    End;
Run;
Data TrialMARcat; Set Trial;
    pMis=1/(1+exp(-0.2*BaseyBin+0.1*group));       * probability of missing
at Visit 4;
    If Rand("UNIFORM")<pMis And visit=4 Then Do;
         yCat=.; yBin=.;
    End;
Run;
Data TrialMNARcat; Set Trial;
 Tox=0.2*group-0.3*Visit*Rand("UNIFORM"); * Tox=unobserved toxicity at
Visit 4;
 pMis=1/(1+exp(-Tox));
    If Rand("UNIFORM")<pMis And visit=4 Then Do;
         yCat=.; yBin=.;
    End;
Run;
```

Lastly. we want to create monotonic missing patterns of y and chgy for later use in the weighted GEE (WGEE).

```
Data TrialMCARMon; set Trial; drop pMis;
pMis=0.3; * pMis= assumed proportion of missings;
If Rand("UNIFORM")<=pMis And Visit=4 Then Do; y=.; chgy=.; End;
Run;
Data TrialMARMon; set Trial;
* pMis= prob. of missings;
pMis=1/(1+exp(-0.2*Basey+0.1*group));
if Rand("UNIFORM")<=pMis And Visit=4 Then Do; y=.; chgy=.; End;
Run;

Data TrialMNARMon; set Trial;
Tox=0.2*group-0.3*Visit*Rand("UNIFORM"); * Tox=unobserved toxicity;
pMis=1/(1+exp(-Tox));
If Rand("UNIFORM")<=pMis And Visit=4 Then Do; y=.; chgy=.; End;
Run;
```

Table 8.3 is a snapshot of MNAR dataset, TrialMNAR.

TABLE 8.3

Snapshot of MNAR dataset, TrialMNAR.

Obs	Pid	y	Chgy	visit	group	basey	sex	Tox	pMis
1	1	-0.99735	0.39504	2	1	-1.39239	Male	0.86946	0.33862
2	1	-2.16058	-0.76819	3	1	-1.39239	Male	0.73997	0.36820
3	1	.	.	4	1	-1.39239	Female	0.36690	0.45837
4	2	1.58284	0.04262	2	1	1.54022	Male	0.22595	0.49351
5	2	0.70399	-0.83624	3	1	1.54022	female	0.79194	0.35619

8.2.2   Single Imputation Methods

As mentioned earlier, the completer analysis is often not preferable. There are several commonly used simple methods that deal with missing data. An example would be the last-observation-carried-forward (LOCF), in which the missing value will be implemented by the previous observation. LOCF is not unbiased even under MCAR assumption (Little, et al. 2010). The LOCF can produce better or worse results for the two groups. If the timings of the two withdrawals are different (e.g., some may withdraw when drug effect starts to decline, others may withdraw when the efficacy is still present, yet others may withdraw from the study due to side-effects or the baseline covariates may differ between the treatment groups. In these instances, bias can occur. Other examples of simple implementation methods, as cited in the CHMP guidance (2009), include replacing the unobserved measurements by values derived from other sources such as information from the same subject collected before withdrawal, from other subjects with similar baseline characteristics, a predicted value from an empirically developed model, and historical data. Examples of empirically developed models are unconditional and conditional mean imputation and best and worst case imputation (assigning the worst possible value of the outcome to dropouts for a negative reason and the best possible value to positive dropouts) are also mentioned in the guidance.

The completer analysis and LOCF analysis are straightforward as shown in the following examples with SAS.

(1) Completer Analysis

This method is straightforward: remove all missing records and then apply the analysis.

```
Data MisIDs; Set TrialMCAR; keep GrpPt MisID;
      misID="XXXXXXXX"; If y =. Then misID=GrpPt;
      If misID = "XXXXXXXX" Then delete;
Run;
Data CompleterMCAR; Merge TrialMCAR MisIDs; by GrpPt;
      If misID=GrpPt Then delete;
Run;
```

An example of completer analysis is provided below with MLE approach.

```
Proc Mixed Data=CompleterMCAR method = ml;
    Class visit group GrpPt;
    Model y= group visit group*visit basey / s;
    Repeated / type=CS subject=GrpPt r;
Run;
```

The simulation data changes every time. One of the simulations, the CompleterMCAR has 177 observations. The outputs of the Proc Mixed show a group effect of 0.154 with p=0.1912. However, this is just one simulation for the trial with MCAR. To evaluate the performance of the method, the simulation has to be performed many times for different covariance structures (e.g., unstructured) and different mechanisms of missingness. We will discuss this more later.

(2) LOCF Implementation

There is a traditional way to implement LOCF in SAS. However, the DO loop of Whitlock (DOW) is innovative, it is unusual to put the SET statement inside a DO UNTIL (LAST.PT) loop. The DOW was originally described by Ian Whitlock at SAS-L sometime in 1999-2000 (Venky Chakravarthy, Ann Arbor, MI, 2001).

No baseline value will be carried forward to the postbaseline. Therefore, if y and chgy are missing at Visit 2, they will be still missing. The following SAS code implements the DOW method for variable y and *chgy*. The where statement controls when the LOCF applies. For example, if the baseline is defined as value at Visit 3, and if it is missing, Visit 2 value will be used; if Visit 2 value is also missing, Visit 1 value will be used as the baseline. However, if Visit 1 value is also missing, the baseline is missing. In this case the statement should be "where = (visit <= 3)." If we want to implement LOCF between Visit 4 and Visit 7, the relevant statement should be "where = (4<= visit <= 7)." The variables $(y, chgy)$ before LOCF and the variables $(LOCFy, LOCFchgy)$ after LOCF are shown in Table 8.4.

```
Data TrialLOCF ;
    Do until ( last.GrpPt ) ;
    Set TrialMCAR( where = ( visit > 0 ) ) ;
    By GrpPt ;
    If y ^= . Then LOCFy = y ;
        If chgy ^= . Then LOCFchgy = chgy ;
    Output ;
    End ; Run ;
```

Now applied the mixed-effect model analysis for repeated measures with LOCF:

```
Proc Mixed Data =TrialLOCF method = ml;
    Class visit group GrpPt;
    Model LOCFy= group visit group*visit basey /s;
    Repeated / type=CS subject=GrpPt r;
Run;
```

TABLE 8.4
Variables before LOCF and after LOCF.

Obs	Pid	y	chgy	visit	group	basey	GrpPT	sex	pMis	LOCFy	LOCFchgy
1	1	-0.99735	0.39504	2	1	-1.39239	01-00001	male	0.5	-0.99735	0.39504
2	1	.	.	3	1	-1.39239	01-00001	female	0.5	-0.99735	0.39504
3	1	0.66978	2.06217	4	1	-1.39239	01-00001	male	0.5	0.66978	2.06217
4	2	1.58284	0.04262	2	1	1.54022	01-00002	male	0.5	1.58284	0.04262
5	2	.	.	3	1	1.54022	01-00002	female	0.5	1.58284	0.04262
6	2	.	.	4	1	1.54022	01-00002	male	0.5	1.58284	0.04262
7	3	1.27915	1.65012	2	1	-0.37097	01-00003	male	0.5	1.27915	1.65012

For the same set of simulated data as for the completer analysis, the outputs from the LOCF analysis show the estimated group effect of 0.2241 with p-value <0.001.

For categorical data (binary, ordinal, count, nominal), GEE can be used. See Section 8.3.2.

8.2.3 Methods without Specified Mechanics of Missing Data

Some statistical approaches to handling missing data do not employ any explicit missing-imputation. Those methods are usually maximum likelihood-based approaches. Generalized estimating equations (GEE) for categorical endpoints and general linear mixed models (GLMM) for normal endpoints are examples of such models. They are usually valid under MCAR and if weights are chosen appropriately they are also valid under MAR assumptions, while the general linear model (GLM) is only valid under MCAR. This is because subjects with missing values are removed from the GLM analysis, i.e., completer analysis, while GLMM utilizes all the observed data. GEE and GLMM can be used for data with repeated measures.

The general linear mixed model's family is given by

$$Y_i = X_i\beta + Z_i\gamma_i + \varepsilon_i, \tag{8.6}$$

where Y_i is response vector, X_i is fixed effects with the associated unknown parameters β , Z_i is random effects with the associated parameters $\gamma_i \sim N(0, G)$, and the random error term $\varepsilon_i \sim N(0, \Sigma_i)$. It is assumed that γ_i and ε_i are independent.

The fitting of a linear model is usually based on the marginal model that, for subject i, is multivariate normal with mean $X_i\beta$ and covariance $V_i(\alpha) = Z_i G Z_i' + \Sigma_i$. The parameter in α is usually called "variance components." The common approach to estimation and inference is based on maximum likelihood (ML) or likelihood. Assuming independence across subjects, the likelihood takes the form

$$L\left(\boldsymbol{\theta}\right) = \prod_{i=1}^{n} \frac{\exp\left[-\frac{1}{2}\left(\boldsymbol{Y}_i - X_i\boldsymbol{\beta}\right)' V_i^{-1}\left(\boldsymbol{\alpha}\right)\left(\boldsymbol{Y}_i - X_i\boldsymbol{\beta}\right)\right]}{\left(2\pi\right)^{n_i/2}\sqrt{|V_i\left(\boldsymbol{\alpha}\right)|}}. \qquad (8.7)$$

After ignoring a constant, the log-likelihood is given by

$$LL = -\frac{n}{2}\ln|V_i\left(\boldsymbol{\alpha}\right)| - \sum_{i=1}^{n}\left[-\frac{1}{2}\left(\boldsymbol{Y}_i - X_i\boldsymbol{\beta}\right)' V_i^{-1}\left(\boldsymbol{\alpha}\right)\left(\boldsymbol{Y}_i - X_i\boldsymbol{\beta}\right)\right]. \qquad (8.8)$$

For the linear mixed model case, inference is conventionally based on the marginal model for $\boldsymbol{Y}_i$, which is obtained from integrating out the random effects. The likelihood contribution for subject i then becomes

$$f_i\left(\boldsymbol{y}_i|\boldsymbol{\beta}, G, \phi\right) = \int \prod_{j=1}^{n_j} f_{ij}\left(y_{ij}|\boldsymbol{\gamma}_i, \boldsymbol{\beta}, \phi\right) f\left(\boldsymbol{\gamma}_i|G\right) d\boldsymbol{\gamma}_i. \qquad (8.9)$$

Based on (8.9) the likelihood for $\boldsymbol{\beta}, G$, and ϕ can be derived as

$$
\begin{aligned}
L\left(\boldsymbol{\beta}, G, \phi\right) &= \prod_{i=1}^{n} f_i\left(\boldsymbol{y}_i|\boldsymbol{\beta}, G, \phi\right) \\
&= \prod_{i=1}^{n} \int \prod_{j=1}^{n_j} f_{ij}\left(y_{ij}|\boldsymbol{\gamma}_i, \boldsymbol{\beta}, \phi\right) f\left(\boldsymbol{\gamma}_i|G\right) d\boldsymbol{\gamma}_i. \qquad (8.1)
\end{aligned}
$$

The exponential-family distributions are often used in conditional form:

$$f_i\left(y_{ij}|\boldsymbol{\gamma}_i, \boldsymbol{\beta}, \phi\right) = \exp\left(\frac{y_{ij}\theta_{ij} - \psi\left(\theta_{ij}\right)}{\phi} - c\left(y_{ij}, \phi\right)\right), \qquad (8.11)$$

with a link-function $g\left(\mu_{ij}\right) = g\left(E\left(Y_{ij}|\boldsymbol{\gamma}_i\right)\right) = \boldsymbol{x}_{ij}'\boldsymbol{\beta} + \boldsymbol{z}_{ij}'\boldsymbol{\gamma}_i$, where $\boldsymbol{x}_{ij}$ and $\boldsymbol{z}_{ij}$ are p-dimensional and q-dimensional vectors of known covariate values, vector $\boldsymbol{\beta} =$ unknown fixed regression coefficients, $\phi =$ scale parameter and, θ_{ij} the canonical parameter. Further, let $f\left(\boldsymbol{\gamma}_i|G\right)$ be the density of the $N\left(\boldsymbol{0}, G\right)$ distribution for the random effects $\boldsymbol{\gamma}_i$. Various covariance structures, such as the compound-symmetric, first-order autoregressive, and unstructured structures, can be used for G.

The solution to maximize likelihood (8.10) is challenging because of the presence of n integrals over the high-dimensional random effects. Monte Carlo simulation may be used since the efficiency of Monte Carlo for integrals is independent of the dimensionality. Other numerical approximations and quasi-likelihood estimates are also proposed.

If the endpoint is not normal, such as count, binary, or ordinal endpoints, GEE and weighted GEE can be used. The GEE procedure implements the generalized estimating equations (GEE) approach (Liang and Zeger 1986), which

TABLE 8.5
Proc GEE Distributions and Default Link Functions.

DIST=	Distribution	Default Link Function
BINOMIAL I BIN I B	Binomial	Logit
GAMMA I GAM I G	Gamma	Reciprocal
IGAUSSIAN I IG	Inverse Gaussian	Reciprocal square
MULTINOMIAL I MULT	Multinomial	Cumulative logit
NEGBIN I NB	Negative binomial	Log
NORMAL I NOR I N	Normal	Identity
POISSON I POI I P	Poisson	Log

extends the generalized linear model to handle longitudinal data (Stokes, Davis, and Koch 2012; Fitzmaurice, Laird, and Ware 2011; Diggle et al. 2002). For longitudinal studies, missing data are common, and they can be caused by dropouts or skipped visits. If missing responses depend on previous responses, the usual GEE approach can lead to biased estimates. So the GEE procedure also implements the weighted GEE method to handle missing responses that are caused by dropouts in longitudinal studies (Robins and Rotnitzky 1995; Preisser, Lohman, and Rathouz 2002). At the moment, SAS' Proc GEE feature only supports monotonic missing cases. The GEE method is a marginal model to longitudinal data. The regression parameters in the marginal model are interpreted as population-averaged.

SAS Proc GEE implements the GEE model. DIST = keyword specifies the built-in probability distribution to use in the model. The default link functions are displayed in Table 8.5. If neither the DIST= option nor the LINK= option is specified, then the GEE procedure defaults to the normal distribution with the identity link function. TYPE= or CORR= specifies the structure of the working correlation matrix that is used to model the correlation of the responses from subjects for ordinary GEEs (Table 8.6). For ordinal multinomial data, only the exchangeable regression structure that is specified by

TABLE 8.6
Log Odds Ratio Regression Structures.

Keyword	Log Odds Ratio Regression Structure
EXCH	Exchangeable
FULLCLUST	Fully parameterized clusters
LOGORVAR(*variable*)	Indicator variable for specifying block effects
NESTK	*k*-nested
NEST1	1-nested
ZFULL	Fully specified z matrix specified in ZDATA= data set
ZREP	Single cluster specification for replicated z matrix specified in ZDATA= data set
ZREP(*matrix*)	Single cluster specification for replicated z matrix

LOGOR=EXCH is supported. Either the LOGOR= or TYPE= option should be specified, but not both.

Let's now discuss some simple examples of using Proc Mixed and Proc GEE.

(1) For a normal endpoint, the analysis using SAS PROC MIXED is straightforward. The order of the measurements should be correctly specified, which can be done by supplying records with missing data in the input data set.

Here is the SAS code using Proc Mixed for the TrialMAR dataset.

```
Proc Mixed Data=TrialMAR Method = ml;
 Class pID visit group;
 Model y= group visit group*visit basey / s;
 Repeated / type=CS subject=pID r;
Run;
```

We can also use Proc GEE as shown below:

```
Proc GEE Data=TrialMCARcat descending;
     Class GrpPt group Visit;
     Model y=group Visit group*Visit / dist=normal;
     Repeated Subject=GrpPt/ corr=cs;
Run;
```

(2) For a binary endpoint, ordinal, multiple nominal, and count Endpoints, GEE can be used, which are implemented in Proc SAS.

```
* Proc GEE for MCAR data with binary endpoint;
Proc GEE Data=TrialMCARcat descending;
 Class GrpPt group Visit;
 Model yBin=group Visit group*Visit / dist=bin link=logit;
 Repeated Subject=GrpPt/ corr=cs;
Run;
```

```
* Proc GEE for MCAR data and ordinal endpoint;
 Proc GEE Data=TrialMCARcat descending;
 Class GrpPt group Visit;
 Model yCat=group Visit group*Visit / dist=multinomial link=cumlogit;
 Repeated Subject=GrpPtt;
Run;
```

Expectation-Maximization Algorithm

For a complex model, the MLE is often found using the so-called expectation-maximization (EM) algorithm. The EM is an iterative algorithm

used to calculate maximum likelihood estimates in parametric models in cases
of missing data. After the initial values are chosen, the iterations involve two
steps: the expectation step or E-step and the maximization step or M-step.
The condition for the EM algorithm to be valid, in its basic form, is ignorability and hence MAR.

In the implementation of the EM algorithm, before the E-step and M-
step begin, the choice of an initial value of parameter $\theta^{(0)}$ is important since
it will affect the speed of convergence. The commonly used value for $\theta^{(0)}$ is the
solution from the complete case (completer) analysis or some simple methods
of imputation.

(1) The E-step

Given the values at the kth iteration $\theta^{(k)}$ for the parameters, the E-step
computes the objective function:

$$Q\left(\theta\mid\theta^{(k)}\right) = \int L\left(\theta\mid y\right) f\left(y_{mis}\mid y_{obs}, \theta^{(k)}\right) dy_{mis} = E\left[L\left(\theta\mid y\right)\mid y_{obs}, \theta^{(k)}\right].$$
(8.12)

(2) The M-step

In the M-step, $\theta^{(k+1)}$ is calculated to maximize the log-likelihood of the
imputed data (or the imputed log-likelihood). Formally, $\theta^{(k+1)}$ satisfies

$$\theta^{(k+1)} = \arg\max_{\theta\in\Theta} Q\left(\theta\mid\theta^{(k)}\right).$$
(8.13)

The EM algorithm can converge to a local maximum if the initial values
are chosen inappropriately, and the speed of convergence can be slow.

The MI procedure in SAS provides EM algorithms for both multivariate
normal and categorical data by means of MCMC imputation method (for general nonmonotonic settings). Proc MI uses the means and standard deviations
from the available cases as the initial estimates for the EM algorithm.

Data A1(rename=(y=Age8)) A2(rename=(y=Age12)) A3(rename=(y=Age16));

Set TrialMCAR;
If Visit=2 Then Output A1;
If Visit=3 Then Output A2;
If Visit=4 Then Output A3;
Run;

Next, we create hypothetical monotonic missing.

Data Growth; Merge A1-A3; by GrpPt;
 drop pMis chgy visit basey;
 If Age8=. Then Do; Age12=.; Age16=.; End;
 If Age12=. Then Age16=.;
Run;

TABLE 8.7

Snapshot of the Growth Data with Monotonic Missing.

Obs	Pid	Age8	group	GrpPT	sex	Age12	Age16
1	1	-0.99735	1	01-00001	female	-2.16058	0.66978
2	3	.	1	01-00003	female		
3	6	0.68051	1	01-00006	female		

Table 8.7 is a snapshot of the Growth dataset with a monotonic missing pattern.

EM Algorithm Using Proc MI

Proc MI Data = Growth seed = 273 Simple nimpute = 0;
  Em itprint outem = growthem;
  Var Age8 Age12 Age16;
  By group;
  Run;

For a time-to-event endpoint with gamma distribution, we can use Proc GEE with a gamma distribution to handle the censoring.

8.2.4   Inverse-Probability Weighting (IPW) Method

We have discussed the IPW in Chapter 7 for time-to-event data with censors. If we can predict the probability of missing correctly, we can use IPW regardless of missing patterns. For nonrandomized trials, propensity score (PS) weighting can be used to adjust treatment imbalance.

When data are MAR but not MCAR, a modification of complete-case analysis can assign a missingness weight to the complete cases so that bias may be reduced. Suppose in the complete dataset, there are 10 counts for $y = 1$, but only 7 of them are actually observed (70% observed, 30% missing). So, we weigh these observations by the inverse of proportion of observed (70%), making it equivalent to 10 observations for the estimation of the mean. However, the proportion of being observed is random variable; practically we use the probability of being observed. That is the basic idea behind the IPW method.

Consider the simple case in which the intended outcome is Y, the design variables are X (can also include auxiliary available). Define a response indicator, $R = 1$ when Y is observed and $R = 0$ when it is missing. An IPW estimator for the mean of Y can be computed as follows:

1. Specify an appropriate model (e.g., logistic model) $\pi(X, \theta) = P_\theta(R = 1|X)$.

2. Estimate the mean of Y using the weighted average

$$\hat{\mu} = \frac{1}{n} \sum_{i=1}^{n} \frac{R_i Y_i}{\pi\left(X_i, \hat{\theta}\right)}. \tag{8.14}$$

That is, the average of the observed Y inflated by the inverse probability of being observed.

For large samples, this method properly adjusts for bias when the data are MAR (Little, et al. 2010), provided the model for $\pi(X, \theta)$ is correctly specified. In finite samples, the method can yield mean estimates that have high variance when some individual-specific weights are high when π is close to zero. To avoid the high variance, we can lower the limit for the weights, making a trade-off between bias and variance. That is why it is important to collect outcome data after individuals withdraw from treatment.

In theory, IPW can also be used for any missing data, even for MNAR as long the missing mechanics can be correctly specified $\pi\left(X_i, Y_i, \hat{\theta}, U\right)$ and the missing probability can be calculated correctly, where U observed data. For example, when a machine is continuously used for a long period, it can overheat and measurements may become difficult and often be missed. In this case, the missing measurements are dependent on the temperature that are not observed. In clinical trials, missing data can relate to the toxicity that might not have been collected or other information outside of the trial. Therefore, $\pi\left(X_i, Y_i, \hat{\theta}, U\right)$ is difficult to know exactly.

The GEE and GENMOD procedures both implement the standard generalized estimating equation approach for longitudinal data; this approach is appropriate for complete data or when data are missing completely at random (MCAR). When the data are missing at random (MAR), the weighted GEE method produces valid inference. Molenberghs and Kenward (2007); Fitzmaurice, Laird, and Ware (2011); Mallinckrodt (2013); O'Kelly and Ratitch (2014) describe the weighted GEE method. The GEE procedure includes alternating logistic regression (Carey, Zeger, and Diggle, 1993; Heagerty and Zeger, 1996) analysis for binary, ordinal, and norminal responses. In ordinary GEEs, the association between pairs of responses association is modeled with correlations. The ALR approach provides an alternative by using the log odds ratio to model the association between pairs. An ordinary GEE with the independent working correlation structure is also available for both nominal and ordinal multinomial data.

SAS Proc GEE provides an IPW method to handle MCAR with the Missmodel statement that requests a weighted GEE analysis. It specifies a logistic regression that is used to estimate the weights under the MAR assumption. If the pattern of missing data is intermittent (not dropout), the GEE procedure terminates and does not perform an analysis.

An example of Proc GEE for normal and binary endpoints is shown below:

Proc GEE Data=TrialMAR descending;
Class GrpPt group Visit ;
Missmodel group Basey; * missingness model;
Model y=group Visit group*Visit / dist=normal;
Repeated Subject=GrpPt/ corr=cs;
Run;
Proc GEE Data=TrialMARcat descending;
Class GrpPt group Visit baseyBin;
Missmodel group BaseyBin; * missingness model;
Model yBin=group Visit group*Visit / dist=bin link=logit;
Repeated Subject=GrpPt/ corr=cs;
Run;

* IPW method with Proc GEE with MNAR data and binary endpoint;
Proc GEE Data=TrialMNARcat descending;
Class pID GrpPt group Visit baseyBin;
Missmodel group BaseyBin; * missingness model;
Model yBin=group Visit group*Visit / dist=bin link=logit;
Repeated Subject=GrpPt/ corr=cs;
Run;

Note that the Missmodel in Proc GEE is experimental as the software menu claimed, we suggest using Proc GENMOD.

Weighted Generalized Estimating Equations

The weighted GEE (WGEE) model is described as marginal for the response Y_{ij} ($j = 1, ..., n_i, i = 1, ..., n$, and $\Sigma_{i=1}^{n} n_i = N$). The parameter vector β is obtained through solving the equation system:

$$S(\beta) = \sum_{i=1}^{n} \frac{\partial \mu_i}{\partial \beta'} [V_i(\alpha)]^{-1} (y_i - \mu_i) = 0, \tag{8.15}$$

where mean $\mu_i = E(Y_i)$, the marginal covariance matrix

$$V_i(\alpha) = \phi A_i^{1/2} W_i^{-1/2} C_i(\alpha) W_i^{-1/2} A_i^{1/2}, \tag{8.16}$$

in which the variance matrix for repeated measures on subject i is $\phi A_i = \phi diag[v(\mu_{i1}), ..., v(\mu_{iT})]$ with ϕ being the unknown dispersion parameter, $C_i(\alpha)$ is the so the called $n_i \times n_i$ working matrix for the ith subject. If $C_i(\alpha)$ is the true correlation matrix of Y_i, then $V_i(\alpha)$ is the true covariance matrix of Y_i.

With the logistic dropout model, the weight is given by (SAS Stat User's Guide, 2006, p. 1681):

$$\frac{1}{w_i} = (1 - \lambda_{im})^{I(m \leq T)} \prod_{j=2}^{m-1} \lambda_{ij}, \tag{8.17}$$

TABLE 8.8

Proc GENMOD Distributions and Default Link Functions.

DIST-	Distribution	Default Link Function
BINOMIAL|BIN|B	Binomial	Logit
GAMMA|GAM|G	Gamma	Inverse (power(-1))
GEOMETRIC|GEOM	Geometric	Log
IGAUSSIAN|IG	Inverse Gaussian	Inverse squared (power(-2))
MULTINOMIAL|MULT	multinomial	Cumulative logit
NEGBIN|NB	Negative binomial	Log
NORMAL|NOR|N	normal	Identity
POISSON|POI|P	Poisson	log

where $\lambda_{ij} = P\left(r_{ij} = 1 | r_{i,j-1} = 1, X_i, Y_{i,j-1}\right)$, m is the time of dropout for the ith subject $(2 \leq m < T - 1)$, and the indicator $I\left(m \leq T\right) = 1$ if $m \leq T$; otherwise $I\left(m \leq T\right) = 0$. When the elements of the weight matrix $W_i =$ identity matrix, WGEE reduces to regular GEE. Unlike classic GLM, GEE uses all data available in the pairwise fashion as defined in the estimates for $\hat{\alpha}$ and $\hat{\beta}$.

Proc GENMOD can be used for the analyses of various endpoints with different distribution (Table 8.8). DIST = keyword specifies the built-in probability distribution to use in the model. If you specify the DIST= option and you omit a user-defined link function, a default link function is chosen as displayed in the Table 8.9. If you specify no distribution and no link function, then the GENMOD procedure defaults to the normal distribution with the identity link function.

There are three steps involved in using WGEE: (1) create missing indicator variable R, (2) create weights based on the model of missing and (2) model the data using the obtained weights. Here is an example of using Proc GENMOD:

```
* Create missing indicator, Rbin;
Data TrialRbin; Set TrialMARcat;
Rbin=1; If yBin=. Then Rbin=0;
Run;
```

```
* Model Missings;
Proc GenMod Data=TrialRbin Descending;
Class group;
Model Rbin = group baseyBin/Pred Dist=b;
Output Out=WGEEbin p=pred;
Run;
```

TABLE 8.9
Parameter Estimates from Imputed Data Sets.

Obs	_Imputation_	_TYPE_	_NAME_	Intercept	group	basey
1	1	PARMS		-0.17029	0.17639	0.20965
2	1	COV	Intercept	0.02453	-0.01471	-0.00017
3	1	COV	group	-0.01471	0.00981	-0.00000
4	1	COV	basey	-0.00017	-0.00000	0.00230
5	2	PARMS		-0.22035	0.23631	0.24016
6	2	COV	Intercept	0.02438	-0.01462	-0.00017
7	2	COV	group	-0.01462	0.00975	-0.00000
8	2	COV	basey	-0.00017	-0.00000	0.00229

```
Data WGEEbin; set WGEEbin; Wt=1/pred; Run;

*Fit WGEE for binary endpoint;
 Proc GenMod Data=WGEEbin Descending;
 Weight wt;
 Class GrpPt group Visit;
 Model yBin=group Visit group*Visit / dist=bin link=logit;
 Repeated Subject=GrpPt/ corr=cs;
 Run;

*Fit WGEE for normal endpoint;
 Proc GenMod Data=WGEEbin Descending;
 Weight wt;
 Class GrpPt group Visit;
 Model y=group Visit group*Visit / dist=normal;
 Repeated Subject=GrpPt/ corr=cs;
 Run;
```

In a nonrandomized experiment, propensity scores (the probability of assigning a treatment given the covariates) may be used for adjusting the treatment imbalance. In this case, we need to create a treatment indicator instead of missingness indicator and the logistic model it uses. After the propensity scores are estimated, the weight is defined as, if treatment = 1, wt=1/ (PS for treatment 1); if treatment = 0, wt=1/(PS for treatment 0).

Missing data can cause unbalance of confounders between treatment groups and bias the estimate of treatment effect. The approaches to confounding control include propensity score control, matching, and stratification, multivariate regression, and inverse probability weighting. Propensity score (PS) methods are weight technique based on causes of the treatment (they mimic randomization). A weight is assigned to each person according to the conditional probability of exposure given the confounder(s). After estimating PS for each person, use it to control confounding by: (1) adjusting for the PS as a covariate, (2) stratifying the effect estimate by the PS, (3) matching group 1 and group 2 people by PS, and (4) use PS as weight. Inverse probability weighting (IPW) is a weight technique that is based on the cause of outcome missing.

8.2.5   Multiple Imputation Method

Multiple imputation (MI) methods generate multiple copies of the "complete data set" by replacing missing values with randomly generated values using Bayesian or other methods, and analyze them as complete sets. MI does not model the dropout process but requires a correct specification of the model that relates the distribution of missing responses to the observed data, known as the imputation model.

According to Rubin (1987), MI involves three distinct tasks:

1. The missing values are filled in M times to generate M complete data sets.

2. The M complete data sets are analyzed by using the standard procedure.

3. The results from the M analyses are combined into a single inference.

The first step is the key. Consider a Bayesian joint model for the complete data and the missingness

$$f\left(Y_{mis}|Y_{obs}\right) = \int f\left(Y_{mis}|Y_{obs}\right) f\left(\theta|Y_{obs}\right) d\theta \qquad (8.18)$$

where

$$f(\theta|Y_{obs}) \propto f\left(\theta\right) \int f\left(Y_{obs}, Y_{mis}|\theta\right) dY_{mis}. \qquad (8.19)$$

MCMC is often used as a missing-imputation algorithm.

Ignorability is the weakest general condition under which the distribution of missingness does not need to be taken into account when making likelihood-based or Bayesian inferences (Rubin 1987). Without ignorability, MIs would have to be drawn from (8.19).

Because MI uses Bayesian method to generate missing values, how to have a valid frequentist inference is an interesting topic. Rubin (1976) describes conditions under which the following asymptotic result holds in a frequentist sense, i.e., the test statistic has a t-distribution.

To estimate β, we can use the weighting average of the M estimates:

$$\hat{\beta} = \sum_{m=1}^{M} w_m \hat{\beta}^{(m)} \qquad (8.20)$$

with variance

$$\hat{V} = W + \left(\frac{M+1}{M}\right) B, \qquad (8.21)$$

where

$$\begin{cases} W = \sum_{m=1}^{M} w_m \hat{V}^{(m)} \\ B = \sum_{m=1}^{M} w_m \left(\hat{\beta}^{(m)} - \hat{\beta}\right)\left(\hat{\beta}^{(m)} - \beta\right)'. \end{cases} \qquad (8.22)$$

Under MAR, $w_m = 1$. Under MNAR, weight w_m can be calculated by using sensitivity methods (Carpenter and Kenward, 2008).

A multiple imputation method using SAS involves two steps: data imputation and analysis. We illustrate the process with the TrialMAR dataset. We assume the primary endpoint is y at Visit 4.

Data Multiple Imputation Step

```
Data TrialMARv4; Set TrialMAR; If Visit=4; Run;
Proc MI data=TrialMARv4 seed=3731 nImpute=6 noprint Out=outmi;
Var y chgy basey;
by group;
Run;
```

```
proc print data=outmi(obs=20); run;
```

The MI procedure creates missing-imputed data sets and stores them in the Outmi dataset. The option nImpute specifies the number of imputed datasets. The default value is 5. The variable named _Imputation_ indicates the imputation numbers.

Based on m imputations, m different sets of the point and variance estimates for a parameter can be computed. The following statements generate regression coefficients for each of the six imputed datasets:

```
Proc Sort data=outmi; By _Imputation_; Run;
Proc Reg Data=outmi Outest=outreg covout noprint;
```

TABLE 8.10

Proc MIanalyze Variance Information.

Variance Information (6 Imputations)							
	Variance				Relative Increase	Fraction Missing	Relative
Parameter	Between	Within	Total	DF	in Variance	Information	Efficiency
Intercept	0.009341	0.025209	0.036107	54.885	0.432309	0.325949	0.948474
group	0.002389	0.010078	0.012865	106.56	0.276517	0.230919	0.962940
basey	0.001638	0.002368	0.004279	25.059	0.807289	0.486124	0.925052

     Model y= group basey;
     By _Imputation_;
     run;
     Proc Print data=outreg(obs=8);
     Var _Imputation_ _Type_ _Name_
     Intercept group basey;
     Title 'Parameter Estimates from Imputed Data Sets';
     Run;

The output dataset, outreg, includes parameter estimates and covariance matrices as shown in Table 8.9.

The following statements combine the six datasets of regression coefficients:

     Proc MIanalyze data=outreg;
     Modeleffects Intercept group basey;
     Run;

Table 8.10 displays variance information (between, within and total) for combining complete-data inferences. It also displays the degrees of freedom for the total variance, the relative increase in variance due to missing values, the fraction of missing information, and the relative efficiency for each parameter estimate.

Table 8.11 displays a combined estimate and standard error for each regression coefficient (parameter). Inferences are based on t distributions. The table displays a 95% confidence interval and a t test with the associated p-value for the hypothesis that the parameter is equal to the value specified with the THETA0= option (in this case, zero by default). The minimum and maximum parameter estimates from the imputed data sets are also displayed.

TABLE 8.11

Proc MIanalyze Parameter Estimates.

Parameter Estimates (6 Imputations)										
Parameter	Estimate	Std Error	95% Confidence Limits		DF	Minimum	Maximum	Theta0	t for H0: Parameter=Theta0	Pr > |t|
Intercept	-0.291385	0.234684	-0.78686	0.204091	16.85	-0.432206	-0.058169	0	-1.24	0.2314
group	0.262190	0.145386	-0.04314	0.567525	18.091	0.144364	0.376424	0	1.80	0.0880
basey	0.212913	0.068694	0.06959	0.356240	19.926	0.150769	0.262454	0	3.10	0.0057

Simulation Algorithm for Comparisons of Different Methods

1. Create response data for the two treatment groups

2. Create missings using missingness mechanism

3. Apply analysis methods

4. Repeat Steps 1-3 and combine and summarize results

8.2.6   Tipping Point Analysis for MNAR

Suppose the data contain a set of fully observed variables X and a variable Y that contains missing observations. The missingness indicator, $R = 0$ if Y is missing and 1 if observed. The MAR assumption is defined as $\Pr(R|X,Y) = \Pr(R|X)$, which implies that $\Pr(Y|X,R) = \Pr(Y|X)$. However, under MNAR assumption, $\Pr(R|X,Y) \neq \Pr(R|X)$, which implies that $\Pr(Y|X,R=0) \neq \Pr(Y|X,R=1)$.

A straightforward sensitivity analysis for the MAR assumption in multiple imputation is based on the pattern-mixture model approach (Little 1993; Molenberghs and Kenward 2007, pp. 30, 34–37), which models the distribution of a response as the mixture of a distribution of the observed responses and a distribution of the missing responses:

$$\begin{aligned} \Pr(Y, X, R) &= \Pr(Y, X|R)\Pr(R) \\ &= \Pr(Y, X|R = 0)\Pr(R = 0) + \Pr(Y, X|R = 1)\Pr(R = 1) \end{aligned}$$

Assuming $X = (Trt, Y_0)$, where Trt is treatment indicator and Y_0 represents baseline variables, one commonly used MNAR assumption for two-group clinical trials is that the missing value in the test group is systematically worse a constant δ than the control group. That is,

$$\Pr(Y = y|trt = 1, Y_0 = y_0, R = 1) = \Pr(Y = y - \delta|trt = 1, Y_0 = y_0, R = 0). \tag{8.23}$$

The implementation of this missingness mechanism is straightforward when the MI method is used, that is, subtracting a value of δ from the test group when a set of the imputation of missing data are generated under MAR. The smallest value of δ that tips the result from significant to non-significant regarding the treatment effect is called tipping point, denoted by δ_{tp}. The value of δ_{tp} can be found numerically through simulations in combination with a search method (e.g., binary search).

In the SAS MI procedure, the new MNAR statement imputes missing values by using the pattern-mixture model approach, assuming the missing data are MNAR. The two main options in the MNAR statement are MODEL and ADJUST. The MODEL option specifies a subset of observations from which imputation models are to be derived for specified variables. The ADJUST option specifies an imputed variable and adjustment parameters (such as shift and scale) for adjusting the imputed variable values of a specified subset of observations. The MNAR statement is applicable only if it is used along with a MONOTONE statement or an FCS statement.

8.2.7   Mixture of Paired and Unpaired Data

In this section, we discuss an optimal approach. For a clinical trial design with paired data, it often involves missing observations. In such case, the data from the trial become a mixture of paired and unpaired data. In case of MCAR, the completer analysis can be used but is inefficient when the proportion of missing data is large. The ignorable MLE-based analyses can be also used. However, we will discuss a simple but optimal approach for dealing with such a missing data problem (Chang and Wang, 2015).

Normal Endpoint

Let $x_{ts} \sim N\left(\mu_t, \sigma_X^2\right)$ be the response of the sth subject in treatment group t, $s = 1, ..., n_p$ for paired data, and $s = 1, ..., n_{tu}$ for unpaired data. Assume the first n_p of x_{1i} and x_{2i} are the paired data. For paired data, let the treatment difference $\hat{\delta}_p = \frac{1}{n_p} \sum_{i=1}^{n_p} (x_{2i} - x_{1i})$; for unpaired data, the treatment difference is estimated by $\hat{\delta}_u = \frac{1}{n_{1u}} \sum_{i=n_p+1}^{n_{1u}+n_p} x_{2i} - \frac{1}{n_{2u}} \sum_{i=n_p+1}^{n_{2u}+n_p} x_{1i}$.

We now propose the estimator for the treatment difference using a linear combination of δ_p and δ_u,

$$\hat{\delta} = w_p \hat{\delta}_p + w_u \hat{\delta}_u \tag{8.24}$$

where the prefixed weight $w_p + w_u = 1$. Assume the missing values are MCAR. In such case, the both estimators $\hat{\delta}_p$ and $\hat{\delta}_u$ of the treatment difference δ are unbiased and will also be an unbiased estimator of δ:

$$E\hat{\delta} = w_p E\hat{\delta}_p + w_u E\hat{\delta}_u = \delta. \tag{8.25}$$

The variance of $\hat{\delta}$ is given by

$$\sigma_{\hat{\delta}}^2 = w_p^2 \sigma_{\delta_p}^2 + (1 - w_p)^2 \sigma_{\delta_u}^2. \tag{8.26}$$

The weights w_p and w_u can be chosen such that the variance σ_δ^2 is minimized. This can be accomplished by letting $\frac{\partial \sigma_\delta^2}{\partial w_p} = 0$, which leads to

$$w_p = \frac{\sigma_{\delta_u}^2}{\sigma_{\delta_p}^2 + \sigma_{\delta_u}^2}. \tag{8.27}$$

Using the weight in (8.27), the minimum variance can be expressed as

$$\sigma_\delta^2 = \frac{\sigma_{\delta_p}^2 \sigma_{\delta_u}^2}{\sigma_{\delta_p}^2 + \sigma_{\delta_u}^2}. \tag{8.28}$$

The confidence interval constructed using this minimum variance will give the narrowest confidence interval.

For normal endpoint denoted by ρ, the correlation coefficient between matched pairs is:

$$\sigma_{\delta_p}^2 = 2(1-\rho)\frac{\sigma_x^2}{n_p}, \tag{8.29}$$

$$\sigma_{\delta_u}^2 = \left(\frac{1}{n_{1u}} + \frac{1}{n_{2u}}\right)\sigma_x^2. \tag{8.30}$$

Substituting (8.29) and (8.30) into (8.27) and (8.28), we obtain

$$w_p = \frac{1}{1 + 2(1-\rho)\frac{f_{1u}f_{2u}}{f_p(f_{1u}+f_{2u})}} \tag{8.31}$$

and

$$\sigma_\delta^2 = \frac{\sigma_*^2}{n} \tag{8.32}$$

where $n = n_p + n_{1u} + n_{2u}$, $f_p = n_p/n$, $f_{iu} = n_{iu}/n$, $(i = 1, 2)$, and the *equivalent variance* for the normal endpoint

$$\sigma_*^2 = \frac{2(1-\rho)\frac{1}{f_p}\left(\frac{1}{f_{1u}} + \frac{1}{f_{2u}}\right)}{2(1-\rho)\frac{1}{f_p} + \left(\frac{1}{f_{1u}} + \frac{1}{f_{2u}}\right)}\sigma_x^2. \tag{8.33}$$

The introduction of equivalent variance will provide a convenience when designing a classical or adaptive trial (the details will be discussed later with examples). When $n_{1u} = n_{2u} = n_u$, the weight becomes

$$w_p = \frac{1}{1 + (1-\rho)\frac{n_u}{n_p}}. \tag{8.34}$$

It is helpful to look into some special cases: (1) for paired data only, $n_u = 0$, and thus $w_p = 1$ and $w_u = 0$; (2) for independent data, $n_p = 0$, and thus $w_p = 0$ and $w_u = 1$; (3) when $\rho > 0$, $w_p > n_p/(n_p + n_u)$, when $\rho < 0$, $w_p < n_p/(n_p + n_u)$, and as $\rho \to 0$, $w_p \to n_p/(n_p + n_u)$.

Based on the derivation above, the correlation coefficient ρ should be determined independent of the current data. However, if ρ is (approximately) independent of $\hat{\delta}_u$ and $\hat{\delta}_p$ such as when n is large, ρ can be estimated from the data. The Pearson correlation coefficient is defined as

$$\hat{\rho} = \frac{\Sigma_i \left(x_{1i} - \bar{x}_1\right)\left(x_{2i} - \bar{x}_2\right)}{\sqrt{\Sigma_i \left(x_{1i} - \bar{x}_1\right)^2 \Sigma_i \left(x_{2i} - \bar{x}_2\right)^2}} \tag{8.35}$$

Binary Endpoint

For binary endpoint, let $x_{ts} = 1$ if subject s responds to treatment t and $x_{ts} = 0$ if subject s does not respond to treatment t. Using that notation, we can write $\hat{\delta}_p = \frac{1}{n_p}\sum_{i=1}^{n_p}(x_{2i} - x_{1i})$ and $\hat{\delta}_u = \hat{\delta}_{1u} - \hat{\delta}_{2u}$ for the observed proportion (treatment) difference for paired and unpaired data, respectively. Here $\hat{\delta}_{1u} = \frac{1}{n_{1u}}\sum_{i=n_p+1}^{n_{1u}+n_p} x_{1i}$ and $\hat{\delta}_{2u} = \frac{1}{n_{2u}}\sum_{i=n_p+1}^{n_{2u}+n_p} x_{2i}$. Thus, equations (8.24) through (8.35) are still applicable for a binary endpoint. However, the standard deviation is determined by

$$\hat{\sigma}_x^2 = \frac{1}{n_p + n_{1u}}\sum_{i=1}^{n_p+n_{1u}}(x_{1i} - \bar{x}_1)^2 + \frac{1}{n_p + n_{2u}}\sum_{i=1}^{n_p+n_{2u}}(x_{2i} - \bar{x}_2)^2. \tag{8.36}$$

The phi coefficient (mean square contingency coefficient), which is computationally equivalent to the Pearson correlation coefficient in the 2×2 case (i.e., $\hat{\rho} = \hat{\phi}$), is

$$\hat{\phi} = \frac{m_{11}m_{00} - m_{10}m_{01}}{\sqrt{\Sigma_j m_{1j}\Sigma_j m_{0j}\Sigma_i m_{i0}\Sigma_i m_{i1}}},$$

where m_{ij} represents the number of counts the 2×2 contingency table.

Alternatively, the variance for the paired mean difference is given by

$$\sigma_{\delta_p}^2 = \frac{\delta_d}{n_p}, \tag{8.37}$$

where δ_d is the proportion of discordant pairs, which can be estimated by

$$\hat{\delta}_d = \frac{1}{n_p}\sum_{i=1}^{n_p}[(1 - x_{2i})x_{1i} + (1 - x_{1i})x_{2i}]. \tag{8.38}$$

The variance for the unpaired mean difference is given by

$$\sigma_{\delta_u}^2 = \frac{\delta_{1u}(1 - \delta_{1u})}{n_{1u}} + \frac{\delta_{2u}(1 - \delta_{2u})}{n_{2u}}. \tag{8.39}$$

Since the correlation coefficient, ρ, is usually unknown, we can estimate it using data from current experiment. However, such a case, the weight w_p is not really constant (especially when the sample size is small). We will study the impact of such approximation on the coverage probability of the confidence interval and type-I error of a hypothesis test using simulations for both normal and binary endpoints. Similar to normal endpoint, we can express the variance as

$$\sigma_\delta^2 = \frac{\sigma_*^2}{n},$$

where the equivalent variance σ_*^2 can be estimated by

$$\hat{\sigma}_*^2 = \frac{\frac{\hat{\delta}_d}{f_p}\left[\frac{\hat{\delta}_{1u}\left(1-\hat{\delta}_{1u}\right)}{f_{1u}} + \frac{\hat{\delta}_{2u}\left(1-\hat{\delta}_{2u}\right)}{f_{2u}}\right]}{\frac{\hat{\delta}_d}{f_p} + \frac{\hat{\delta}_{1u}\left(1-\hat{\delta}_{1u}\right)}{f_{1u}} + \frac{\hat{\delta}_{2u}\left(1-\hat{\delta}_{2u}\right)}{f_{2u}}}. \tag{8.40}$$

Power and Sample Size for Hypothesis Test

If we denote the treatment difference by δ, we can write the typical hypothesis test for either normal or binary endpoint as,

$$H_o : \delta \le 0 \text{ versus } H_a : \delta > 0, \tag{8.41}$$

and define the test statistic as (for large sample size n)

$$T = \frac{\hat{\delta}}{\hat{\sigma}_\delta} \sim N\left(\frac{\delta}{\sigma_\delta}, 1\right) = N\left(\frac{\delta\sqrt{n}}{\sigma_*}, 1\right) \tag{8.42}$$

When $\delta = 0$, T has the standard normal distribution: $T \sim N(0, 1)$.

The two-sided $(1 - \alpha)\, 100\%$ confidence interval for treatment difference δ is given by

$$w_p \delta_p + (1 - w_p)\, \delta_u \pm z_{1-\alpha/2} \frac{\sigma_*}{\sqrt{n}}, \tag{8.43}$$

where w_p is given by (8.31).

This confidence interval can be used for the analysis of non-inferiority trials.

If both pairs are missing, we have to replace the missing observations. Therefore, for simplicity, we assume there are no such cases.

For the hypothesis test (18), the power for the classical design is given by

$$1 - \beta = \Phi\left(\frac{\delta}{\sigma_\delta} - z_{1-\alpha}\right).$$

The overall sample size for superiority test is given by

$$n^* = \left[\frac{(z_{1-\alpha} + z_{1-\beta})}{\delta}\right]^2 \sigma_*^2 \tag{8.44}$$

where σ_*^2 is given in (8.33) and (8.40) for normal and binary endpoints, respectively.

For normal endpoint, when $n_{1u} = n_{2u} = n_u$, then $n_p + 2n_u = n$ (total sample size) and $f_u = \frac{n_u}{n}$. Thus, from (8.33), we obtain

$$\sigma_*^2 = 2\sigma_x^2 \frac{1-\rho}{1-(1+\rho)f_u}. \tag{8.45}$$

In case there is no missing ($f_u = 0$), the sample size required for paired design is

$$n = \left[\frac{(z_{1-\alpha} + z_{1-\beta})}{\delta}\right]^2 2\sigma_x^2(1-\rho).$$

If the missing data are ignored, the sample size required for the target power $1 - \beta$ will be inflated by a factor of $1 - 2f_u$, i.e.,

$$\tilde{n} = \frac{n}{1-2f_u}. \tag{8.46}$$

Since the sample size n is proportional to the equivalent variance σ_*^2, the ratio of the sample size n^* with missing data included (8.44, 8.45) to the sample size with missing data excluded (Eq. 8.23) is

$$R = \frac{n^*}{\tilde{n}} = \frac{1-2f_u}{1-(1+\rho)f_u} \tag{8.47}$$

when $\rho = 0$ (independent), $R = \frac{1-2f_u}{1-f_u}$. When $\rho \to 1$, $R \to 100\%$ and $n \to 0$. From (8.47), we can see that the relative impact (R) of missing data increases when the correlation coefficient (ρ) increases. For example, if $\rho = 0.8$ and $f_u = 0.2$ (40% missing), $R = \frac{0.6}{1-(1.8)0.2} = 93.8\%$. That is, a 40% missing leads to a 6.2% savings in sample size. For $\rho = 0.5$ and $f_u = 0.2$, $R = \frac{0.6}{1-(1.5)0.2} = 85.7\%$, leading to a 14.3% savings. For $\rho = 0$ and $f_u = 0.2$, $R = 75\%$, it leads to a 25% savings. For $\rho = 0.5$ and $f_u = 0.3$ (60% missing), $R = \frac{0.4}{1-(1.5)0.3} = 72.7\%$, leading to 27.3% savings.

8.2.8   Comparisons of Different Methods

Single-imputation methods such as LOCF are simple to implement, but they generally do not conform to well-recognized statistical principles for drawing inference, and often lead to a biased estimate. The minimum variable approach for mixed paired and unpaired data is a special method applicable to MCAR.

Maximum likelihood approaches under ignorable missingness provide valid inferences. Random effects models can be very useful to simplify a highly multivariate distribution with a few parameters. However, when missingness is not ignorable, the impact is difficult to assess.

The IPW method is simple to implement when the missing values have a monotone pattern, and can be carried out in software packages that allow weighted analyses. The IPW method allows the inclusion of auxiliary variables such as previously observed outcomes. There are potential instabilities of? large weights, leading to high variance in finite samples, especially when the missingness model is incorrectly specified. Methods that yield valid inferences when either one or the other of the outcome regression or the missingness model is correct are said to have a double-robustness property. In a missing data model, an estimator is DR if it remains consistent when either (but not necessarily both) a model for the missingness mechanism or a model for the distribution of the complete data is correctly specified (Bang and Robin, 2005).

Multiple imputation methods explicitly specify the missing data assumptions and allows the use of large amounts of auxiliary information. They can be relatively straightforward to implement, without special programming needs, and can handle arbitrary patterns of missing data.

The exact pattern of missing is impossible to know. Sensitivity analyses with different missingness assumptions are necessary when missing data are extensive. The tipping-point analysis is a commonly used method in the sensitivity analysis.

Recently, Permutt and Li (2016) propose an exact test of the hypothesis of no drug effect, taking all randomized patients into account, based on a readily interpretable statistic. The method also copes with a drug that is toxic in some patients but beneficial to others, a difficult problem for standard methods. A robust conclusion of efficacy can be drawn without missing pattern assumptions.

8.2.9 Regulatory and Operational Perspectives

CHMP, the European health authority (2009) states "Missing data are a potential source of bias when analyzing clinical trials... A critical discussion of the number, timing, pattern, reason for and possible implications of missing values in efficacy and safety assessments should be included in the clinical report as a matter of routine... It should be noted that just ignoring missing data is not an acceptable option when planning, conducting or interpreting the analysis of a confirmatory clinical trial...The justification for selecting a particular method should not be based primarily on the properties of the method under particular assumptions (for example MAR or MCAR) but on whether it will provide an appropriately conservative estimate for the comparison of primary regulatory interest in the circumstances of the trial under consideration." The agency notes that using completer analysis as the sole means to address missing data (completer analyses) may violate the strict ITT principle, which requires measurement of all patient outcomes regardless of the protocol adherence. This principle is of critical importance as confirmatory clinical trials should estimate the effect of the experimental intervention in the population of patients with greatest external validity.

There are many factors that can affect missingness: (1) the complexity of the measurements, (2) the frequency of measurements, (3) self-reported versus in-clinic measure by clinicians, (4) the nature of the outcome variable, such as modality versus morbidity, (5) the treatment modalities such as surgical versus medical treatment, (6) frequency of the treatment, (7) the benefit-risk profile of the treatment, (8) duration of the clinical trial since a longer trial will likely have a larger proportion of missing data than a shorter trial, (9) the therapeutic indication: missing values are more frequent in those diseases where the adherence of patients to the study protocol is usually low (e.g. psychiatric disorders), (10) data entry error, some numbers may be easier to missight than others, and (11) the design and conduct of the experiment.

A reduction in missing data can be achieved by paying careful attention to clinical trial designs, strengthening data collection, and whenever possible, collecting outcome data after withdrawal. To minimize potential bias, CHMP (2009) recommends that a detailed description of the pre-planned methods used for handling missing data, any amendments of that plan and a justification for the amendment should be included in the clinical study report. A critical discussion of the number, timing, pattern, and reasons for and possible implications of missing values in efficacy and safety assessments should be included in the clinical report as a matter of routine. Because of the unpredictability of some problems, authorities sometimes allow in the study protocol the possibility of updating the strategy for dealing with missing values in the statistical analysis plan, or during the blind review of the data at the end of the trial.

At the request of FDA, the National Research Council convened the Panel on the Handling of Missing Data in Clinical Trials, under the Committee on National Statistics, to prepare "a report with recommendations that would be useful for FDA's development of a guidance for clinical trials on appropriate study designs and follow-up methods to reduce missing data and appropriate statistical methods to address missing data for analysis of results." The panel developed an excellent report titled "The prevention and treatment of missing data in clinical trials" (Little, et al. 2010). The panel consisted of a group of academic statisticians, however there is evidence that there was also some interaction with industry statisticians as indicated in the acknowledgments. Among many useful suggestions, they recommended the following.

Clinical Trial Design

Investigators, sponsors, and regulators should design clinical trials consistent with the goal of maximizing the number of participants who are maintained on the protocol-specified intervention until the outcome data are collected.

The techniques to reduce the occurrence of missingness include (1) adding run-in periods before randomization to identify who can tolerate or respond to the study treatment, (2) using flexible-dose (titration), (3) restricting trial to target population for whom treatment is indicated, (4) adding the study treatment to a standard treatment, (5) reducing length of follow-up period, (6) allowing rescue medication in the event of poor response, and (7) defining outcomes that can be ascertained in a high proportion of participants. Of course, benefits of these options need to be weighed against costs.

Clinical Trial Conduct

Trial sponsors should continue to collect information on key outcomes on participants who discontinue their protocol-specified intervention during the course of the study, except in those cases for which a compelling cost-benefit analysis argues otherwise, and this information should be recorded and used in the analysis.

The techniques to limit the amount of missing data include (1) choices of study sites, investigators, participants, study outcomes, time in study and times of measurement, and the nature and frequency of follow-up to limit the amount of missing data, (2) limiting participant burden in other ways, such as making follow-up visits easy in terms of travel and childcare, (3) providing frequent reminders of study visits, (4) training of investigators on the importance of avoiding missing data, (5) providing incentives to investigators and participants to limit dropouts, and (6) monitoring of adherence and in other ways dealing with participants who cannot tolerate or do not adequately respond to treatment.

The panel recommends that study sponsors should explicitly anticipate potential problems of missing data. In particular, the trial protocol should contain a section that addresses missing data issues, including the anticipated amount of missing data, and steps taken in trial design and trial conduct to monitor and limit the impact of missing data.

Trial Data Analysis

There is no universal method for handling incomplete data in a clinical trial. Despite difference among the trials, there are common principles that can be applied in a wide variety of settings as suggested by the panel:

1. A basic assumption is that missingness of a particular value hides a true underlying value that is meaningful for analysis.

2. The analysis must be formulated to draw inference about an appropriate and well-defined causal estimand.

3. Reasons for missing data must be documented as much as possible.

4. The trial designers should decide on a primary set of assumptions about the missing data mechanism. Those primary assumptions then serve as an anchor point for the sensitivity analyses.

5. The trial sponsors should conduct a statistically valid analysis under the primary missing data assumptions.

6. The analysts should assess the robustness of the treatment effect inferences by conducting a sensitivity analysis.

Despite efforts to minimize missing data in the design and conduct of clinical trials, the statistical analysis often has to deal with a nontrivial amount of missing data. There is no single correct method for handling missing data. As such, the panel recommends that statistical methods for handling missing data should be specified by clinical trial sponsors in study protocols, and their associated assumptions stated in a way that can be understood by clinicians. Single imputation methods like last observation carried forward and baseline observation carried forward should not be used as the primary approach to the treatment of missing data unless the assumptions that underlie them are scientifically justified. Sensitivity analyses should be part of the primary reporting of findings from clinical trials. Examining sensitivity to the assumptions about the missing data mechanism should be a mandatory component of reporting.

Bibliography

Bang, H., Robins, J.M. (2005). Doubly robust estimation in missing data and causal inference models. Biometrics. 2005 Dec;61(4):962-73.

Carey, V., Zeger, S. L., and Diggle, P. J. (1993), "Modelling Multivariate Binary Data with Alternating Logistic Regressions." Biometrika 80:517–526.

Chang, M. and Wang, J. (2015). Trial Design and Analysis with Incomplete Paired Data. American Journal of Biostatistics, American Journal of Biostatistics, Volume 5, Issue 2, Pages 61-68

CHMP (2009). Guideline on missing data in confirmatory clinical trials/1776/99 Rev. 1.

Fitzmaurice, G. M., Laird, N. M., and Ware, J. H. (2011). Applied Longitudinal Analysis. John Wiley & Sons, New York.

Heagerty, P., and Zeger, S. L. (1996). "Marginal Regression Models for Clustered Ordinal Measurements." Journal of the American Statistical Association 91:1024–1036.

Little, R.J. (1993). Pattern-mixture models for multivariate incomplete data. Journal of the American Statistical Association 88, 125-134.

Little, R.J. et al. (2010). Panel on Handling Missing Data in Clinical Trial. The prevention and treatment of missing data in clinical trials. The National Academies Press. Washington, D.C.

Little, R.J. and Rubin, D.B. (2002). Statistical Analysis with Missing Data (2nd edn). John Wiley & Sons, New York.

Mallinckrodt, C. (2013). Preventing and Treating Missing Data in Longitudinal Clinical Trials: A Practical Guide. Cambridge: Cambridge University Press.

Molenberghs, G. and Kenward, M.G. (2008). Missing data in clinical studies. John Wiley & Sons, New York.

O'Kelly, M., and Ratitch, B. (2014). Clinical Trials with Missing Data: A Guide for Practitioners. John Wiley & Sons, New York.

Permutt, T. and Li, F. (2016). Trimmed means for symptom trials with dropouts. Pharmaceut. Statist. 2017, 16 20–28

Rubin, D.B. (1976). Inference and missing data. Biometrika 1976; 63:581–592.

Rubin, D.B. (1987). Multiple Imputation for Nonresponse in Surveys. John Wiley & Sons, New York.

SAS Institute (2006). SAS/STAT 9.1 User's Guide, Volumes 1-7. 2006. SAS Institute, Gary, NC.

9

Special Issues and Resolutions

9.1 Overview

In this chapter, special issues that come up in clinical trials are identified along with solutions or paths for consideration.

9.2 Drop-Loser Design Based on Efficacy and Safety

9.2.1 Multi-Stage Design with Treatment Selection

The comparison of several distinct treatments with a common control occurs frequently in clinical trials. To optimize and potentially limit sample size, adaptive designs with the ability to evaluate interim efficacy and/or safety data and also potentially drop inferior arms are often proposed. The pick-the-winner design discussed in Chapter 4 is an example of multiple-arm adaptive design. The methods are based on efficacy criteria in order to preserve the type-I error. Thall et al. (1988, 1989) proposed a design only allowing one treatment to continue beyond the first interim. Stallard and Friede (2008) proposed a more general design with prespecified number of treatments at each stage. Follmann et al. (1994) considered a design in which treatments are only dropped at interim if found significantly inferior to control.

However, drug toxicities also have to be considered in selecting treatments and thus require more flexible mechanics for dropping losers while controlling type-1 error rate. More flexible two-stage designs have been proposed by several authors (Schmidli et al., 2006; Bretz et al., 2006). These designs used closed testing procedures and/or combination tests to control the probability of making a type-I error whilst allowing many modifications to be made at the interim.

Magirr et al. (2012) extend Dunnett's multiple-testing procedure to multiple stages, which allows interim efficacy or futility claims as long as the trial crosses the corresponding efficacy or futility boundaries (Wason et al., 2017). Chang and Jing (2015) study multiple arm design with treatment selection by adding-arm or dropping-arm mechanics. In this design both efficacy and toxicity can be considered. Hampson and Koenig (2017) studied the many-to-one comparisons after safety selection in multi-arm clinical trials. They conclude that the adjusted Dunnett critical values can be further modified based on the number of arms remaining as long as the correlation between toxicity and efficacy is nonnegative. However, these trial designs have not considered the early loser dropping.

Deng and Chang (2018) consider the two drop-loser designs with sufficient flexibility to consider the safety information in treatment selection, but at the same time retain reasonably high power. The drop-loser design can have sample-size adjustment mechanics. In all cases they considered, it is assumed that due to the requirement for a minimum number of subjects to be included in the safety database, the trial does not allow early stoppage for an interim efficacy claim (not enough sample size for safety evaluation), but the trial can stop earlier due to safety concerns or lack of efficacy. The nonbinding futility rule is applied for determining the critical values in the hypothesis testing at the final analysis.

9.2.2 Dunnett Test with Drop-Losers

It is important that a trial can be flexible enough to allow to drop losers based on other factors in addition to the efficacy criterion. The critical values for the classical Dunnett's pairwise tests are applied to the classical dose-finding studies with the common control. When these critical values are applied to a drop-loser design without rejection of any null hypothesis in the pairwise comparisons at interim analyses, the FWER can be controlled or can be even more conservative. This is because when losers are dropped, the numbers of pairwise comparison will reduce and thus reduce the chance of making type-I errors. Therefore, this is a conservative approach, but the design provides great flexibility allowing for any number of analyses performed at any time to drop any number of arms based on any criteria (efficacy, safety etc. without prespecifications). This design will save sample size if some treatment arms are dropped at interim analyses. However, the design may not be very efficient in some scenarios. We designate it the drop-loser design with Dunnett's test (DLDDT). The Dunnett test critical values will depend on the number of comparisons and can be obtained through numerical integrations or simulations (See Chapter 4).

The mathematical proof of FWER with DLDDT is straightforward:

$$
\begin{aligned}
\alpha &= \sup \Pr\left(\text{Reject at least one } H_k | H_0\right) = \sup \Pr\left(\cup_{k=1}^{K} t_k \geq \mu_\alpha | H_0\right) \\
&\geq \sup \Pr\left(\cup_{k=1}^{L} t_k \geq \mu_\alpha | H_0\right) = \sup \Pr\left(\cup_{k=1}^{L} t_k \geq \mu_\alpha | H_{0L}\right),
\end{aligned}
$$

where L is the number of remaining arms in the final stage, H_{0L} is the set of hypotheses for those remaining arms, which belong to H_0. The inequality is due to the removal of some union sets. Because Dunnett's test controls FWER, for other configurations of null hypothesis, it can be shown (Xuan,

2018 and below) that the error of testing remaining arms is smaller than the error of traditional Dunnett test in the similar manner.

This design is not only a conservative approach, but also it provides flexibility allowing for any number of interim analyses performed at any time, and any number of arms may be dropped without pre-specifying criteria in advance. DLDDT could also save sample size if some treatment arms are dropped in the interim stages compared to the fixed sample size Dunnett test.

The following is a proof of FWER control with DLDGKP:

$$\sup \Pr\left(\text{reject at least on } H_k | H_{oL}\right) \leq \sup \Pr\left(\text{reject at least on } H_k | H_{oK}\right)$$
$$= \sup \Pr\left(p_w \leq \alpha^*_{\tau_{\max},K} | H_{ow}\right) \leq \alpha,$$

where H_{oK} is the all subsets of hypotheses for all K arms, H_{oL} is the all subsets of hypotheses for all remaining arms in the final stage, p_w is the p-value for the winner arm in the final stage and H_{ow} is the null hypothesis for the winner arm. Note that $\tau_{\max}$ and K are prefixed at design stage.

9.2.3 Drop-Loser Design with Gatekeeping Procedure

The second approach, drop-loser design with gatekeeping procedure (DLDGKP), is proposed by Deng and Chang (2018) to improve efficiency of the design by sacrificing some not very useful flexibility, that is, allowing for any number of analyses performed at any time no later than $\tau_{\max}$ to drop any number of arms based on flexible criteria don't have to be fully prespecified, but a non-negative correlation is required between the final test statistic and the statistic at the IA for dropping the losers. Furthermore, at the final analysis, the hypothesis testing for the pairwise comparisons will be performed in a gatekeeping fashion as described below. We assume the drop-loser decisions are made by the independent data monitor committee (IDMC).

(1) The efficacy winner was dropped due to safety issue. If the efficacy winner has dropped from at an interim and not included in the final analysis, then we will use the Dunnett critical value $\alpha_{1,K-1}$ for m pairwise comparisons ($m < K$), where m is the number of active arms at the final analysis. The critical values $\alpha_{\tau,K}$ for the pick-the-winner design and $\alpha_{1,K-1}$ for Dunnett's test can be found in Table 9.1. The critical value for the Dunnett test with a drop-loser mechanism is a special case of the pick-the-winner design when $\tau = 1$. We can see that the critical values for DLDGKP, $\alpha^*_{\tau_{\max},K} \geq \alpha_{1,K}$, less stringent than that for the Dunnett test in this case.

(2) The efficacy winner was not dropped due to safety issue. When the efficacy winner has not been dropped at an interim due to a safety issue, it will be included in the final analysis even if the efficacy winner has a safety issue at the final analysis. The efficacy winner is selected at the last interim analysis performed at time $\tau \leq \tau_{\max}$. Note that the winner may not be the best efficacy arm in terms of data from the final cumulative data. The critical value for pick-the-winner design will depend on the number of comparisons and can be obtained through numerical integrations or simulations (see Chapter 4).

TABLE 9.1

Critical Values, $\alpha_{\tau,K}$ for Pick-the-Winner Design.

τ	Number of Active Arms, K						
	1	2	3	4	5	6	7
0.5	0.025	0.0151	0.0114	0.0093	0.0080	0.0071	0.0064
0.7	0.025	0.0143	0.0104	0.0082	0.0069	0.0060	0.0054
1.0	0.025	0.0135	0.0094	0.0073	0.0060	0.0051	0.0045

Note: if p-value $\leq \alpha_{\tau,K}$, reject the hypothesis test. FWER=0.025.

Examples of critical values with a larger sample size assumption are presented in Table 9.1. To control FWER, the winner will be tested against critical value $\alpha_{\tau_{\max},K}$. If not significant, no further pairwise test will be performed. If significant, the remaining pairwise comparisons will be performed against $\alpha_{1,K-1}$. This is because we need to control type-I error in the following two scenarios: (1) under global H_0 using $\alpha_{\tau_{\max},K}$ and (2) when winner is very effective and all others are not effective using $\alpha_{1,K-1}$.

Optimal Design

The optimal (largest) $\tau_{\max}$ should be chosen so that $\alpha_{\tau_{\max},K} = \alpha_{1,K-1}$. This way, no α will be wasted. In other words, we can use Dunnett critical value $\alpha_{\tau,K-1}$ and find the latest possible time to drop losers, $\tau_{\max}$, so that $\alpha_{\tau_{\max},K} = \alpha_{\tau,K} = \alpha_{1,K-1}$. Examples of optimal $\tau_{\max}$ are presented in Table 9.2.

Remark: it is important (for controlling FWER) to be sure the reason to drop the winner is due to safety reasons and has nothing to do with the relative effectiveness between the arms. If the winner has not been dropped, the gatekeeping procedure has to be applied, even when the winner arm is too toxic at the final analysis or has a low utility value.

The proof of FWER control of DLDGKP will be somewhat more involved:

(1) For independent case: The FWER of DLDGKP is also strongly controlled if the treatment selection rule is independent from the efficacy data. To show this, let $D = 1$ when the winner arm in the interim is dropped and $D = 0$ otherwise; $L \leq K$ be the number of remaining arms in the final stage; H_{0L} be the set of hypotheses for those remaining arms, which belongs to H_0; p_w be the p-value for testing the interim selected winner arm versus control

TABLE 9.2

Optimal Critical Values, $\alpha^*_{\tau_{\max},K}$ for DLDGKP.

	Number of Active Arms, K				
	3	4	5	6	7
$\alpha^*_{\tau_{\max},K}$	0.0135	0.0094	0.0073	0.0060	0.0051
$\tau_{\max}$	0.2850	0.4920	0.6250	0.7150	0.7750

Note: if p-value $\leq \alpha_{\tau,K}$, reject the hypothesis at $\alpha = 0.025$.

group in the final stage. Then,

$$\sup \Pr \left(\text{Reject at least on } H_k | H_{0L} \right)$$

$$= \quad \sup \Pr \left(D = 1 \cap \min_{l \in \{1,\ldots,L\}} (p_l) \le \alpha_{\tau_{\max}, K} | H_{0L} \right)$$

$$+ \sup \Pr \left(D = 0 \cap p_w \le \alpha_{\tau_{\max}, K} | H_{0L} \right)$$

$$= \quad \sup \Pr \left(D = 1 \right) \Pr \left(\min_{l \in \{1,\ldots,L\}} (p_l) \le \alpha_{\tau_{\max}, K} | H_{0L} \right)$$

$$+ \sup \Pr \left(D = 0 \right) \Pr \left(p_w \le \alpha_{\tau_{\max}, K} | H_{0L} \right)$$

$$\le \quad \Pr \left(D = 1 \right) \alpha + \Pr \left(D = 0 \right) \alpha = \alpha,$$

where the inequality is because of

$$\Pr \left(\min_{l \in \{1,\ldots,L\}} (p_l) \le \alpha_{\tau_{\max}, K} | H_{0L} \right) \le \Pr \left(\min_{l \in \{1,\ldots,K\}} (p_l) \le \alpha_{\tau_{\max}, K} | H_{0,(K-1)} \right),$$

and $H_{0,(K-1)}$ is the set of hypotheses for the arms excluding the interim selected winner arm.

(2) For dependent case, see Deng and Chang (2018) for a proof of FWER. The basic idea in the proof is to show the error rate under a positive correlation condition is no larger than the error rate under independent case.

9.2.4   Drop-Loser Design with Adjustable Sample Size

We emphasize here that allowing multiple arms to carry forward to the final analysis is often important because the more efficacious arms may also be associated with greater toxicity. However, sometimes the highest efficacy arm has to be dropped at an interim analysis because intolerable toxicities are observed. When this happens, the power may not be as high as expected. To retain the power, we can modify the design allowing for increase in sample size for the next most efficacious arm or all remaining arms when the most effective arm is dropped. The sample size adjustment does not depend on effect size of any arm, that is, the sample size will increase by $x\%$ as long as the efficacy winner is dropped at an interim analysis due to toxicity. The final sample size of the trial is not a function of efficacy data at the previous stages. This makes the type I error control and power similation much simpler since the same critical values for DLDGKP can be used for the DLDGKP with the design with adjustable sample size.

9.2.5   Drop-Loser Rules in Terms of Efficacy and Safety

Method 1: define the rules of dropping a loser based on safety and efficacy separately:

1. If the toxicity (active arm i versus the control) $\varsigma_i > \varsigma_{\max}$ (the maximum tolerated odd ratio or rate), the corresponding arm will be dropped.

2. If the efficacy of active arm i, $\delta_i < r\delta_{max}$, arm i will be dropped. Here, δ_{max} is the maximum observed effect for the arms without safety concerns.

This method can be used with or without the sample size adjustment method discussed above. No change is necessary for the critical values if the sample size adjustment is independent of effect size of the arms. Here is a proposed algorithm for sample size reestimation: If the best efficacy arm (based on the last interim efficacy data) is dropped, the sample size will increase by $x\%$ for each of the remaining arms, where x can be any number as long as it is independent of efficacy of the remaining arms.

Method 2: define the rules of dropping loser based on a utility function that incorporates safety and efficacy:

1. Define the utility as

$$U = U_{eff} - U_{Tox}, \tag{9.1}$$

and

$$\begin{cases} U_{eff} = (1 + 100\exp(-\frac{b_E}{\delta_{min}}x))^{-1}, \\ U_{Tox} = (1 + 100\exp(-\frac{b_T}{\varsigma_{max}}x))^{-1} \end{cases} \tag{9.2}$$

where we suggest $b_E = b_T = 1$ to 10. If ς_{max} is very large ($\to \infty$), the toxicity issue is ignored and the utility, $U = U_{eff} + 1/101$, is only based on efficacy. Similarly, if δ_{min} is very larger ($\to \infty$), the utility is dependent on the toxicity only.

2. If the utility $U_i - U_{Placebo} < 0.8U_{min}$ or $U_i < 0.5U_{max}$, arm i ($i = 1, ..., K$) will be dropped, where U_{min} is the minimum utility value required beyond the control and U_{max} is the maximum observed utility among all arms at an interim analysis.

9.2.6   Simulation Study

We will use simulation to compare the efficiencies of the two designs: drop-loser-design with Dunnett's Test and drop-loser-design with gatekeeping procedure. First, we set up the response curves for the normal efficacy endpoint and the binary toxicity endpoint. For each of the endpoints, the same four different curves are considered as indicated in Table 9.3.

SAS Macros 9.1 were developed for the drop-loser design with Dunnett's test (DLDDT) and drop-loser design with gatekeeping procedure (DLDGKP), respectively. In the following simulations, assume the minimum effect size required is $\delta_{min} = 0.15$ and the maximum tolerated toxicity rate is $\varsigma_{max} = 0.15$, and constants $b_E = b_T = 3$ in the utility definition. The interim analysis is performed at optimal information time $\tau = 0.625$ ($n_1 = 320$/arm, $n_2 = 192$/arm) and $U_{min} = 0.01$ for the both methods DLDDT and DLDGKP.

TABLE 9.3

Response Curves of Efficacy and Toxicity

Scenario	Arm				
	1	2	3	4	5
Low flat	0.1	0.1	0.1	0.1	0.1
High flat	0.2	0.2	0.2	0.2	0.2
Linear	0.05	0.1	0.15	0.2	0.25
S-Shape	0.1	0.1	0.15	0.2	0.2

Note: normal efficacy endpoint μ/σ and binary toxicity endpoint.

An example of invoking the macro is:

Title "Power for linear efficacy & S-Shape toxicity"; run;
Data dInput;
 Array us{6}(0,0.05,0.1,0.15,0.2,0.25);
  Array ps{6}(0.000001,0.1,0.1,0.15,0.2,0.2);
%DrpLsrDTGKP(nSims=100000,nArms=6, MTTR=0.15);

There are $4 \times 4 = 16$ efficacy-toxicity scenarios simulated. The simulation results include the probability of success for each active arm and overall probability of success (PoS) defined as at least one active arm is successful. The power of pick-the-winner is that only one arm or the winner is carried to the final design for the hypothesis test without considering safety issues. Table 9.4 show partial results from the simulations.

From the simulation results, we can see that the overall power is similar for the DLDDT and DLDGKP when the response curves are flat. However, DLDDT has a higher power for flat dose-response curves, while DLDGKP has higher power for uneven dose-response curves. This is understandable since optimal DLDGKP uses the pick-the-winner mechanics to have larger critical value 0.0073 versus 0.006 for the DLDDT method. DLDGKP requires that the interim winner be tested first in the final analysis; if the winner is not the best arm in the final analysis DLDGKP will reduce the power, which will often be the case when the dose-response curve is flat or all doses are equally good.

9.3 Clinical Trial Interim Analysis with Survival Endpoint

9.3.1 Hazard Ratio versus Number of Deaths

The logrank test is a commonly used method for testing survival difference between two groups in classical and adaptive clinical trials. The stopping rules and conditional power at an interim analysis of an adaptive trial are

TABLE 9.4
Power of Drop-Loser Design with Utility Stopping Rule.

Efficacy μ/σ	Toxicity p	Drop-Loser Design			PWD	
		Dun Pow	GKP Pow	Ave N	Power	Ave N
Low flat	low flat	0.407	0.409	2367	0.415	2304
	high flat	0.122	0.128	2151		
	linear	0.314	0.331	2309		
	S-Shape	0.312	0.329	2281		
Ligh flat	low flat	0.958	0.939	2611	0.939	2304
	high flat	0.909	0.907	2412		
	linear	0.935	0.932	2493		
	S-Shape	0.944	0.937	2511		
Linear	low flat	0.956	0.945	2439	0.945	2304
	high flat	0.871	0.872	2333		
	linear	0.774	0.784	2371		
	S-Shape	0.884	0.888	2382		
S-Shape	low flat	0.885	0.867	2455	0.867	2304
	high flat	0.716	0.721	2299		
	linear	0.686	0.701	2375		
	S-Shape	0.763	0.773	2379		

Note: PWD = pick-the-winner design without toxicity consideration.

conventionally specified in terms of logrank statistic or p-value. However, study statisticians are often asked to explain a value of the p-value or logrank statistic in terms of hazard ratio and a difference in median time. To answer the question, we have to look into the relationship of those quantities (Table 9.4).

In Chapter 7, we discussed the logrank test. If the two groups have the same survival function, the logrank statistic is approximately standard normal. A one-sided level α test will reject the null hypothesis if $Z > z_{1-\alpha}$. If there are n total subjects with the hazard ratio θ and the probability a subject in either group will have an event is d (thus the expected number of events is $D = nd$), then the logrank statistic is approximately normally distributed:

$$Z \tilde{} N\left(\log\theta\sqrt{f_1 f_2 D}, 1\right), \tag{9.3}$$

where f_1 and f_2 are the sample size for the two groups (Schoenfeld, 1981).

There is no one-to-one relationship between logrank statistic (or p-value) and median survival difference (or hazard ratio), we can derive the relationship using some reasonable assumptions.

We know that for a balanced design, logrank statistic is asymptotically normal, that is,

$$Z \tilde{} N\left(\log\theta\sqrt{D/4}, 1\right). \tag{9.4}$$

Therefore, under the large sample size assumption, Z is a good estimator of $\log \theta \sqrt{D/4}$, where θ is hazard ratio between the two groups and D is the expected total number of events. The expected value of the test statistic

$$\bar{z} = \log \theta \sqrt{\frac{D}{4}}. \tag{9.5}$$

To relate the test statistic to the hazard ratio, answer the above question, we derive an approximate relation association from (9.5) by replacing the expected values with the observed value, that is,

$$\hat{\theta} \approx \exp\left(z\sqrt{\frac{4}{D}}\right). \tag{9.6}$$

Example 9.1: Suppose logrank statistic $z = 0.5$ with $D = 100$ events observed, the estimated hazard ratio is $\hat{\theta} = \exp\left(0.5\sqrt{\frac{4}{100}}\right) = 1.105\,2$. If we further assume an exponential survival model, then $\hat{\theta} = \frac{T_{1median}}{T_{2median}}$, where $T_{1median}$ and $T_{2median}$ are median times for the two groups, respectively. If $T_{2median} = 9.2$ months, then $T_{1median} = \hat{\theta}T_{2median} = 1.1052 * 9.2 = 10.\,168$ months.

9.3.2 Conditional Power

Given the interim decision rules, continue to the second stage if at the interim analysis $\alpha_1 < p_1 \leq \beta_1$ and at the final analysis reject H_0 if the final p-value $p \leq \alpha_2$.

The conditional power for a balanced two-stage group sequential design with is

$$\Pr(p \leq \alpha_2 | N_2, p_1; \delta, \sigma) = \Phi\left[\frac{\delta}{\sigma}\sqrt{\frac{N_2}{4}} - \frac{z_{1-\alpha_2} - \sqrt{1-\tau_1}z_{1-p_1}}{\sqrt{\tau_1}}\right], \alpha_1 < p_1 \leq \beta_1, \tag{9.7}$$

where N_2 is the total sample size of the two groups (not cumulative sample size) for the second stage, the information time $\tau_1 = \frac{N_1}{N_1+N_2}$ is the sample size fraction at the interim analysis. Practically, we use the interim observed value $\frac{\hat{\delta}_1}{\hat{\sigma}_1}$ to replace the parameter of the standardized effect size $\frac{\delta}{\sigma}$ in the above formulation. For survival endpoint, $\delta/\sigma = \ln\hat{\theta}$, the log hazard ratio and N_1 and N_2 are the numbers of events for the two stages.

For example, if the interim analysis is performed on 50% events, $\tau_1 = 0.5$, assuming logrank statistic $z = 0.5$, and $N_1 = D = 100 = N_2$, and $\ln\hat{\theta} = 0.5\sqrt{\frac{4}{100}} = 0.1$ as in Example 9.1, and $\alpha_2 = 0.024$ or $z_{1-\alpha_2} = 1.977$, then the conditional power $\Pr(p \leq \alpha_2 | p_1) = 1 - \Phi\left(\frac{1.977-0.5\sqrt{0.5}}{\sqrt{0.5}} - 0.1\sqrt{\frac{100}{4}}\right) = 0.036$.

The conditional calculation is implemented in SAS Macro 9.1 in Appendix 12.7. Here is example of invoking the macro.

```
%ConPower(alpha2=0.024,  ux=0.2, uy=0.3, sigma=1, p1=0.3085, N1=100,
N2=100);
```

9.3.3   Prediction of Timing for Target Number of Events

Suppose the cdf or failure function is $F(T)$, where T is failure time. For instantaneous enrollment of N patients, the expected number (K_t) of events at time t is

$$K_t = N \cdot F(t). \tag{9.8}$$

If the N patients are enrolled or going to be enrolled at different time, $\tau_{1,...,N}$, then

$$K_t = \sum_{i=1}^{N} F(t - \tau_i) I(t > \tau_i), \tag{9.9}$$

where indicator function $I(t > \tau_i) = 1$ if $t > \tau_i$; otherwise 0.

At the interim monitoring time τ with K_τ deaths observed, if we know the set of associated enrollment time $D = \{\tau_{i_1}, \tau_{i_2}, ..., \tau_{i_{K_t}}\}$, then the expected time t for additional k deaths is the solution of the following equation:

$$k = \sum_{\tau_i \notin D} F(t - \tau_i) I(t > \tau_i). \tag{9.10}$$

In practice, we usually don't know the associated enrollment time set D. In such a case, we can assume patients who enrolled early will die early, thus, $D = \{\tau_1, \tau_2, ..., \tau_{K_\tau}\}$, where enrollment time $\tau_1 \leq \tau_2 \leq \cdots \leq \tau_{K_\tau} \leq \tau_{K_\tau + 1} \leq \cdots \leq \tau_N$.

This algorithm (9.10) is implemented in SAS Macro 9.2 in Appendix 12.7.

Here is an example of invoking the macro with a dummy patient enrollment data.

```
Data PtsEnroll;
    Input Month NewPts @@;
 * for more precise, one can use weekly enrollment instead of monthly;
datalines;
 1 5 2 8 3 7 4 8 5 8 6 8 7 8 8 8 9 8 10 8 11 8 12 8 13 6
14 6 15 0 16 0 17 0 18 0 19 0 20 0 21 0 22 0 23 0 24 0
;
run;
Title "Exponential model"; run;
%PredDeaths(Model="EXPONENTIAL", a=0.8, b=0.5, TotDeaths=12, t=8);
Title "Lognormal model"; run;
%PredDeaths(Model="LOGNORMAL", a=0.8, b=0.5, TotDeaths=12, t=8);
Title "Gamma model"; run;
```

The distribution of $F(T)$ can be determined and/or updated through modeling as the data (death and enrollment) accumulate. The commonly used survival destitutions are exponential, lognormal, Weibull, and gamma curves. The model fitting tests can be done using SAS Proc Univariate or other procedures.

Here is an example with dummy enrollment time (*enrolled*) and time-to-event (*tte*) data.

Alternatively, we can use a simulation method. Given the observed deaths, simulate the additional time needed for have total deaths required from the time of last death observed. The algorithms are:

1. Simulate survival time for all patients.

2. Merge with enrollment data to get calendar time of death: survival time + time of enrollment.

3. Sort the merged dataset by the calendar time of death.

4. Get the calendar time for the last observed death and predicted death time for the target number of deaths.

5. The difference between the two death times is additional time needed to have the target number of deaths.

See SAS Macro 9.x in Appendix 12.7. Here is an example to invoke the SAS macro to get the additional time needed for the targeted number of deaths.

```
Data PtsEnroll;
  Input EnDay @@; * Day on which each patient enrolled or are expected to
enroll;
  datalines;
  1 5 10 14 21 25 30 33 40 44 51 55 60 65 70 75 80 85 90 95 100
  ;
  * if the enrollment times for future patients are simulated, the enrollment vari-
ability can be considered in a certain degree;
  run;
Data PtsEnroll; set PtsEnroll; iPt=_N_; run;
%PredTime(nSims=10, Model="EXPONENTIAL", scale=0.2, nPts=21, obsd-
Deaths=3, DeathsNeed=18);
```

Example 9.2: Fitting Lognormal, Weibull, and Gamma Curves

The following is the dummy data and SAS code to select the best fitting model. The dummy data will be replaced with the real data once they become available.

```
data PtsEnroll;
  do n = 1 to 205;
   enrolled = int (24*ranuni(1) + 1);
    tte = 5*rangam(1, 1);
    duration = enrolled + int (tte);
    output;
  end;
  run;
proc univariate data=PtsEnroll;
```

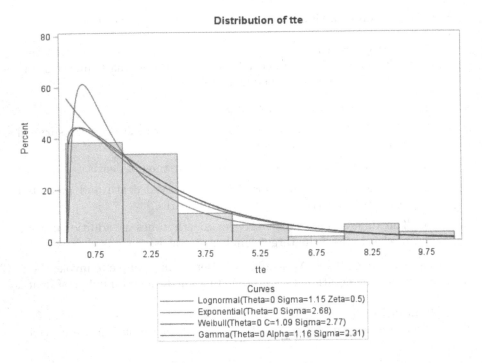

FIGURE 9.1
Four-Model Fitting Information.

```
    var tte;
      where duration LE 12;
      histogram / exponential gamma lognormal weibull;
      ods output GoodnessOfFit=fit;
    run;
```

The key outputs for the goodness-of-fit tests are Kolmogorove-Smirnov, Cramer-von Mises, and Anderson-Darling tests. A larger *p*-value indicates a better fit. See Figure 9.1 for four different curve-fittings.

A general simulation approach to this type of problem is:

1. Generate dataset without any condition (e.g., survival time as a random variable under the null or alternative hypothesis).

2. Apply the condition (e.g., given the number of events observed, the timing of the last event, or combination of the two, or certain baseline characteristics, enrollment pattern and so on) to extract the subset from the dataset.

3. Calculate the quantities we need from the subset of the simulated data.

Alternatively, we can simulate the data using conditional distribution:

1. For patients who are enrolled using the conditional survival function to generate the survival time.

2. For patients to be enrolled, the enrollment times will be generated, and their survival times will be generated based on unconditional survival distribution.

3. The distribution of the survival time of the nth death + enrollment date is the calendar time that can be obtained through many simulations, where n is the additional number of patients required for the study.

Alternatively, we can use a conditional distribution approach to do the simulation, that is, using conditional distribution of the survival time for who were enrolled but still alive at the time of prediction. See the SAS code in Appendix 12.7.

9.4 Power and Sample Size for One-Arm Survival Trial Design

The one-sample logrank test was first introduced by Breslow (1975) and studied by Hyde (1977), Gill and Ware (1979). and Anderson et al. (1993). Study designs using the one-sample logrank test were considered by Woolson (1981), Finkelstein, et al. (2003), Kwak and Jung (2014), Jung (2013), Sun et al. (2011), and Wu (2014a, 2014b).

We can imagine that a one-arm study is a generation of a two-arm study with the control arm having infinitely large sample size (so that the interesting observed values become constant), thus, the power and the sample size are in the test group is what we are interested in. In fact, when $N = N_1 + N_2 \to \infty$ and N_1 is kept constant, $N_j \to \infty$, $(1 - N_{1j}/N_j) \to 0$, $(N_j - O_j)/(N_j - 1) \to 1$, $O_j/N_j \to \lambda_j$ (hazard rate at time j), and $O_j(N_{1j}/N_j) = \lambda_j N_{1j} = E_{1j} =$ the number of expected deaths at time j. In other words, V_j from Eq. (**9.1**) is equal to E_{1j} when $N_2 \to \infty$ and $N_1 = $ constant. Therefore, for a large one-arm survival trial, the test statistic is the limit of (9.2):

$$Z = \lim_{N_j \to \infty} \frac{\sum_{j=1}^{J} (O_{1j} - E_{1j})}{\sqrt{\sum_{j=1}^{J} V_j}} = \frac{O - E}{\sqrt{E}}, \tag{9.11}$$

where O is the cumulative observed deaths and E is the expected total number of deaths. Under the null hypothesis of no treatment effect, Z has the standard normal distribution.

Wu (2014b) also proved that for larger sample size, the following test statistic Z^* has the standard normal distribution under the null hypothesis.

$$Z^* = \frac{O - E}{\sqrt{(E + O)/2}}. \tag{9.12}$$

By a closed inspection, Z is a linear transformation of O, therefore they should have the same type of distribution. Note that Eq (9.12) is only applicable to larger sample size. For a small sample size, it can fail terribly. For instance, using two-arm design analogy to obtain one-arm adaptive design (exponential survival, uniform enrollment): From the software (using two-arm design analogy, sample-size ratio = 10000, enroll time = 18 month, total study time = 36, $\lambda_1 = 0.770$ and $\lambda_2 = 0.0462$), 33 patients and 25 events are needed for 80% power at one sided α−level = 0.025. However, given $O = 25$ events and sample size 33, the smallest value of the test statistics (when all patients die in the expected value E) $Z = \frac{25-33}{\sqrt{33}} = -1.392\,6 > -z_\alpha = -1.96$. Thus, we fail to reject H_0. In other words, with 33 patients and 25 targeted events, there is no chance to reject H_0 if Wu's formulation ($Z = \frac{O-E}{\sqrt{E}}$) is used.

9.5 Estimation of Treatment Effect with Interim Blinded Data

9.5.1 Likelihood

Keeping trial data blinding is important to the validity and integrity for a pivotal phase III clinical trial. However, the sponsor often wants to know more about the treatment effect after seeing the interim blinded data for the decision-making. In this section, we will discuss how to use the blinded information to update the knowledge about the treatment effect using the maximum likelihood method (MLE) and Bayesian Method (marginal posterior distribution). Both methods require likelihood functions.

There are types of different likelihood: In addition to the basic likelihood function, the maximum, partial, profile, and marginal are other types. They are described below.

Denote the model parameters of primary interest by μ and the parameters that are not of primary interest as θ. A likelihood function is a joint probability of the data given μ and θ, but is viewed as a function of μ and θ given data. Denote the (standard) likelihood by $L(\mu, \theta|data)$.

Maximum Likelihood: the estimation of μ and θ that maximizes $L(\mu, \theta|data)$.

Partial Likelihood: Since we are only interested in μ, if the likelihood function is separable or $L(\mu, \theta|data) = L_1(\mu|data)L_2(\theta|data)$, then an estimate of μ can be obtained by maximizing $L_1(\mu|data)$.

Profile Likelihood: If θ can be expressed as a function of μ, $\theta = g(\mu)$, then θ can replace by $g(\mu)$ and an estimate of μ can be obtained by maximizing $L(\mu, g(\mu)|data)$.

Marginal Likelihood: To obtain the likelihood function of μ, we integrate out θ from the likelihood function, $L_0(\mu) = \int L(\mu, \theta|data)d\theta$.

Given data $x_1, x_2, ..., x_n$ from distribution $f(x)$ for continuous variable, the likelihood function is

$$L(\mu, \theta) = \prod_{i=1}^{n} f(x_i). \tag{9.13}$$

Given k out n responses for a binary endpoint with success rate p, the likelihood is

$$L(p) = \prod_{i=1}^{k} \binom{n}{i} p^i (1-p)^{n-i}. \tag{9.14}$$

For time-to-event variables, the likelihood given by Eq. (6.3) in Chapter 6 and for a special case with right-censoring,

$$L(\boldsymbol{\theta}) = \prod_{t_i \in \Omega_U} P(T = t_i|\boldsymbol{\theta}) \prod_{t_k \in \Omega_R} P(T > t_k|\boldsymbol{\theta}) \tag{9.15}$$

where Ω_U and Ω_R are the sets for uncensored and right-censored data, respectively.

9.5.2 MLE Method

If the distribution of the response variable Y for treatment 1 is $f_1(y; \mu_1)$ or treatment 2 is $f_2(y; \mu_2)$, the blinded data (pooled data) will have a mixture of the two distributions (Figure 9.2)

$$Y \sim w_1 f_1(y) + w_2 f_2(y), \tag{9.16}$$

where w_1 and w_2 are the sample size fractions of the two groups.

Note that (9.16) is not a distribution of sum of the two response variables Y_1 and Y_2 for the two treatment groups. The distribution of variable $Z = Y_1 + Y_2$ is obtained by the convolution

$$f_Z(z) = \int_{-\infty}^{\infty} f_1(t) f_2(z-t) dt. \tag{9.17}$$

The distribution of variable $T = Y_2 - Y_1 = Y_2 + (-Y_1)$ is obtained from (9.17) by replacing Y_1 with $-Y_1$, that is,

$$f_Z(z) = \int_{-\infty}^{\infty} f_1(-t) f_2(z+t) dt. \tag{9.18}$$

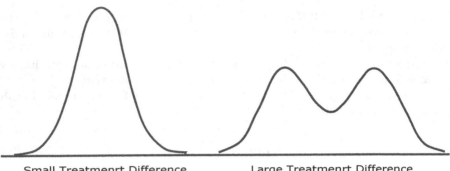

Small Treatmenrt Difference   Large Treatmenrt Difference

FIGURE 9.2
Mixture of Two Normal Distributions (small δ vs large δ).

The MLEs of all parameters (μ_1, μ_2) of the mixed distribution can be obtained by maximizing the likelihood using EM algorithm. The treatment difference can be obtained using

$$\hat{\delta} = \hat{\mu}_{2MLE} - \hat{\mu}_{1MLE} \tag{9.19}$$

Example 9.3: In the case of a mixture of two normal endpoint with a known common variance, the following R code is an example of computing the treatment effect (difference) and drawing histogram of the blinded responses. The R program uses EM algorithm to estimate the parameter by means of normalmixEM function from the mixtools package.

```
library(mixtools)
# MLE of treatment effect using EM algorithm
# y= rnorm(n, mu, sigma)
y0= rnorm(1000, 0, 1.0)      #Response in Placebo group
y1= rnorm(1000, 1.9, 1.1)   #Response in Test group
y=c(y0, y1)                  #Pooled response
EstParms=normalmixEM(y, lambda = .5, mu = c(0, 1), sigma =c(1.2, 1.2))
trtEffect=EstParms$mu[2]-EstParms$mu[1]
trtEffect
hist(y)
```

This MLE approach for mixed normal distribution is not applicable to a binary endpoint.

9.5.3 Bayesian Posterior

However, given the effect size in clinical trials, MLE requires a very large sample size to obtain an estimate with a reasonable precision. We have to use theUsing prior information, better estimates can be obtained to get better estimates, especially for phase III trials since there are usually larger data available on the test drug and control from previous studies.

$$f(\mu_1, \mu_2|y) = cL(y|\mu_1, \mu_2)\pi(\mu_1, \mu_2) \tag{9.20}$$

where c = normalization constant, $L(\mu_1, \mu_2)$ = likelihood, the prior $\pi(\mu_1, \mu_2)$ can often be $\pi(\mu_1, \mu_2) = \pi_1(\mu_1)\pi_2(\mu_2)$.

The posteriors of μ_1 and μ_2 are, respectively,

$$f_1(\mu_1|y) = \int c_1 L(y|\mu_1, \mu_2)\pi(\mu_1, \mu_2)\, d\mu_2 \tag{9.21}$$

and

$$f_2(\mu_2|y) = \int c_2 L(y|\mu_1, \mu_2)\pi(\mu_1, \mu_2)\, d\mu_1 \tag{9.22}$$

where c_1 and c_2 are normalization factors. The posterior distribution of $\Delta = \mu_2 - \mu_1$ is the convolution:

$$f_\Delta(\Delta = \delta|y) = \int_{-\infty}^{\infty} f_1(-t|y) f_2(\delta + t|y)\, dt. \tag{9.23}$$

This Bayesian approach can be applied to different endpoints.

Note that this posterior distribution (9.23) is different from the posterior distribution using unblinded data with $\pi_1(\mu_1)$ and $\pi_2(\mu_2)$ even when $\pi(\mu_1, \mu_2) = \pi_1(\mu_1)\pi_2(\mu_2)$. The posterior for treatment 1, $f_1(\mu_1|y)$, will relate not only to the data and prior $\pi_1(\mu_1)$ for treatment 1, but also to the data and prior in the other treatment group. In general, the posteriors, (9.21) and (9.22), put more weights weights on prior values with the unblinded corresponding posteriors. This is because pooled data contain less information than the unblinded data.

9.6 Analysis of Toxicology Study with Unexpected Deaths

Description of Problem

Consider a preclinical study using mice as the animal model with 2 groups and 25 mice in each group. Half of each group were dosed with study drug (genetically modified human stem cells) and the control group was not treated. The mice were kept in cages (5 in each cage), separated by treatment group, so 5 cages were utilized for each group of 25. The study duration was 170 days. At Day 57, all 5 mice in one of the treated group cages died over a 24-hour period. During the rest of the study, 3 more mice in the treated group died at Days 77, 162, and 163. Apparently in this mouse model the researchers expect somewhere around 15-20% of all mice to die. They checked one of the 5 mice that died and found no sign of infection. Their hypothesis is that the particular cage may have had some hygiene problem or the mice received no water, and that these first 5 deaths happened very early in the experiment and were not related to the drug. They believe that if the deaths were drug-related, that the deaths would have been distributed randomly among the 5 cages.

Questions to answer: Are these 5 deaths are likely related to the drug? How should the death rate be estimated?

If we excluded the cage with the 5 mice that died, the result is 0 of 25 deaths in the control group compared to 3 of 20 in the treated group. The 3 of 20 (15%) rate difference is considered acceptable in this mouse model.

Statistical Analysis

A key question to answer is that given the death rate in the treated group of 20 % as the maximum death rate suspected as the research, what is the probability of having 5 deaths in a single group of the 5 groups. If this probability is low, we can conclude that there must be some other reason(s). Otherwise, we will need to conclude that the reason is that the deaths are likely related to the treatment.

To calculate the probability, imagine that we label $1, 2, \ldots, 5$ for the mice in the first cage, $6, .7 \ldots, 10$ for the second cage,$\ldots$, and $21, 22, \ldots, 25$ for the mice in the 5th cage.

Given the 15% death rate if the 5 early deaths are excluded and we denote by D_i the deaths of 5 mice in cage i, the probability that the first 5 deaths will occur in one cage is:

$$P = \sum_{i=1}^{5} \Pr(D_i) = 5(0.15^5) = 0.0004,$$

a very small value. Even when the death rate is 8 of 25 (32%) to include all the deaths, the probability of first 5 animals in the same cage dying is $P = 5 \times 0.32^5 = 0.0168$, less than 2%. Therefore, the 5 deaths in that cage are very likely due to causes other than the drug or at least it is unlikely that the drug is the main reason. Also, the 5 deaths are much closer timewise than other three deaths. This is also an indication of another cause of death. Thus, the first 5 deaths should be excluded in the death rate estimation for the drug, leading to an estimated death rate of 15% (3 mice of 20).

Since this is a post-data analysis, the conclusion may not as robust as for a prespecified hypothesis test. Patterns other than "first 5 deaths in a cage " can be chosen. For example, specifying "5 deaths in a cage," may or may not lead different conclusions. When we specify a very specific pattern (involving, e.g., particular weight, age, color) the probability will be very low, and we will likely draw a different conclusion about the cause of the deaths

TABLE 9.5

2 × 2 Table for Binary Endpoint.

	Control	Test	
Response	a	b	$m_1 = a + b$
Non-response	c	d	$m_0 = c + d$
	$n_0 = a + c$	$n_1 = b + d$	$n_0 + n_1 = m_0 + m_1 = N$

9.7 Fisher's versus Barnard's Exact Test Methods

9.7.1 Wald Statistic

There are two fundamentally different exact tests for comparing the equality of two binomial probabilities – Fisher's exact test (Fisher, 1925), and Barnard's exact test (Barnard, 1945).

Given total sample size $a + c$ and $b + d$ in the control and test groups, and total response $a + b$, the probability of obtaining any such set of values in Table 9.5 is a hypergeometric distribution:

$$P(a, b, c, d | m_1, n_0, n_1) = \frac{\binom{n_0}{a} \binom{n_1}{b}}{\binom{N}{m_1}} \tag{9.24}$$

The test statistic for an exact test is based on the Wald statistic

$$T(\mathbf{X}) = \frac{P_1 - P_0}{\sqrt{\frac{P_1(1-P_1)}{n_1} = \frac{P_0(1-P_0)}{n_0}}} \tag{9.25}$$

The p-value is defined as the probability

$$p(P) = \sum_{T(\mathbf{X}) \geq T(\mathbf{X}_{obs})} \Pr(X|P) \tag{9.26}$$

9.7.2 Fisher's Conditional Exact Test p-Value

Fisher's exact test is often used to conduct one-sided hypothesis test, $H_0 : P_1 = P_0$ versus $H_a : P_1 > P_0$, where P_0 and P_1 are the response rates for the control and test group, respectively. Fisher's exact test is conditional on the overall number of responses observed.

Under the null hypothesis, and conditional on the marginal response m_1, each table has a hypergeometric probability that no longer depends on the nuisance parameter P.

The Fisher P-value defined as the probability of getting equal or more extreme values than the observed data (assume more response better) is,

$$P_{Fisher} = \sum_{k=0}^{m_1} \frac{\binom{n_0}{k}\binom{n_1}{m_1-k}}{\binom{N}{m_1}} = \sum_{k=0}^{m_1} \frac{(k+1)\cdots n_0 \cdot (m_1-k+1)\cdots n_1 \cdot m_1!}{k!(m_1-k)!N(N-1)\cdots(m_1+1)}$$

(9.27)

Fisher's exact test is available in SAS Proc Freq. However, for clinical trial simulations, using Proc Freq often slows down the process. Therefore, we developed a SAS macro to perform the Fisher's exact test for clinical trial simulations.

Note that the test statistic of Fisher's conditional exact test is not symmetric, therefore, a two-sided test at 2α level is not equivalent to a one-sided test at α level. For a clinical trial we should use the one-sided test since we are more interested in a better response rate than the control rate than the control in most situations. Also, due to the discrete nature of the exact test statistic, power is not a monotonic function in N (sample size) when N is small.

9.7.3   Barnard's Unconditional Exact Test p-Value

Barnard's exact test is an unconditional test. It generates the exact distribution of $T(X)$ by considering all possible configurations of the 2×2 the tables, and rather than just the tables with fixed m_1. We can set Barnard's probability under the null hypothesis proportion P as:

$$P_B(P) = \sum_{T(X) \geq T(X_{obs})} \binom{n_0}{x_a}\binom{n_1}{x_b} P^{x_a+x_b}(1-P)^{N-x_a-x_b}$$

(9.28)

Because $P_B(P)$ is a function of unknown parameter P, the p-value is conservatively taken as

$$p(P) = \sup_{P_0 \in (0,1)} P_B(P)$$

(9.29)

Figure 9.3 shows how Barnard probability varies as the null hypothesis proportion, P varies for different observed responses in the two groups and different sample sizes, where the legend $P_B(n_0, n_1, N = 15)$ is the Barnard probability for responses n_0 and n_1 in the two groups and sample size 15 per group.

9.7.4   Power Comparisons of Fisher's versus Barnard's Tests

Before we compare the power of the two methods, we check the type-I error rates. From Table 9.6, we can see that the Fisher's exact test is much more

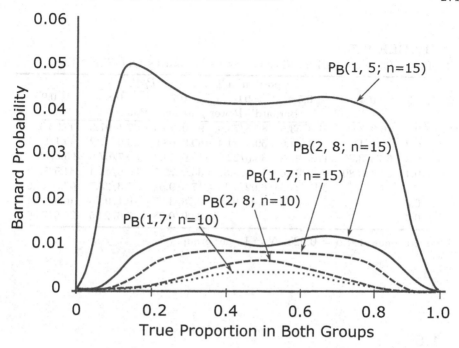

FIGURE 9.3
Barnard Probability versus Proportion under Null Hypothesis.

conservative than Barnard's test in terms of α. This because Fisher's test has (1) discrete nature of the test statistic and (2) control of the error rate under the conditional basis. Barnard's test usually does not control type-I error at exact α level neither for a given $H_0 : P$. This is because Barnard's test has (1) discrete nature of the test statistic and (2) control type-I error rate over the entire range $P \in (0, 1)$.

The power comparisons (numerically calculated from the above formulations) are presented in Table 9.7. In all cases we have investigated, Barnard's method is more powerful than Fisher's method. Power of Fisher's test is not monotonic in sample size when sample size is small, whereas power from Barnard's test is almost monotonic (Figure 9.4).

In some situations with an unbalanced design, the p-value from Fisher's

TABLE 9.6
Actual Type-I Error Rate with Target One-Sided $\alpha = 0.025$.

True P	0.1	0.2	0.3	0.4	0.5	0.6	0.7
Fisher α	.00273	.00837	.00849	.00804	.00825	.00786	.00681
Barnard α	.01222	.02163	.01996	.02041	.02153	.02041	.01996

TABLE 9.7
Power (%) Comparison Fisher's versus Barnard's One-Sided Test.

P_c	Proportion in Test group, P_t					
	0.4	0.5	0.6	0.7	0.8	0.9
	Barnard's Power / Fisher's Power					
0.1	46.3/32.5	67.3/53.6	84.5/73.9	95.0/89.4	99.1/97.5	99.96/99.8
0.2	19.1/11.1	37.3/24.6	59.9/44.4	80.9/68.0	93.9/87.2	99.1/97.5
0.3	6.78/3.26	17.6/9.63	35.9/22.7	59.0/43.4	80.7/67.9	95.0/89.1
0.4	2.04/0.80	69.2/31.6	17.7/9.52	35.9/22.7	59.9/44.4	84.5/72.2
0.5		2.15/0.83	6.92/3.15	17.6/9.52	37.3/23.7	67.3/48.6
0.6			2.04/0.79	6.78/3.07	19.1/9.76	46.3/24.4
0.7				2.00/0.68	7.76/2.65	25.6/7.66

Note: one-sided $\alpha = 0.025$, $N = 15$ per group.

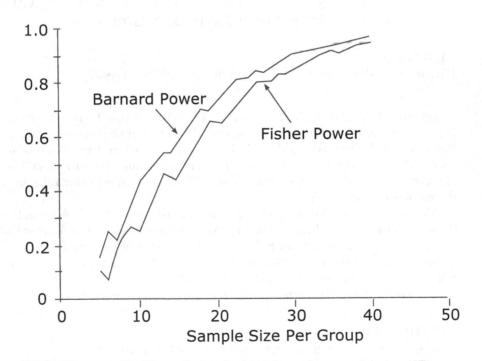

FIGURE 9.4
Saw-Shaped Fisher and Barnard Power Curves.

TABLE 9.8
Results of Comparison of Fisher's and Barnard's p-Values.

Sample Size		Number of responses		Barnard	Fisher
Group 1	Group 2	Group 1	Group 2	p-value	p-value
		0	5	0.00727	0.00593
		0	6	0.00175	0.00156
14	10	0	7	0.00039	0.00035
		3	4	0.31486	0.29596
		7	7	0.31486	0.28985

test can be smaller than the p-value from Barnard's test (see Table 9.8), but Barnard's test is still period at end of sentence.

Because Fisher's test has a lower type-I error rate than the nominal α, the critical value for the Fisher exact test can be inflated using simulations unconditionally without fixing the total number of responses. However, the error control must be performed for all values of the proportion $P \in (0, 1)$. As a result, the critical value may appear to be larger than α even though the family-wise error is controlled at α level [2,4]. The error rate with normality-based method not only depends on the sample size, but also depends on the proportion under null condition (show examples, curves).

In actual trials, experiment-wise type-I error for the Fisher exact test is control unconditionally. The conditional and unconditional error rates are different. Simulations show that the Fisher test is usually very conservative and has been criticized (Andres, 1995, Andres and Tejecdor, 2009; Grans and Shuster, 2008). This conservative approach comes from two sources: (1) the difference between the conditional and unconditional tests and (2) the discrete nature of the test statistic and p-value with small sample size.

Based on extensive simulations with different treatment effects, bal- anced and unbalanced sample sizes, Barnard's exact test is more pow- erful than the Fisher test. In a balanced design, we didn't find any case that for given observed rates P_1 and P_2 the p-value from Barnard's test is larger than the p-value from Fisher's test. However, for unbalanced designs, we did find some observed pairs of responses in the two groups, for which the Fisher test p-value can be smaller than the Barnard test p-value, even though the latter is more powerful. Therefore, from a power per- spective, we recommend the Barnard test rather than the popular Fisher test without any reservation.

9.8 Adaptive Design with Mixed Endpoints

It is not uncommon in an adaptive design that the short-term endpoint at interim analysis and long-term primary endpoint for the final analysis are of different types. For instance, in an oncology adaptive trial, the tumor response rate might be used for interim decision-making and survival or progression-free survival might be the primary endpoint for the final analysis. How do we design an adaptive trial with such mixed endpoints?

To determine the efficacy stopping boundaries, we have to conservatively assume a perfect correlation $\rho = 1$ because exact ρ is unknown. In other words, the efficacy stopping boundaries will be the same as if the same primary endpoint has been used for the interim and the final analyses.

However, in power calculation or simulation, an estimation of effect size of the interim and final endpoints and their correlation is important. Such estimation can be based on data from a previous trial.

The Spearman correlation coefficient ρ is often used for ordinal data, whereas Pearson's bivariate correlation coefficient r is used for continuous-level (ratio or scale) data. The point-Biserial correlation Coefficient, η, is a correlation measure of the strength of association between a continuous-level variable (ratio or interval data) and a binary variable. The Kendall τ_b correlation coefficient is a nonparametric measure of association based on the number of concordances and discordances in paired observations.

Like others correlation coefficients (e.g. Pearson's r, Spearman's ρ), the point-biserial correlation coefficient measures the strength of association of two variables in a single measure ranging from -1 to $+1$, where -1 indicates a perfect negative association, $+1$ indicates a perfect positive association and 0 indicates no association at all. All correlation coefficients are interdependency measures that do not express a causal relationship. Mathematically, the point-biserial correlation coefficient is calculated just as the pearson's bivariate correlation coefficient would be calculated, wherein the dichotomous variable of the two variables is either 0 or 1.

9.9 Summary

This chapter provided a brief overview of special issues that may arise in clinical trials. While variations of these issues may also be seen, the solutions proposed are intended to provide a basis for understanding and an initial step towards resolution of these challenges.

In practice, the decision of dropping losers is often based on both efficacy and safety. The simple Dunnett-test-based drop-loser design is a good solution in many cases. The drop-loser design with gatekeeping approach (include the optimal design) is an alternative solution, especially when toxicity is low and only one arm is effective.

Interim decision rules are often defined based on the p-value or test statistic, z. To explain to a nonstatistician using a hazard ratio or median time in survival trial we can use the approximate relationship between z (or p-value) and the number of deaths, D, between D and hazard ratio, and hazard rate and median time under an exponential distribution, equations (9.5) and (9.6).

Projecting the times when target numbers or events will be reached is of interest in a clinical trial with a time-to-event endpoint. The projection of time can be done either through numerical or simulation methods.

One-group survival trials are not very common since reliable historical data is often not available. The method described in Section 9.4 should be used with caution when the trial is small since the normality assumption can be seriously violated.

Estimation of treatment effect in an adaptive design using blinded data can be of great interest to the sponsor's decision-making. Two methods that can be used are the maximum likelihood estimate using the EM algorithm and the Bayesian approach. The former requires a large sample size to provide a good estimate. The latter will heavily rely on a prior distribution or knowledge.

In preclinical and clinical experiments, sometimes unexpected events happen, such as sudden deaths as discussed in Section 9.6. There are ways to statistically analyze whether the events are likely a result of the medical intervention or not. However, such a post hoc analysis should be used with caution.

Fisher's exact tests for two groups are commonly used in NDA submissions when the sample size is relatively small. Fisher exact test is known to be very conservative, while test is much more powerful.

There are many more practical issues in clinical trials that require a biostatistician's innovative thinking and choosing the most appropriate methods for the design and analyses as the examples discussed in the chapter are just a few cases we have encountered.

Bibliography

Andrés, A.M. (1991). A review of classic non-asymptotic methods for comparing two proportions by means of independent samples. Statistics: Simulation and Computation, 1991; 20(2&3):551-583.

Andrés, A.M., Tejedor, H.I. (1995). Is Fisher's exact test very conservative? Computational Statistics and Data Analysis 1995; 19:579-591.

Andrés, A.M. and Tejedor, I.H. (2009). Comments on "How conservative is Fisher exact test?" A quantitative evaluation of the two-sample comparative binomial trial' by G. G. Crans and J. J. Shuster, Statistics in Medicine, Jan 2009.

Barnard, G.A. (1945). A new test for 2 × 2 tables. Nature 156:177.

Barnard, G.A. (1947). Significance tests for 2×2 tables. Biometrika 1947; 34:123-138.

Berger, R,L., Boos, D.D. (1994). P values maximized over a confidence set for the nuisance parameter. Journal of the American Statistical Association 1994; 89(427):1012-1016.

Boschloo, R.D. (1970). Raised conditional level of significance for the 2×2 table when testing the equality of two probabilities. Statistica Neerlandica 1970; 24(1):1-35.

Bretz, F., Schmidli, H., Konig, F., et al. (2006). Confirmatory seamless phase II/III clinical trials with hypotheses selection at interim: general concepts. Biom J 2006; 48: 623–634.

Chan, I. (1998). Exact tests of equivalence and efficacy with a non-zero lower bound for comparative studies. Statistics in Medicine 17, 1403-1413.

Chang, M., Wang, J. (2015). The Add-Arm Design for Unimodal Response Curve with Unknown Mode. Journal of Biopharmaceutical Statistics 2015;25(5):1039-64.

Deng, X. and Chang, M. (2018). Flexible drop-loser design considering efficacy and safety. Biometrical, Submitted.

Finkelstein, D.M., Muzikansky, A., Schoenfeld, D.A. (2003). Comparing survival of a sample to that of a standard population. Journal of the National Cancer Institute 95: 1434-1439.

Fisher, R.A. (1925). Statistical Methods for Research Workers. Oliver and Boyd Edinburgh.

Follmann, D., Proschan, M. and Geller, N. (1994). Monitoring pairwise comparisons in multi-armed clinical trials. Biometrics 50, 325–36.

Grans, G.G. and Shuster, J.J. (2008). How conservative is Fisher's exact test? A quantitative evaluation of the two-sample comparative binomial trial. Statistics in Medicine. 2008; 27: 3598–3611

Hlavin, G., Hampson, L.V., Koenig, F. (2017). Many-to-one comparisons after safety selection in multi-arm clinical trials. PLoS ONE 12(6).

Jung, S.H. (2013). Randomized phase II cancer clinical trial. CRC Press: Chapman & Hall.

Kwak, M., Jung, S.H. (2014). Phase II clinical trials with time-to-event endpoints: optimal two-stage designs with one-sample log-rank test. Statistics in Medicine 33: 2004-2016.

Magirr, D., Jaki, T., and Whitedead, J. (2012). A generalized Dunnett test for multi-arm multi-stage clinical studies with treatment selection. Biometrika (2012), pp. 1–8.

Mansmann, R.J. Unconditional non-asymptotic one-sided tests for independent binomial proportions when the interest lies in showing non-inferiority and/or superiority. Biometrical Journal 1999; 41(2):149-170.

McDonald, L.L., Davis, B.M., Milliken, G.A. (1977). A non-randomized unconditional test for comparing two proportions in a 2×2 contingency table. Technometrics 1977; 19:145-150.

Mehta, C.R., Hilton, J.F. (1993). Exact power of conditional and unconditional tests: going beyond the 2×2 contingency table. American Statistician, 47:91-98.

Sampson, A. and Sill, M. (2005). Drop-the-losers design: Normal case. Biometrical Journal 2005; 47: 257–268.

Schmidli, H., Bretz, F., Racine, A., Maur, W. (2006). Confirmatory Seamless Phase II/III Clinical Trials with Hypotheses Selection at Interim: Applications and Practical Considerations. Biometrical, Volume 48, Issue 4 August 2006. 635–643.

Schoenfeld, D. (1981). The asymptotic properties of nonparametric tests for comparing survival distributions. Biometrika, Volume 68, Issue 1, 1 April 1981, 316–319.

Stallard, N. and Friede, T. (2008). A group-sequential design for clinical trials with treatment selection. Statistics in Medicine 27, 6209–27.

Sun, X., Peng, P., Tu, D. (2011) Phase II cancer clinical trials with a one-sample log-rank test and its corrections based on the Edgeworth expansion. Contemporary Clinical Trials 32: 108-113.

Thall, P.F., Simon, R. and Ellenberg, S.S. (1989). A two-stage design for choosing among several experimental treatments and a control in clinical trials. Biometrics 1989; 45: 537–547.

Thall, P., Simon, R. and Ellenberg, S. (1988). Two-stage selection and testing designs for comparitive clinical trials. Biometrika 75, 303–10.

Wason, J., Stallard, N., et al. (2017). A multi-stage drop-the-losers design for multi-arm clinical trials. Statistical Methods in Medical Research 2017, Vol. 26(1) 508–524.

Woolson, R.F. (1981). Rank-tests and a one-sample log-rank test for comparing observed survival-data to a standard population. Biometrics 37: 687-696.

Wu, J. (2014a). Sample size calculation for the one-sample log-rank test. Pharmaceutical Statistics. Volume 14, Issue 1, 2015 Pages 26–33.

Wu, J. (2014b). A New One-Sample Log-Rank Test.

10

Issues and Concepts of Data Monitoring Committees

In this chapter we will provide a brief overview of the basic methods and operation of a data monitoring committee (DMC), relying on the many excellent publications that contain the standard, proven elements of the set-up and conduct of the DMC (Calis, et al, 2017; Herson, 2016; Ellenberg, Fleming, and DeMets, 2002). This overview will set the stage for several advanced topics, including the application of meta-analysis in safety assessment, Bayesian monitoring and simulations for positioning of both safety and efficacy results.

The primary responsibility of a DMC (sometimes referred to as a data safety monitoring board or committee, when restricted primarily to trial safety considerations) is to alert the sponsor of a clinical trial to any issues that could compromise the safety of clinical trial participants, and to weigh safety concerns against efficacy in many trials, thereby representing the interests of trial participants by assessing the risk and benefit ratio in ongoing trials. As noted in the FDA Guidance for Data Monitoring Committees (FDA, 2006), "A clinical trial DMC is a group of individuals with pertinent expertise that reviews on a regular basis accumulating data from one or more ongoing clinical trials. The DMC advises the sponsor regarding the continuing safety of trial subjects and those yet to be recruited to the trial, as well as the continuing validity and scientific merit of the trial."

Data monitoring committees thus have a valuable contribution to make in the drug development process, and their purview covers many concepts of safety, efficacy and therefore clinical benefit. The importance of a DMC for trials in which the safety of patients may be compromised by the therapeutic agent is well recognized, but the contribution of the DMC to the overall development process may not be as clear. Further, the benefits of having a DMC as an integral part of the development process has become more acute in recent years, with the proliferation of programs of study to establish effective and safe therapies for an ever-increasing number of rare diseases. This in turn has induced a variety of constraints on the operations of the DMC, as therapies become increasingly targeted and sample sizes are often too small to rely on large-sample statistical methods.

10.1   Overview of DMC

The initial step in establishing a DMC is to develop the formal charter that will be used to describe the organizational structure of the DMC, the number, type and qualifications of the DMC members, the training that may be required for the members in the therapeutic area of the study, the frequency of meetings, the nature and format of the statistical and descriptive output to be reviewed, and the guidelines the DMC will use to determine any recommendations for modifying or terminating the trial. A thorough review of the study protocol, followed by careful review, discussion at the (preferably face to face) organizational DMC meeting and subsequent approval of the DMC charter by the DMC members, is essential to the proper functioning of the DMC.

It is critical that the integrity of the trial be protected, that bias is not introduced and therefore it must be clear who has access to information relative to the safety and efficacy outcomes of the trial. It is commonly accepted that the DMC must have access to the unblinded data results in a blinded trial, in order to properly determine the risk-benefit profile of the therapeutic entity under consideration. Therefore, maintaining trial integrity is also the primary reason why the DMC must maintain independence from those responsible for the day to day conduct of the trial.

Members of the DSMB typically include clinical trial experts, including physicians with the appropriate training in the therapeutic area being studied, at least one biostatistician and possibly other specialists, such as biomedical ethics, preclinical, pharmacology, and law experts.

The role of chairperson is particularly important, requiring experience in clinical trial design, monitoring and interpretation of analyses; the chairperson will often need to provide the final evaluation based on the opinions and judgments of the other members. The DMC chair ensures that the DMC is operating in a manner consistent with the requirements of the charter, and will call for the meetings, propose and review and approve agendas, and ensure that the meeting minutes and recommendation letters are prepared. The chair will decide if unscheduled meetings are to be called, based on the information received from the trial sponsor or designated data coordination center, and also ensure that all necessary communications among all DMC members and the support staff take place.

Support staff typically include personnel from a data processing center and an unblinded, support statistician to conduct the analyses of safety and efficacy, to prepare the report to guide the DMC members through the output, and to be on-hand to explain how the data were processed and the statistical methods used. Typically, these personnel are either employees of a contract research organization engaged by the sponsor to be responsible for the execution of the trial and/or employees of the sponsor company.

In many cases, the DMC receives reports in two parts: an open section, which presents data only in aggregate and focuses on trial conduct issues such as accrual and dropout rates, timeliness of data submission, eligibility rates and reasons for ineligibility; and a closed section, in which the comparative outcome data are presented. The open section of these reports is usually provided to sponsors, who may convey any relevant information in these reports to investigators, IRBs, and other interested parties, as the data presented in the open section are not likely to bias the future conduct of the trial and are often important for improving trial management (FDA, 2006). The data presented in the open section are typically blinded, whereas data discussed in the closed section can be unblinded, especially for a phase III trial DMC.

10.2 Operation of DMC

A DMC will conduct an organizational meeting, preferably with all members present, to outline the operational aspects of DMC meetings. Subsequent meeting frequency is typically based on achievement of specific enrollment goals with allowance for data processing time; note that completely cleaned data is rarely available, therefore the DMC members and support analysts must be aware of data anomalies that could skew results. Critical data elements should be cleaned to the extent feasible.

DMC has a number of functions and activities, which include administrative work, safety data monitoring, and interim analysis for efficacy and to determine whether the trial can demonstrate a reasonable risk-benefit ratio. Specific data items reviewed by the DMC include but are not limited to:

- Interim and cumulative data that will be evaluated for evidence of study-related adverse events or other safety issues, such as abnormal laboratory values;

- Interim data for evidence of efficacy according to pre-established statistical guidelines, if appropriate;

- Data quality, completeness, and timeliness, including an assessment of the performance of individual centers as appropriate;

- Adequacy of compliance with goals for recruitment and retention, including those related to the participation of women and minorities;

- Any obvious non-adherence to the protocol or other study requirements;

- Factors that might affect the study outcome or compromise the confidentiality of the trial data (such as protocol violations, unmasking of a blinded trial, etc.); and,

- Factors external to the study such as scientific or therapeutic developments that may impact participant safety or the ethics of the study. The trial sponsor bears equal responsibility to ensure that all such scientific information related to either safety or efficacy of the therapeutic product under study is made available to the DMC in a timely manner.

10.3   Role of DMC Biostatistician

The DMC biostatistician must be knowledgeable about statistical methods for clinical trials and sequential analysis of trial data, preferably with experience in the therapeutic area under study, but also with a varied background in general methods used in all phases of clinical trials of all sample sizes.

A good synopsis of the general role of the DMC statistician was provided by John Whitehead: "The major concerns that the statistician should have are the following. The pre-trial planning should be done carefully and will require the time of all DMC members. However, it is the statistician who can perhaps best foresee the dangers of reaching conclusions in an unstructured way and who has the most to gain by paying attention to design. The statistician will also have the greatest influence on the format of the reports received by the DMC. Thought and effort at the time when these are being devised will bring benefits of clarity and efficiency at the interim reviews. The statistician must be prepared to explain the methods of analysis, and also simple concepts such as the dangers of repetition and multiplicity of data analyses." (Whitehead, 1999).

For an adaptive design, the statistician must fully understand the trial design and explain to the other DMC members what adaptations are allowed and why. He or she must emphasize the importance to adhere to the planned adaptations and not make ad hoc changes. The statistician should be able to articulate the technical terms in layman terms so that non-statistician members can understand these issues well. He or she should also ensure "maximal blinding" of data and integrity of firewalls to preserve the integrity of a trial. Ideally, the DMC statistician should also be the main author of the DMC charter, or at a minimum be involved in the review of the document.

10.4   Need for DMC

When should a DMC be used for a given study? The specific methods for safety monitoring of a clinical trial are related to both the degree of risk involved to study participants and to the size and complexity of the study. However, previous notions that the primary use of a DMC is in the area of larger, phase III multicenter trials are rapidly changing in the era of increasing study of rare diseases. Further, it has become evident that the safety and efficacy of a therapeutic option must be considered as a totality to determine the proper risk to efficacy balance, that is, to properly determine clinical benefit to patients. Finally, as more adaptive trial designs are used, the DMC may become an even more integral partner in the decisions to stop for futility, re-assess sample size, conclude efficacy has been established at an interim or to continue the trial as planned. Thus, the appropriate monitoring plan for a particular study can range from episodic or continuous monitoring by the PI or steering committee, to the more rigorous monitoring by an independent DMC.

It should be noted that there are no absolute or well-defined criteria for determining the need for a DMC for any specific study or development program. There are potentially many reasons for establishing a DMC for a particular study, as noted in the FDA Guidance and in the many recent published articles on the use of a DMC:

- The study endpoint is such that a highly favorable or unfavorable result, or even a finding of futility, at an interim analysis might ethically require termination of the study before its planned completion. This may result in the DMC overseeing the specific adaptive design used.

- There are a priori reasons for a particular safety concern, as, for example, if the procedure for administering the treatment is particularly invasive, or the therapy is in a class of drugs known to have particular side effects of concern.

- There is prior information suggesting the possibility of serious toxicity with the study treatment. It will be noted further in this chapter that this possibility may provide a significant rationale for the use of Bayesian methods to incorporate prior information into the safety monitoring.

- The study is being performed in a potentially fragile population such as children, children, pregnant women, the very elderly, or other vulnerable populations, such as those who are terminally ill or of diminished mental capacity.

- The study is being performed in a population at elevated risk of death or other serious outcomes, even when the study objective addresses a lesser endpoint.

- The study is large, of long duration, and multi-centered. Note however that more and more studies are being conducted in rare diseases, where the use of large study populations and multiple centers may not be the rule, and yet a DMC could be critical to the safety and efficacy monitoring of the trial.

10.5   Use of DMC in Rare Disease Studies

There can be a number of conceptual and operational differences in clinical trials in rare conditions in contrast to trials in non-rare conditions. However, the extent and nature of these differences are not entirely understood. While it is desirable to apply the same standards of inference to rare and non-rare disease studies, there are often daunting restrictions on the study of rare diseases related to sample size, ethics of the use of placebo controls, ready availability of study sites to patients, and lack of commercial enthusiasm due to an oft-perceived small market opportunity. Individual rare diseases are by nature uncommon in the general population, however, in total there are thousands of conditions that could be classified as rare. This means about 60 million people are affected by at least one of these rare diseases in the United States and EU alone (Gagne et al, 2014; Bell and Smith, 2014). Rare diseases can afflict various organ systems, organ systems, have mutational causes, produce wide ranging and often poor prognoses, and exhibit varying prevalence. There are numerous methodological and data constraints that limit the ability to generate evidence on patient health outcomes. Often there is no consensus on the efficacy endpoints that are most sensitive to detecting changes in disease progression or improvement. A particular issue in the study of rare degenerative diseases is that the rate of progression is often unknown and likely is rarely linear with respect to the primary endpoint(s) under study.

The most obvious challenge to conducting research that is analogous to the study of non-rare disease is the small number of eligible participants for a given study. Researchers often face a lack of knowledge about the clinical course of a disease and few comparator treatments to assess. Fortunately, in some cases there exist registries, or natural history studies, that should be used both in study design and to inform the assessments of a DMC for both efficacy and safety. In cases where such registries and natural history studies do not exist, sponsors must often conduct studies to obtain such information before starting or in parallel with a clinical trial. Biostatisticians engaged in the trial must also be familiar with the designs of the additional studies.

A comprehensive study was done wherein a search of the ClinicalTrials.gov registry revealed a total of 24,088 Interventional trials registered after January 1, 2006, conducted in the United States, Canada and/or the European Union that were categorized as rare or non-rare Bell and Smith, 2014). The authors discovered that rare disease trials cited in the database generally had smaller target and obtained sample size, they are more likely to be early-phase, more likely to recruit to a single arm, more likely to be non-randomized, and more likely to be unblinded. The authors found that rare disease studies employed a DMC more frequently than non-rare disease studies. Clinical trials were phase II or earlier in 69.9% of the rare disease studies, with 63% being single-arm studies, in contrast to 36.6% of non-rare disease trials being phase II or earlier and only 29.6% being single-arm. Clearly these major design differences need to be accounted for in the operation and deliberations of the DMC in rare disease studies, where 53.2% of these studies include a DMC in contrast to 40.9% of non-rare disease trials (Beoll and Smith, 2014). These differences make the clinical judgment of the DMC, aided by proper statistical presentation of results, more likely to involve subjective elements and more dependent on historical or literature sources of comparative data.

10.6   Statistical Methods for Safety Monitoring

The evaluation of safety data by the DMC is usually performed through the use of by-subject data listings and summary tabulations, through observation and informal comparison among treatment groups for trials with multiple treatment groups (including placebo or other controls) and by implicit comparisons to expected rates of safety issues for single-arm trials. Formal analysis of rates of adverse effects are typically restricted to Phase II or later phase trials, for endpoints such as serious or more severe events, adverse events of special interest (AESI), or rates of events for specific body systems.

Many Phase II and III clinical trials have treatment efficacy as the primary objectives, but generally have safety assessment as a key secondary objective. The inclusion of safety assessment criteria in addition to the analysis of efficacy allows an evaluation of overall patient clinical benefit by the DMC to be made. It is important for the DMC members to be informed as to any preliminary information regarding the safety profile based on the mechanism of action of the drug or based on data from preclinical/animal testing, previous trials or data from drugs in a similar class. Safety monitoring criteria should be employed, even when the trial is not comparative. Since the DMC safety analyses are inherently sequential, safety analysis may be performed using such methods as sequential probability ratio tests (SPRT) or Bayesian methods. The crossing of pre-defined safety boundaries may be analyzed using either overall blinded data, which would be similar to an analysis of data from a single-arm trial, or an unblinded comparative analysis. (Yao et al, 2013).

10.7   Statistical Methods for Interim Efficacy Analysis

For efficacy monitoring of an adaptive trial, the prespecified rules should be followed to preserve the integrity and validity of the trial. Family-wise error rate control is currently considered a key to maintain the trial validity for late phase trials.

In the trial protocol and DMC charter, roles for adaptations are specified. The trial monitoring statistician will indicate the adaptation(s) to utilize based on the interim data analysis results and adaptation rules. Such an adaptation may include early stopping of the trial for efficacy or futility (Section 4.3.2), adjusting sample size (Section 4.3), dropping losers or picking the winner (Section 4.4 and 9.2), selecting an optimal subpopulation (Sections 5.3 and 5.4). The decision may involve predicting future results and thus simulations can be powerful tools.

For a group sequential trial with error-spending, the rules are specified by Eq. (4.2) or (4.3), where the stopping boundary should be recalculated based on the actual interim analysis time (information time). Calculation or recalculation of stopping boundaries can be performed using commercial software or simulation programs discussed in Chapter 4 and SAS macros in the Chapter 12 appendices. If no change in interim analysis time was observed, then the stopping boundaries specified in the protocol or DMC charter can be used directly for the decision-making. Table 4.1 shows examples of stopping boundaries.

For adaptive trial with sample size reestimation, the adaptation rules are specified in Eq. (4.12). At the interim analysis, calculations of conditional power and new sample size are often required. The conditional power can be calculated using Eq. (4.13) based on the sample sizes n_1 and n_2, and the observed test statistic at stage 1, z_1. The new sample size calculation is also straight forward based on Eq. (4.14). Note that for logrank test of survival endpoint, a normal approximation is used, in which the treatment size is based on log hazard ratio with a standard deviation of 1. The sample size is based on number of events instead of number patients.

For pick-winner or drop-loser design, the winner can be the arm with best observed response rate, the critical value for the rejection is dependent on the timing of interim analysis as shown in Table 4.2. When the winner is determined not solely by efficacy or including other factors. For the later, the FWER can be smaller than the nominal level.

For biomarker-adaptive winner design, Table 5.1 provides samples of critical values for rejection of null hypothesis of no treatment effect. The best subpopulation is identified by the effect size.

For optimal drop-loser design with Dunnett's test, the critical value and optimal time for the last interim analysis can be found in Tables 9.1 and 9.2. The stopping rule and be established base efficacy, safety and other critical without inflating the FWER.

For Bayesian continual reassessment dose-escalation design, the Bayesian posterior distribution for the maximum tolerable dose (MTD) is calculated when new data become available. The details can be found in the books by Chang (2007, 2014) and Berry (2010).

10.8 Summary and Discussion

The DMC plays a critical role in monitoring clinical trials. Three key aspects, safety, efficacy, and data integrity need to be considered in trial monitoring. he "benefit-to-risk" term is a common composite criterion used to assist in decision-making.

There are common issues that affect a DMC's decision, such as short-term versus long-term treatment effects, early termination philosophies, responses to early beneficial trends, responses to early unfavorable trends, and responses where there are no apparent trends. A balance must be struck between well-being of the trial participants and potential benefits to future patients, however, the safety of trial subjects must always be the paramount consideration. According to the World Medical Association Declaration of Helsinki, the rights, safety, and well-being of the trial subjects are the most important considerations and should prevail over interests of science and society. FDA's 2006 Guidance: "Establishment & Operation of Clinical Trial Data Monitoring Committees" can be used in principle for the trial monitoring; however, it is not enough for adaptive trial monitoring. The statistical tools/methods provided in chapters of this book can assist DMCs to accomplish their duties.

It is desirable to be able to predict with reasonable certainty the likelihood of success of the trial given the interim current data. The frequentists use conditional power, whereas Bayesian statisticians use predictive power.

There are controversial views on whether or how much the sponsor and DMC can be involved in the unblinded interim data review. From the scientific perspective, the sponsor and KOLs are most knowledgeable about the disease and the test drug; therefore, they are the most suitable experts to be responsible for the interim decision. However, there is a significant concern of conflict of interests, which is why it is particularly important to have an independent DMC reviewing the data and making the recommendations, and it is rare for sponsors to disagree with DMC recommendations for this reason.

Bibliography

Bell. S.A. and Smith, C.T. (2014). A comparison of interventional clinical trials in rare versus non-rare diseases: an analysis of ClinicalTrials.gov, Orphanet Journal of Rare Diseases 2014, 9:170.

Calis, et al, (2017). Recommendations for data monitoring committees from the Clinical Trials Transformation Initiative, Clinical Trials, 2017, Vol. 14(4) 342–348.

Dominguez-Urban (1997) Harmonization in the regulation of pharmaceutical research and human rights: the need to think globally. Cornell International Law Journal 30: 245-286.

Ellenberg, S.S., Fleming, T.R., and DeMets, D.L. (2002). Data Monitoring Committees in Clinical Trials – A Practical Perspective, John Wiley and Sons, New York.

FDA (2006). Guidance for Clinical Trial Sponsors Establishment and Operation of Clinical Trial Data Monitoring Committees. https://www.fda.gov/downloads/regulatoryinformation/guidances/ucm127073.pdf

FDA (2016). Adaptive Designs for Medical Device Clinical Studies Guidance for Industry and Food and Drug Administration Staff. https://www.fda.gov/downloads/medicaldevices/deviceregulationandguidance/ guidancedocuments/ucm446729.pdf

Gagne et al, (2014). Innovative research methods for studying treatments for rare diseases: methodological review, British Medical Journal 2014;349.

Herson. J. (2016). Data and Safety Monitoring Committees in Clinical Trials, 2nd Edition. Taylor & Francis, Boca Raton, FL.

Proschan, M.A., Lan, K.K.G. and Wittes, J.T. (2006). Statistical Monitoring of Clinical Trials, a uniform approach. Springer, New York.

Wandile, P. and Ghooi, R. (2017). A Role of ICH- GCP in Clinical Trial Conduct. Journal of Clinical Research & Bioethics. Journal of Clinical Research & Bioethics 2017, 8:1.

Whitehead, J. (1999). On being the statistician on a data and safety monitoring board, Statist. Med. 18, 3425-3434.

Yao et al, (2013). Safety Monitoring in Clinical Trials, Pharmaceutics 2013, 5, 94-106.

11

Controversies in Statistical Science

11.1 What is a Science?

To put it simply, a science is mainly a set of investigations of so-called scientific laws that characterize causal relationships within a field of study. When the relationships address the underlying problems in physics, society, or psychology, we have different sciences that sometimes entail different methodologies.

Any proposed law of science or hypothesis must involve testable predictions. This implies that (1) science is a study of (ideally) repeated events, and (2) an essential role of science is to make predictions, so that we can act early and wisely and verify what we believe to be true. The reason we study history and experimentation is to "discover" the law that can be used to predict the future when the cause repeats. However, we like to think (even if it would be difficult to prove) that there is a single history, and everything is unique at the moment and over time.

When we slice history into pieces and judge two pieces to be the same, we intentionally or unintentionally ignore their differences; at least we ignore the different "neighboring pieces" in the chain of history. Such slicing and grouping of similar pieces artificially create repetitions of events that we consider to be the same even if they aren't, and allows us to discover natural laws or causalities. In this sense, a natural law is firstly invention (grouping the similar pieces), and then pattern discovery.

However, the grouping of similar things is often done implicitly and subjectively, which inevitably creates intangible controversies in scientific inference. For example, if you are a tall man, from which of the following four groups do you infer your characteristics (e.g., longevity, the likelihood of being successful in career, or the chance of having cancer): all men, tall people, tall men, or the entire population (Chang, 2014)?

11.2 Similarity Principle

The notion behind prediction is causality, whereas causality is based on the similarity principle (Chang 2012, 2014): similar conditions will likely result in the same or similar outcomes. The principle can be stated differently for better understanding depending on the problem. For example, we might state: "similar things will behave similarly." In a sense, the similarity principle is the most fundamental belief we hold in scientific communities, but is not explicitly expressed.

A scientific law states that a certain (same) condition will lead to a certain (same) consequence. But no two dynamics are exactly the same. "Same" means similar in this context. When we say "the same," we ignore the differences that might be hidden and contradict scientific law that seems to apply. Once such a contradiction is uncovered, an exception to the law is observed which may require some modification of the law. In other words, at some point in the future, any scientific law may be reduced to an approximation or even be proven false.

As to how the similarity principle is used in scientific discovery, or even in daily life, let's look at a few examples.

When investigating human or animal populations we often divide the study population into different groups based on age, gender, race, and the like. This is done because we think subjects in each group are similar in terms of the causal relationship we are investigating. But each subject is unique, thus such grouping is subjective. In psychological settings we may study a person's behavior using the knowledge we have from similar subjects whom we have studied. In doing this we have put the subject into a group and applied the similarity principle.

Drug discovery and development constitute a stepwise process: a new chemical compound is tested on animals first. When the compound shows itself to be efficacious and safe in animals it will be tested in humans in clinical trials. This approach is taken in order to protect patients. The reason we think this stepwise approach works is that we believe the animals are similar to humans, and therefore the drug effects on animals and humans will be similar. Based on the similarity principle: the animal experiment (drug + animal) is similar to the human experiment (drug + human), and therefore its use in humans will likely lead to the same or similar drug effect.

In Bayesian statistics, data on drug effects on animals can be used as prior knowledge in deriving the posterior distribution of the drug's effect on humans. The frequentist statisticians do not use animal data to directly calculate the drug effect on the humans, but animal data is used in the drug development process to help the decision-making: to stop, continue, or modify the existing drug development program.

The grouping that our minds carry out in hand with the similarity principle makes everything happen for a reason, but at the same time, due to the approximation of such grouping, every law or causal relationship has exceptions.

TABLE 11.1

Drug Effects on Male and Female Subjects.

	Drug A	Drug B
Male	200/500	380/1000
Female	300/1000	140/500
Total	500/1500	520/1500

11.3 Simpson's Paradox

Subjectivity in similarity grouping reflects an individual's belief, experience, and knowledge. The controversies caused by similarity grouping can be well illustrated using Simpson's paradox (Simpson 1951).

In probability and statistics, Simpson's paradox, introduced by Colin R. Blyth in 1972, points to apparently contradictory results between aggregate data analysis and analyses from data partitioning. Let's look into an example in drug development.

Suppose two drugs, A and B, are available for treating a disease. The treatment effect (in terms of response rate) is 520/1500 for B, better than 500/1500 for treatment A. Thus, we will prefer treatment B to A. However, after further looking into the data for males and females separately (Table 11.1), we found that the treatment effect in males is 200/500 with A, better than 380/1000 with B, while the treatment effect in females is 300/1000 with A, better than 140/500 with B. Therefore, whether female or male, we will prefer treatment A to B. Should we take treatment A or B?

The problem can be even more controversial. Suppose when we further look further into the young female and old female subcategories (Table 11.2), the direction of treatment effects switches again, i.e., treatment B has better effect than treatment A in both subcategories, consistent with the treatment effect for the overall population. The question is: what prevents one from partitioning the data into arbitrary sub-categories artificially constructed to yield wrong choices of treatments?

People try to resolve this dilemma mathematically, but that is an incorrect solution. One can find a mathematically optimal solution, yet that will not address the underlying issue. The issue here is not to find a single answer that everyone agrees on or one that is scientifically correct, because there is no

TABLE 11.2

Drug Effects on Young and Old female Subjects.

	Drug A	Drug B
Young Female	20/200	40/300
Old Female	280/800	100/200
Total	300/1000	140/500

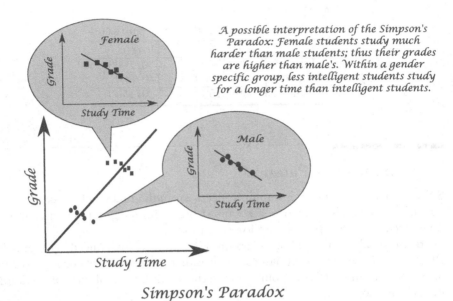

Simpson's Paradox

FIGURE 11.1
Simpson's Effect for Continuous Variable.

single correct answer. The issue is about the fundamental belief inherent in the similarity principle, which comes before any statistical principles or paradigms. The criteria used to group a person with others reflect one's personal belief about which errors can be pooled together meaningfully to minimize the total error in the statistical analysis. Some people may believe that errors about drug effects on all patients, even animal data, can be meaningfully combined; others may believe only patients with, as an example, the same gender, can be combined.

Simpson's paradox is not uncommon if we continue slicing the data into more categories until the paradox appears. In a worldwide drug development program, for example, a drug can appear to be effective globally while its effects in different countries or regions may be very different. The question is how should such a drug be used in different countries or regions?

Furthermore, proportions of patients with certain characteristics in a clinical trial are often purposely handled differently from the main patient population. Thus, if the test drug effects are different for different types of patients, then the sample size mean will be different from the treatment effect for the population. The Simpson paradox can also occur for other types of endpoints (Figure 11.1).

11.4 Causality

Every event is the effect of antecedent events, and these in turn are caused by events antecedent to them, and so on. Human actions are no exception to this rule, including such consequential actions as the choice of committing a crime and the choice of punishing a criminal. In this view, there is no such thing as a choice made primarily of one's own will . However, we, as scientific researchers, always ask why we make certain choices is sufficient. We may ask ourselves: with the ultimate development of neuroscience and understanding of the human brain, how much space remains for free will of choice?

So what does causality really mean if everything is deterministic? The construct that we call causality is a consequence of our belief in the similarity principle. Since our brains cannot deal with everything happening in our lives, we group similar things together and apply, consciously or not, the similarity principle. Only in this way can our brains handle the universe. Only with the similiarity principle can causality make sense scientifically, can scientific laws be derived, can we meaningfully discuss inferences and prediction, will the connotation of "scientific knowledge" become lucid, and can we deal with the concepts of probability and random errors (Chang 2014).

Within the context of scientific discovery, a causal relationship between events A and B means three conditions: (1) A precedes B in time, (2) the law of factor isolation holds: If A then B; if not A then not B, and (3) the relationship is verifiable, at least in principle, which means that condition 2 is persistent over time, which further requires that the events in condition 1 are repeatable. The repetition of events is what gives causality its great usefulness: we use it to make predictions.

So far we have only discussed the possibility that factor A is the sole cause of B. But how do we test the causes when either factor A or C alone can be sufficient cause of B? This issue becomes very complicated. Let us look into the paradox of murder in desert (Smullyan,1976): A caravan of three people (A, B, and C) were going through the Sahara Desert, where one night they pitched tents. A hated C and decided to murder him by putting poison in the water of his canteen (C's only water supply). B, who also wanted to murder C, didn't realize that C's water was already poisoned, and he drilled a small hole in C's canteen so that the water would slowly leak out. As a result, several days later C died of thirst. The question in the court is, who was the murderer, A or B? According to one argument, B was the murderer, since C never drank the poison added to the canteen by A; hence, he would have died even if A hadn't poisoned the water. According to the opposite argument, A was the real murderer, since B's actions had absolutely no effect on the outcome; once A poisoned the water, C was doomed, and hence A would have died even if B had not drilled the hole. Which argument do you agree with?

Another interesting point is the interchangeability of causality and association. We always say that an association between variables is not necessarily causal. Indeed, association is a necessary but not a sufficient condition for causality. But more importantly, an association can become a causal relationship. For instance, data have shown that people who carry matches are more likely to have lung cancer than people who do not carry the matches. That is, there is an association between matches and lung cancer, because smoking cigarettes can cause cancer and smokers usually carry matches. Therefore, carrying matches is not a cause of lung cancer. However, by further inspection, we learn that the direct cause of lung cancer is carcinogens in the cigarette, not the cigarette. If we can extract the carcinogens from cigarettes, then smoking cigarettes will no longer be a cause of lung cancer. On the other hand, a causal relationship can become an association. For example, if only cigarette smokers can carry matches and all cigarettes smokers carry matches, then by extension we can consider matches a cause of lung cancer.

11.5   Type-I Error Rate and False Discovery Rate

Consider the classical experiment of flipping a coin repeatedly. If all the conditions (the force used, the direction of the force,the coin's rigidity, etc.) are precisely the same each time I flip the coin, the result of each flip will also be identical. The so-called random variation is simply caused by hidden variables: the way you flip the coin is in fact slightly different each time. The point is that the randomness is caused by many hidden or unspecified factors. To reduce false findings caused by randomness, we can use the measure of false discovery rate (FDR) defined as the expected proportion of false positive findings among all findings (Chang 2011, p.21; Benjamini and Hochberg, 1995). One way to control FDR is through hypothesis testing, briefly described below.

Suppose we want to test the null hypothesis H_0: drug X is ineffective, versus the alternative hypothesis H_a: drug X is effective. When p-value $\leq \alpha$, a nominal level, we reject H_0 and conclude the drug is effective. Technically, a p-value is the probability of obtaining an effect at least as extreme as the one contained in sample data, assuming the truth of the null hypothesis. Therefore, a p-value does not directly answer the question as to how effective a drug is.

A smaller p-value indicates a discrepancy between the hypothesis and the observed data. In this sense, p-value measures the strength of evidence against the null hypothesis. However, p-value s not a probability that a null hypothesis is true.

A level of significance, $\alpha = 5\%$, does not mean there are 5% false positive findings because the null hypothesis (a condition used to define p-value) is just an assumption. For example, if the null hypotheses under investigation are true, then all positive findings are false, no matter what value of α is used.

In contrast, if all null hypotheses we investigate are in fact false, there will be zero false findings, independent of α.

If some proportion R of all null hypotheses to be investigated are true, we want to control the false findings among these true hypotheses at a rate of α, the significance level of the null hypothesis test. Therefore, α can be interpreted as the expected proportion of false findings among all true null hypotheses. The problem is that we have to apply the same α to all null hypotheses since we don't know which null hypotheses are true. As a consequence, the power of the hypothesis testing is reduced or the ability (probability) of detecting a true positive finding is reduced unless the sample size increases. How can we use a single index to measure both probabilities of correctly identifying positive and negative findings? The false discovery rate is such a measure. The proportion of false positive findings among all findings (FDR) is approximately:

$$FDR = (\alpha \times R)/(\alpha \times R + power \times (1 - R)) \quad (11.1)$$

It is interesting to know that we can control type-I error rate in clinical trials with a simple experiment of flipping coins and conduct a trial with only 2 patients: (1) we recruit 2 patients for testing the drug: one will take placebo and the other will take the test drug. If the treatment difference between the 2 patients is positive (only 50% chance when H_0 is true), then (2) we flip a fair coin 6 times and if all heads, we reject the null hypothesis and claim efficacy of the test drug. times. In this way, we can have unbiased estimate of treatment effect from the two patients and control the type-I error at $\alpha = 0.5^6 = 0.01525$. It is obvious that the clinical trial is very cost effective and can be done quickly since we need only 2 patients and 6 coin flips. If we fail to claim efficacy, we can do the experiment again and again. If we repeat the experiment 100 times with a total of 200 patients (2 for each trial), the chance of claiming efficacy for an ineffective drug will be 88.5%; if we repeat the experiment 150 times with a total of 300 patients, the probability of claiming efficacy for an ineffective drug will be 90%.

We often wish to have a direct answer to the question of the effectiveness of a drug or a clinical intervention. To this end, we can use Bayesian posterior probability, which is a combination of prior knowledge and current experimental data. One common criticism of the Bayesian method is its subjectivity in determining prior knowledge. Such subjectivity combined with a psychological bias, such as anchoring, makes the result more controversial (Lench, Safer, Levine, 2011). Anchoring is a cognitive bias that describes the common human tendency to rely too heavily on the first piece of information offered (the "anchor") when making decisions. We are constantly using the Bayesian notion of learning or reasoning in our scientific research and our daily lives, because every conscious action we take is a utilization of prior relevant experiences or knowledge. The determination of the prior probability is essentially an application of the similarity principle that suffers the same subjectivity issue that affects the determination of a similarity set.

11.6 Multiplicity Challenges

The word *multiplicity* refers to the statistical phenomenon of error inflation in falsely rejecting the null hypothesis when multiple tests are performed without the so-called multiplicity adjustment to the level of significance, α. While this technical definition may pose some initial difficulty to the non-specialist, an understanding can be achieved based on the examples given below.

In a national lottery a few years ago, there was one and only one winning ticket. Ten million people bought one ticket each, so each person had a very small chance of winning—1 out of 10 million. A Mr. Brown was the lucky winner, but he also was the object of a lawsuit charging him with conspiracy. The prosecution argued that the chances of Mr. Brown winning the lottery were so low that, practically speaking, it could not happen unless there was a conspiracy. However, Mr. Brown defended: "There must be a winner whoever he or she might be, regardless of any conspiracy theory." This paradox is a typical multiplicity problem. The multiplicity emerges when we apply the conspiracy theory (the null hypothesis is that there is no conspiracy) to each of the ten million lottery buyers.

Vidakovic (2008) gave the following example of multiplicity problem: Suppose a burglary has been committed in a town, and 10,000 men in the town have their fingerprints compared to a sample from the crime. One of these men has a matching fingerprint, and at his trial it is testified that the probability that two fingerprint profiles match by chance is only 1 in 20,000. However, since 10,000 men had fingerprints taken, there were 10,000 opportunities to find a match by chance; the probability of at least one fingerprint match is 39% calculated from a binomial distribution with true 1/20000 "considerably more than 1 in 20,000.

Now suppose Interpol were going to run a fingerprint check according to the alphabetic order of last names, starting with the letter A, and that the check is to be stopped if and when a match is found. Suppose that the suspect's fingerprints were the very first checked (his last name happened to be Aadland) and that they matched the crime sample. Thus, the probability is 1/20,000. But the suspect could argue that if the agency's check started with last names beginning with Z and even if the agency wanted to check everyone, they would have identified all 0.36 million fingerprint matches in the world population of 7.20 billion before checking on him. Therefore, fingerprints (and similarly, DNA matching) can only be used for excluding suspects, but not for convictions. Do you agree with this argument?

The third controversial example is about how to use clinical trial results for medical decision-making. Suppose you are diagnosed with a rare disease, and the doctor provides you two options: Drug A or Drug B; each has been tested on sets of 100 patients to see if it is better than a control treatment with a known 50% cure rate. In the first clinical trial, 59 of 100 patients treated with

Drug A are cured, which is statistically significant at the one-sided 5% level. In the second clinical trial, 60 patients out of 100 are cured with Drug B. But this is not even statistically significant, because in the second trial there is an interim analysis of the first 50 patients where 30 of them were found cured, and, as we explained in the previous coin-flipping experiments, the hurdles for rejecting the null hypothesis are higher when there are multiple analyses.

Here is the dilemma: Drug B shows a better cure rate of 60% versus Drug A with a 59% cure rate. But Drug A is statistically better than the control and Drug B has not achieved statistical significance in comparison with the control treatment. Which drug do you take? On one hand, you may decide to take Drug A since Drug B does not even achieve statistical significance, implying that Drug B appearing better than the control may just be random chance. On other hand, you may conclude that with or without the interim analysis, the chemical structure of the drug will not change. In this case, you can ignore the interim analysis; a cure rate of 60% is better than 59%, so you should take Drug B. We should know that when there are many interim analyses, a cure rate of 90% may not be statistically significant because the α for each test is adjusted to a very low value.

Here, we can see two different concepts of the effectiveness of a drug. One is the physical properties of the test compound, which will *not* change as the hypothesis test procedure changes (with or without interim analysis). The other is the statistical property will change since it reflects an aggregated attribute of a group of similar results so the statistical property will depend on the choice of similarity groups.

The multiplicity issue does not necessarily explicitly involve multiple hypothesis tests. It can arise from model fitting by trying multiple models, or from analyses performed on the same data by different researchers. Linear regression is one of the most common statistical procedures used in research. For multiple regression, the backward elimination algorithm (BEA) is often applied. The problem with this method is type-I inflation and consequently FDR increases. For example, if there are 10 factors to investigate, in multiple regression with BEA the type-I error is about 40%. This means that a scientist can use any data with 11 variables and perform multiple regression with BEA and have at least a 40% chance of finding at least one model that is significant. As the variables increase, the type-I error rate increases. Therefore, we have to control, or at least assess, the type-I error or FDR. Otherwise, there will be too many false scientific conclusions.

Multiplicity is indeed challenging in scientific discovery: if one research study has a false discovery and other 100 research studies are conducted to confirm it, then we will expect that 5 studies will falsely verify the finding using hypothesis test at 5% significance level. There might be a misconception that if we do the experiment very carefully, the error or false positive findings can be eliminated. But this is just an illusion. The main reason that error is unavoidable is not that our experimental design is poor or the measurements we have taken have errors. Error is unavoidable because of hidden confounders that we cannot know or are unobservable at the moment of experiment.

As data accumulate continually throughout long or serial investigations of medical interventions (and other areas of research), more analyses will be performed on the same data and thus inflate FDRs. On the other hand, since meta-analyses yield more reliable data, the statistical conclusions will be more reliable. How then can we simply dismiss the results from meta-analyses just because we have "spent all α?"

11.7 Regression with Time-Dependent Variables

The principle of factor isolation (PFI) is often used to investigate causality with a single cause in physics. However, in life, social, and medical sciences, there are many other random factors, observable to hidden, simple regression can be viewed as a utilization of PFI in the presence of randomness. In order for the regression to be effective the experiment is often conducted with a control group and randomization to balance out confounding factors. When the causality involves multiple causes, we often use multiple regression or ANCOVA to investigate the main effect and covariate effects. The main effect can often be treatment interventions and the covariates are often confounders.

For a variable to be a confounder in a clinical trial it must satisfy three conditions (Chang 2014):

1. It must be associated with the treatment (the main factor).

2. It must be a predictor (not necessarily a cause) of the outcome being measured.

3. It must not be a consequence of the treatment (the main factor) itself.

A factor is not a confounder if it lies on the causal pathway between the variables of interest. Such a factor can be a direct cause or a mediator. Of course, the causal pathway is often not observable and dependent on our interpretation. It is not always necessary to know the intimate pathway; however, through a hypothetical pathway, we often can often better model the mechanism of a system. Latent variable structure equation modeling is an example of such hidden pathway modeling. Such a technique is often used in sociology, psychology, and econometrics studies. Before we can deal with sophisticated situations, let's just study the challenges imposed by an observable confounder in multiple regression.

The randomized controlled experiment is a great invention, but the analyses of data from such an experiment and the interpretation of results do

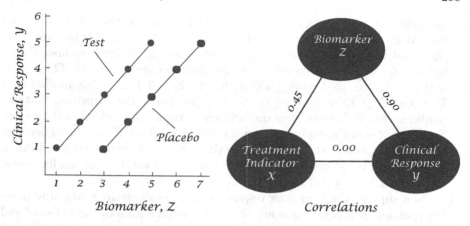

FIGURE 11.2
Paradox of Multiple-Regression.

not lack challenges and controversies. Whether it is an observational or a controlled experiment, multiple regression is a common tool for analyzing the data. For a linear regression model (linear in constants a and b), $Y \approx aX^2 + bX$, we wouldn't say the effect of X on Y is b because a is also a partial indicator of the X effect. However, if we write the equation as $Y = aZ + bX$, and the covariate $Z = X^2$ is not indicated but the correlation $\text{corr}(X, Z) \approx 1$ is observed, then we often mistakenly say the effect of X on Y is b. Here Z is a measured covariate, a confounder, or a mediator. Let's discuss the controversies further through an example provided by Chang (2007, 2011).

Suppose five subjects in each of two treatment groups ($X = 0$ for placebo and $X = 1$ for test drug) in a clinical trial are measured for the primary endpoint Y and biomarker responses Z. We first calculate Pearson's correlations between the variables: the treatment, biomarker, and the primary endpoint. The results are presented in Figure 11.2. We can see that the correlations between them are not transitive. In other words, a correlation between the treatment and the biomarker ($R_{XZ} = 0.45$) and a correlation between the biomarker and the primary endpoint ($R_{YZ} = 0.90$) do not ensure a correlation (R_{XY}) between the treatment and the clinical response.

The average response with the primary endpoint is 4 for each group, which indicates that there is no treatment effect. On the other hand, the average biomarker response is 6 for group B and 4 for group A, which indicates that the drug has effects on the biomarker.

After fitting a linear model with the data we obtain

$$Y \approx Z - 2X \tag{11.2}$$

This model fits the data well based on the model-fitting p-value and R^2. Specifically, R^2 is equal to 1. The p-values for the model and all parameters are equal to 0. The coefficient 2 in the model is the separation between the two lines. Based on the model, we would conclude that the biomarker has a positive effect and the treatment has a negative effect on the clinical response. But in fact the treatment has no effect on the clinical response at all. The reason is that $\bar{Z}$ relates to $\bar{X}$ through their means $\bar{Z} = 3 + 2\bar{X}$. This implies that $\bar{Y} = 3 + 2X - 2X = 3 = 3 + 0 \cdot \bar{X}$. Therefore, it is not surprising that the coefficient for X changes when the different covariate Z is added to the model. Note that Z is not a confounder per our definition since Z is a consequence of treatment X, and thus does not meet criterion 3 in the confounder definition. In most practice, Z and X have a correlation $\rho < 1$ without colinearity issues, but the controversy still exists.

Now suppose the biomarker responses in the example are changed to baseline confounder Z before randomization. We would obtain the same model and the same conclusion that the treatment has a negative effect on the clinical response. We further learn that if we change our similarity grouping to also consider the biomarker value at baseline, then we will select 3 patients (with $z = 3, 4, 5$) in the control and 3 patients with the same biomarker values in the test group. Now there is clearly a treatment effect of -2 for every patient with same baseline value for Z. This is consistent with the multiple regression producing $Y = Z - 2X$ obtained from the data.

From this example we can see that in multiple regression one should use baseline confounders, but not variables that result from treatment (or main effect) as covariates. In general, a different set of variables included in the regression model implies a different similarity grouping for which the similarity principle applies.

We often use an entire dataset for statistical modeling; the resulting model is the consequence of minimizing the total error. But that may not be desirable. For instance, a drug's effect on youth and the elderly can be very different. Thus, what we really want to minimize is the relevant error. What is relevant error? It has to be based on the similarity principle: if you think people with similar ages will have a similar treatment effect, then use that group of people to do modeling to minimize the error of the model within that group. How do we determine such subgroups? It is a trade-off between accuracy and precision. Dividing the sample into many smaller subsamples may allow a researcher to reach accurate conclusions but with poor precision, due to small sample sizes in a subgroup, whereas dividing the sample into a few bigger subsamples may yield conclusions with good precision but inaccuracy because characteristics in the subsample may still be very different.

11.8 Hidden Confounders

When people are studying association relationships, it is important to exclude confounders' effects and get the true relationship between variables of interest.

Classical analysis approaches to deal with confounders include adjustment for confounders and stratified analysis by confounders, etc. Using classical methods, people need to know what the potential confounders are beforehand so that the relevant data can be collected, and adjustment or stratified analysis can be applied or keep study design balanced with regard to confounders. However, in reality, it is sometimes hard to know what the confounders are in a study. In other words, when there is a potential hidden confounder, how can we deal with it? A hidden confounder is unidentified; thus it is unmeasured, or it is an unnamed ghost.

Even though randomization can help alleviate confounding issues, there is no guarantee that all potential confounders are balanced through randomization. Besides, for some studies, for example retrospective studies, randomization is not applicable. So, it is important researchers have tools ready to deal with the confounding issue. .

When exploring the relationship between outcome and predictors of interest, suspected confounders are also added into regression models. This is called adjustment. By adjusting for confounders, the true relationship between outcome and predictors can be obtained. If suspected confounders are categorical, stratified analysis could be used. This means that people can explore the relationship between outcome and predictors of interest within each confounder level. In this way, a confounding effect will be excluded.

Let's study a variable simple case of hidden confounder: analysis of treatment-blinded data can be viewed as a hidden confounder issue; the hidden confounder is the treatment. Assume the response Y is normally distributed within each of the two treatment groups. Therefore, the pooled or blinded data have a mixed normal distribution:

$$f(x) = \sum_{i=1}^{2} w_i f_i\left(x; \mu_i, \sigma_i^2\right), \tag{11.3}$$

where the constant weight $w_i > 0$, $w_1 + w_2 = 1$ ($w_1 : w_2$ is the randomization ratio) and

$$f_i\left(x; \mu_i, \sigma_i^2\right) = \frac{1}{\sqrt{2\pi}\sigma_i} \exp\left(-\frac{(x - \mu_i)^2}{2\sigma_i^2}\right). \tag{11.4}$$

The mean and variance of the mixed distribution are

$$\mu = w_1 \mu_1 + w_2 \mu_2, \tag{11.5}$$

and

$$\sigma^2 = \left(w_1 \sigma_1^2 + w_2 \sigma_2^2\right) + w_1 w_2 \delta^2 \tag{11.6}$$

where treatment difference $\delta = \mu_1 - \mu_2$. For equal variance $\sigma_1^2 = \sigma_2^2 = \sigma_0^2$, we have

$$\sigma^2 = \sigma_0^2 + w_1 w_2 \delta^2. \tag{11.7}$$

The skewness of the mixed distribution is (Casella and Berger, 1990, Wang, 2001, 2006),

$$\Gamma = w_1 w_2 (w_2 - w_1) \delta^3. \tag{11.8}$$

Solving (11.8) for δ^3, we obtain

$$\delta^3 = \frac{\Gamma}{w_1 w_2 (w_2 - w_1)}, \tag{11.9}$$

Therefore, an unbiased estimator for δ^3 is

$$\hat{\delta}^3 = \frac{\hat{\Gamma}}{w_1 w_2 (w_2 - w_1)} \tag{11.10}$$

The sample skewness is

$$\hat{\Gamma} = \frac{1}{n} \sum_{i=1}^{n} (x_i - \bar{x})^3 = \frac{1}{n} \sum_{i=1}^{n} \left(x_i - \frac{1}{n} \sum_{i=1}^{n} x_i \right)^3 \tag{11.11}$$

and the pdf of $\hat{\Gamma}$ is asymptotically a normal distribution (Figure 11.3):

$$f_{\hat{\Gamma}}(x) = \frac{2}{\sqrt{2\pi}\sigma} e^{-\frac{(x-\delta^3)^2}{2\sigma^2}}, (-\infty < x < \infty). \tag{11.12}$$

For small sample size,

$$\hat{\delta} = \left(\frac{\hat{\Gamma}}{w_1 w_2 (w_2 - w_1)} \right)^{1/3} \tag{11.13}$$

is a biased (downwards) estimator of δ. For $w_1 = 1/4$ and $w_2 = 3/4$,

$$\hat{\delta} = 4 \left[\frac{\hat{\Gamma}}{6} \right]^{1/3}$$

Optimally randomization for the purpose of unblinded estimation of treatment effect is $w_1 : w_2 = 3 : 1$ to $4 : 1$. The sample size is approximately 1000 times that required in a clinical trial with 80% to 90% power in order to have a good precision. After obtaining $\hat{\delta}$ for $\mu_1 - \mu_2$, μ_1 and μ_2 can be calculated using $\mu_2 = \hat{\mu} - w_1 \hat{\delta}$ and $\mu_1 = \hat{\mu} + w_2 \hat{\delta}$.

When the treatment difference is small (e.g., $\mu_1 = 2.5$ versus $\mu_2 = 3$), the distribution of $\hat{\delta}$ from (11.13) becomes bimodal, while the distribution $\hat{\Gamma}$ is still approximately normal (Figure 11.3). This implies that even when δ^3 can be estimated precisely, the estimation of δ can still be very inaccurate – a counter-intuitive result. When the treatment difference is large (e.g., $\mu_1 = 0.5$

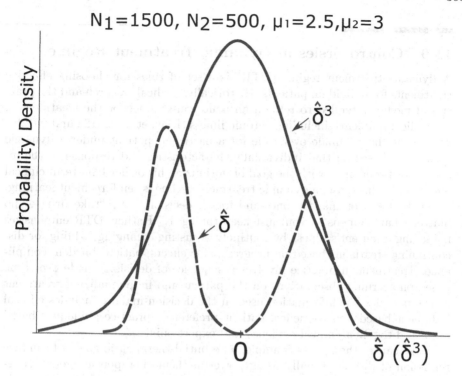

FIGURE 11.3
N1 = 1500, N2 = 500, $\mu_1 = 2.5, \mu_2 = 3$.

versus $\mu_2 = 3$), both distributions of $\hat{\delta}$ and $\hat{\Gamma}$ are normal (Figure 11.3) and the blinded treatment estimation is accurate (see Table 11.3).

From Table 11.3, we can see that, using (11.13) to estimate the treatment effect requires a very large sample size when a hidden confounder is present. A better approach was proposed by Zhao and Chang (2018) using E-M algorithm. The simulation SAS Macro BlindedEstofTrtEffect used to study the effect of a confounder, can be found in the in Appendix 12.8.

TABLE 11.3
Blinded Treatment Effect Estimate Using Skewness Γ.

δ	3	2	1	0.8	0.5	0.3	0.2	0.1	0
$\hat{\delta}^*$	2.997	1.992	0.788	0.460	0.124	0.028	0.008	0.002	0.000
$\sigma_{\hat{\delta}}$	0.094	0.127	0.630	0.764	0.812	0.808	0.805	0.803	0.802
$\hat{\delta}^{**}$	2.999	1.996	0.895	0.559	0.154	0.036	0.009	0	0
$\sigma_{\hat{\delta}}$	0.066	0.089	0.420	0.618	0.719	0.720	0.718	0.716	0.716

Note: for δ^*, N1 = 1000 and N2 = 250; for δ^{**}, N1 = 2000 and N2 = 500.

11.9 Controversies in Dynamic Treatment Regime

A dynamic treatment regime (DTR) is a set of rules for choosing effective treatments for individual patients. Historically, medical research and the practice of medicine tended to rely on an acute care model for the treatment of all medical problems, including chronic illness (Diaz, et al., 2012a and 2012b). Treatment choices made over time for a particular patient under a dynamic regime are based on that individual's characteristics and response to the interventions over time, with the goal of optimizing his or her long-term clinical outcome. In this sense, a dynamic treatment regime is reinforcement learning.

DTR does not make a once-and-for-all decision, e.g., "take drug A no matter what happens to you, just keep taking it." Rather, DTR emphasizes managing a patient's illness by routinely adjusting, changing, adding, or discontinuing treatment based on progress, side effects, patient burden, compliance. Treatment in practice involves a sequence of decisions made over time based on accruing observations on the patient and individualizing treatment to the patient. The information used in the decision-making includes clinical judgment based on experience, patient preference, practice guidelines based on pieced-together clinical evidence and expert opinion.

Take cancer therapy as example. The initial therapeutic goal is to induce remission of disease, usually using powerful chemotherapeutic agents. If remission is obtained, then the goal is to maintain remission as long as possible before relapse/recurrence occurs, e.g., by administering additional agents that intensify or maintain the effects of the initial induction therapy. If the patient does not achieve remission, then another therapy may be tried to induce remission (Figure 11.4). The primary endpoint is a time-to-event, e.g., disease-free survival time or overall survival.

Despite the value of a dynamic treatment regimen, there are controversies surrounding techniques for estimating treatment effects. We will discuss briefly the controversies using the following simple example.

In a study of effectiveness of different interventions on cancer, in Cycle 1, patients are randomized to receive either drug A_1 (Cycle1 = 1) or A_2 (Cycle1 = 0). For simplicity, assume that if a patient survives long enough, he will definitely respond to A_1 or A_2 at time Month 1. Per study design (Figure 11.5), patients who respond will receive treatment B_1 and patients who don't respond will receive treatment B_2. Since all patients who survive longer than 1 month will respond and receive B_1 and other non-responders will receive B_2, we code Cycle2 = 1 for responders and Cycle2 = 0 for no responders.

Assume the overall survival time X has an exponential survival distribution. The analysis will be performed using linear model: $x = a \cdot Cycle1 + b \cdot Cycle2 + \varepsilon$. In what follows, we will show the model postulate a false effect of Cycle 2. We simulate the data so that there is no effect for Cycle 1 and Cycle 2.

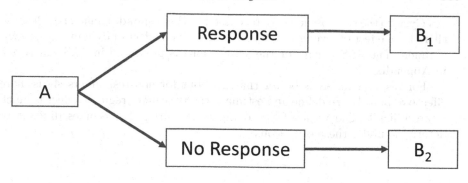

FIGURE 11.4
A Simple Dynamic Treatment Regimen.

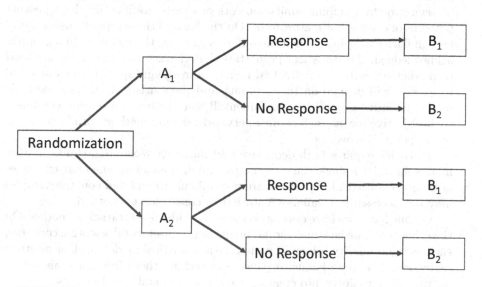

FIGURE 11.5
Sequential Multiple Assignment Randomized Trial (SMART).

We generate survival time X from an exponential distribution for all subjects. To make Cycle1 have no effect on survival time x, we randomly assign 0 or 1 to a subject. To make Cycle 2 have no effect on survival, we code Cycle2 $= 1$ at Month 1 (thus for those died before Month 1, Cycle2 $= 0$) and no change will be made on survival time x. In other words, anyone who survives longer than 1 month will be given ineffective treatment Cycle2. However, the outcomes from the following regression model show that the effect of Cycle2 is significant with p-value <0.0001 with 1000 patients. The bias results from the assignment of Cycle2 because only patients who survive long enough will get Cycle2 (the same issue as we discussed in the responder analysis). Because there is no effect of Cycle1 and Cycle2, there is no effect of dynamic treatment regimen. The SAS macro for the simulations is presented in SAS Macro 9.3 in Appendix 12.7.

For responders, A_1 is better than A_2, but for non-responders A_2 is more effective than A_1. To define and estimate the treatment regimen effect is much more difficult. The value of approving a new drug A_1 becomes difficult to determine under these conditions.

11.10   Summary and Recommendations

Science is a study of (ideally) repeated events. Since everything is unique in its own way, by grouping similar objects or events, we identify the repeating patterns of events that matter to us. On the basis of these repetitions we apply the similarity principle. When the difference among the members in a group is acknowledged, the statistical properties that characterize the group are used to predict properties of individual members in the group. But the statistical properties will depend on the grouping and the statistical analysis methods used. Similarity grouping is fundamentally subjective, but can be combined with objective means such as unsupervised learning methods or clustering in our scientific discoveries.

Statistics requires both deductive and inductive reasoning. Unlike mathematics, in which a single counterexample can dismiss a false theorem, examples of failing a statistical hypothesis are not difficult to find and counterexamples may not necessarily invalidate a statistical conclusion or method.

On one hand, we have developed some very advanced statistical models. On the other hand, we lack understanding of some fundamental scientific concepts, such as the similarity principle, and of basic statistical models such as multiple regression. It is time for us to pause and rethink those fundamentals before putting all our efforts into creating more complex statistical models.

Bibliography

Benjamini, Y. and Hochberg, Y. (1995). Controlling the false discovery rate: A practical and powerful approach to multiple testing. *Journal of the Royal Statistical Society B*, 57(2):289-300.

Chang, M. (2007). *Adaptive Design Theory and Implementation Using SAS and R*. CRC Press/Taylor Francis Group. Boca Raton, FL.

Chang, M. (2011). Modern Issues and Methods in Biostatistics, Springer. New York, New York.

Chang, M. (2012). Paradoxes in Scientific Inferences. CRC Press/Taylor Francis Group. Boca Raton, FL.

Chang, M. (2014). Principles of Scientific methods. CRC Press/Taylor Francis Group. Boca Raton, FL.

Chang, M. and Chang, M. (2017). iWordNet: A New Approach to Cognitive Science and Artificial Intelligence. Advances in Artificial Intelligence. Volume 2017.

Diaz, F.J., Hung-Wen Yeh, Jose de Leon. (2012a). Role of Statistical Random-Effects Linear Models in Personalized Medicine. Volume 10, Issue 1.

Diaz, F.J. et al. (2012b). Drug Dosage Individualization Based on a Random-Effects Linear Model. Journal of Biopharmaceutical Statistics. Volume 22, Issue 3.

Lench, H.C, Safer, M.A., Levine, L.J. (2011). Focalism and the Underestimation of Future Emotion: When It's Worse Than Imagined. Emotion, Vol. 11, No. 2, 278–285.

Lord, F. M. (1967). A paradox in the interpretation of group comparisons. Psychological Bulletin, 68 (5):304—305.

Simpson, E.H. (1951). The Interpretation of Interaction in Contingency Tables. Journal of the Royal Statistical Society, Series B 13: 238–241.

Vidakovic, B. (2008). Bayesian Statistics Class handout. Brhttp://www2.isye.gatech.edu/~brani/isyebayes/handouts.html

Zhao, Q. and Chang, M. (2018). A novel approach to dealing with hidden confounders. JBS. Submitted.

12

Appendix: SAS and R Code

12.1   Chapter 3

SAS Macro 3.1: Simon Two-Stage Design with Single Arm

```
%Macro SimonBinary(nSims=10000, p=0.4, N1=21, N2=29);
* Simon one-arm two-stage with binary endpoint;
Data GSD; Keep FSP AveN Power;
p=&p; N1=&N1; N2=&N2; N=N1+N2;
FSP=0; AveN=0; Power=0;
Do isim=1 To &nSims;
AveN=AveN+N1/&nSims;
m1 = rand('BINOM',p,N1);
If m1<=2 Then FSP=FSP+1/&nSims;
If m1>2 Then Do;
m2 = rand('BINOM',p,N2);
If m2+m1>7 Then Power=Power+1/&nSims;
AveN=AveN+N2/&nSims;
End;
End;
Output;
Run;
Proc Print Data=GSD; Run;
%Mend SimonBinary;
%SimonBinary(nSims=10000, p=0.25, N1=21, N2=29);
run;
```

12.2   Chapter 4

12.2.1   SAS Macro for Group Sequential Design

**SAS Macro 4.1: Two-Stage Group Sequential Design
with Normal Endpoint**

```
%Macro GSDNormal(nSims=10000000, ux=0.4, uy=0.8, sigma=1.2, N1=50,
N2=50, alpha1=0.0025, beta1=1, alpha2=0.024);
* Out pout power, esarly efficay and futility stopping probabilities, average sam-
ple;
* Applicable to any sample size as along as the stopping boundaries are adjusted
to control type-I error rate;
Data GSD; Keep FSP ESP AveN Power;
alpha1=&alpha1; alpha2=&alpha2; beta1=&beta1; ux=&ux; uy=&uy;
sigma=&sigma; N1=&N1; N2=&N2; N=N1+N2;
FSP=0; ESP=0; AveN=0; Power=0;
Do isim=1 To &nSims;
AveN=AveN+N1/&nSims;
ux1 = Rannor(0)*sigma/Sqrt(N1)+ux;
uy1 = Rannor(0)*sigma/Sqrt(N1)+uy;
T1 = (uy1-ux1)*Sqrt(N1/2)/sigma;
p1=1-ProbNorm(T1);
If p1>beta1 Then FSP=FSP+1/&nSims;
If p1<=alpha1 Then do;
Power=Power+1/&nSims; ESP=ESP+1/&nSims;
End;
If alpha1<p1<=beta1 Then Do;
AveN=AveN+N2/&nSims;
ux2 = Rannor(0)*sigma/Sqrt(N2)+ux ;
uy2 = Rannor(0)*sigma/Sqrt(N2)+uy;
Aveux=(ux1*N1+ux2*N2)/N;
Aveuy=(uy1*N1+uy2*N2)/N;
T2 = (Aveuy-Aveux)*Sqrt(N/2)/sigma;
p2=1-ProbNorm(T2);
If .<p2<=alpha2 Then Power=Power+1/&nSims;
End;
End;
Output;
Run;
Proc Print Data=GSD; Run;
%Mend GSDNormal;
```

SAS Macro 4.2: Two-Stage Group Sequential Design with Binary Endpoint

```
%Macro GSDBinary(nSims=1000000, px=0.4, py=0.6, N1=50, N2=50, al-
pha1=0.0025, beta1=1, alpha2=0.024);
* Out pout power, esarly efficay and futility stopping probabilities, average sam-
ple;
* Applicable to any sample size as along as the stopping boundaries are adjusted
to control type-I error rate;
Data GSD; Keep FSP ESP AveN Power;
alpha1=&alpha1; alpha2=&alpha2; beta1=&beta1;
px=&px; py=&py; N1=&N1; N2=&N2; N=N1+N2;
FSP=0; ESP=0; AveN=0; Power=0;
Do isim=1 To &nSims;
AveN=AveN+N1/&nSims;
px1 = rand('BINOM',px,N1)/N1;
py1 = rand('BINOM',py,N1)/N1;
SE=sqrt(px1*(1-px1)/N1+py1*(1-py1)/N1);
T1 = (py1-px1)/SE;
p1=1-ProbNorm(T1);
If p1>beta1 Then FSP=FSP+1/&nSims;
If p1<=alpha1 Then do;
Power=Power+1/&nSims; ESP=ESP+1/&nSims;
End;
If alpha1<p1<=beta1 Then Do;
AveN=AveN+N2/&nSims;
px2 = rand('BINOM',px,N2)/N2;
py2 = rand('BINOM',py,N2)/N2;
avepx=(px1*N1+px2*N2)/N;
avepy=(py1*N1+py2*N2)/N;
SE=sqrt(avepx*(1-avepx)/N+avepy*(1-avepy)/N);
T2 = (Avepy-Avepx)/SE;
p2=1-ProbNorm(T2);
If .<p2<=alpha2 Then Power=Power+1/&nSims;
End;
End;
Output;
Run;
Proc Print Data=GSD; Run;
%Mend GSDBinary;
```

SAS Macro 4.3: Two-Stage Group Sequential Design with Poisson Endpoint

```
%Macro GSDPoisson(nSims=1000000, Lamdax=4, Lamday=6, N1=50, N2=50,
alpha1=0.0025, beta1=1, alpha2=0.024);
* Out pout power, esarly efficay and futility stopping probabilities, average sam-
ple;
```

```
* Applicable to any sample size as along as the stopping boundaries are adjusted
to control type-I error rate;
    Data GSD; Keep FSP ESP AveN Power;
    alpha1=&alpha1; alpha2=&alpha2; beta1=&beta1; Lamdax=&Lamdax;
    Lamday=&Lamday; N1=&N1; N2=&N2; N=N1+N2;
    FSP=0; ESP=0; AveN=0; Power=0;
    Do isim=1 To &nSims;
    AveN=AveN+N1/&nSims;
    Lamdax1Obs=rand('POISSON',N1*Lamdax)/N1;
    Lamday1Obs=rand('POISSON',N1*Lamday)/N1;
    SE=max(0.000000000001, sqrt(Lamdax1Obs/N1+Lamday1Obs/N1));
    T1 = (Lamday1Obs- Lamdax1Obs)/SE;
    p1=1-ProbNorm(T1);
    If p1>beta1 Then FSP=FSP+1/&nSims;
    If .<p1<=alpha1 Then do;
    Power=Power+1/&nSims; ESP=ESP+1/&nSims;
    End;
    If alpha1<p1<=beta1 Then Do;
    AveN=AveN+N2/&nSims;
    Lamdax2Obs=rand('POISSON',N2*Lamdax)/N2;
    Lamday2Obs=rand('POISSON',N2*Lamday)/N2;
    aveLamx=(Lamdax1Obs*N1+Lamdax2Obs*N2)/N;
    aveLamy=(Lamday1Obs*N1+Lamday2Obs*N2)/N;
    SE=max(0.000000000001, sqrt(aveLamx/N+aveLamy/N));
    T2 = (aveLamy - aveLamx)/SE;
    p2=1-ProbNorm(T2);
    If .<p2<=alpha2 Then Power=Power+1/&nSims;
    End;
    End;
    Output;
    Run;
    Proc Print Data=GSD; Run;
    %Mend GSDPoisson;
```

SAS Macro 4.4: Two-Stage Group Sequential Design with Survival Endpoint

%Macro GSDSurvival(nSims=1000000, tStd=12, tAcr=4, Lamdax=0.5, Lam-
day=0.5, N1=50, N2=50, alpha1=0.0025, beta1=1, alpha2=0.024, alpha=0.025);
    * Out pout power, esarly efficay and futility stopping probabilities, average sam-
ple;
    * Applicable to any sample size as along as the stopping boundaries are adjusted
to control type-I error rate;
    * N1, N2 = sample size per group for stage 1 and 2 (not cumulative);
    * nEvents = total number of events, AvenEvents = average number of events;

```
Data GSD; Keep FSP ESP AveN Power nEvents AvenEvents;
alpha=&alpha; alpha1=&alpha1; alpha2=&alpha2; beta1=&beta1;
ux=&Lamdax; uy=&Lamday; N1=&N1; N2=&N2; N=N1+N2;
Expuxd=exp(-ux*&tStd); Expuyd=exp(-uy*&tStd);
sigmax=ux*(1+Expuxd*(1-exp(ux*&tAcr))/(&tAcr*ux))**(-0.5);
sigmay=uy*(1+Expuyd*(1-exp(uy*&tAcr))/(&tAcr*uy))**(-0.5);
sigma=((sigmax**2+sigmay**2)/2)**0.5;
FSP=0; ESP=0; AveN=0; Power=0;
Do isim=1 To &nSims;
AveN=AveN+N1/&nSims;
ux1 = Rannor(0)*sigma/Sqrt(N1)+ux;
uy1 = Rannor(0)*sigma/Sqrt(N1)+uy;
T1 = (uy1-ux1)*Sqrt(N1/2)/sigma;
p1=1-ProbNorm(T1);
If p1>beta1 Then FSP=FSP+1/&nSims;
If p1<=alpha1 Then do;
Power=Power+1/&nSims; ESP=ESP+1/&nSims;
End;
If alpha1<p1<=beta1 Then Do;
AveN=AveN+N2/&nSims;
* Add # of events and aveEvents required;
nEventsx = N/&tAcr*(&tAcr-1/ux*(exp(ux*&tAcr)-1)*Exp(-ux*&tStd));
nEventsy = N/&tAcr*(&tAcr-1/uy*(exp(uy*&tAcr)-1)*Exp(-uy*&tStd));
nEvents=nEventsx+nEventsy;
AvenEvents=AveN/N*nEvents;
ux2 = Rannor(0)*sigma/Sqrt(N2)+ux ;
uy2 = Rannor(0)*sigma/Sqrt(N2)+uy;
Aveux=(ux1*N1+ux2*N2)/N;
Aveuy=(uy1*N1+uy2*N2)/N;
T2 = (Aveuy-Aveux)*Sqrt(N/2)/sigma;
p2=1-ProbNorm(T2);
If .<p2<=alpha2 Then Power=Power+1/&nSims;
End;
End;
Output;
Run;
Proc Print Data=GSD; Run;
%Mend GSDSurvival;
```

12.2.2 SAS Macro for Sample Size Re-estimation

SAS Macro 4.5: Two-Group Two-Stage Sample Size Re-estimation with Promising-zone method for Normal Endpoint

%Macro   SSRTwoGroupDesignNormal(nSims=1000000,   n1=100,   n2=100, N2max=100, u0=0.1, u1=0.25, sigma=1.2, alpha=0.025, TargetPower=0.9, alpha1= 0.00153, alpha2=0.02454, beta1=0.8, PromisingL=0.0213, PromisingU=0.214);

* n1 and n2 = balanced design stagewise sample size per group at stages 1 and 2;

* N2max = maximum allowable sample size per group at stage 2 for SSR;

* Promising zone: $0.0213 < p1 < 0.214$ or $1.206 < z1 < 2.027$ or $0.526 <$ Delta_obs/delta_ini< 0.884 or $0.36 <$conditional power < 0.9;

* Applicable to Larger sample size trials only;

Data MPSSR;

keep u0 u1 sigma alpha alpha1 alpha2 beta1 PromisingL PromisingU ESP FSP Power AveN;

n1=&n1; n2=&n2; u0=&u0; u1=&u1; sigma=σ alpha1=&alpha1; alpha2=&alpha2; beta1=&beta1;

power = 0; AveN = 0; FSP = 0; ESP = 0;

PromisingL=max(alpha1, &PromisingL); * Make sure Promising lower bound > efficacy stopping boundary on p-scale;

PromisingU=min(beta1, &promisingU); * make sure Promising upper bound < futiltiy boundary;

Do iSim = 1 To &nSims;

* Generate data for stage 1;

AveN = AveN + n1/&nSims; * Average sample size per group;

u01 = RAND('Normal')*sigma/sqrt(n1)+u0; * Observed mean response in Control;

u11 = RAND('Normal')*sigma/sqrt(n1)+u1; * Observed mean response in Test;

SE=sigma/sqrt(n1/2); * assume sigma known or large sample assumption;

z1=(u11-u01)/SE;

pv1=1-ProbNorm(z1);

If pv1<=alpha1 Then ESP=ESP+1/&nSims; * Efficacy stopping;

If pv1>beta1 Then FSP=FSP+1/&nSims; * Futility stopping;

If alpha1<pv1<=beta1 Then Do; * Start Stage 2;

n2=&n2; n02=&n2;

If PromisingL<pv1<PromisingU Then Do; * Sample size estimation within promising zone;

If z1 NE 0 Then n2=round((n1/z1**2)*((Probit(1-&alpha)*sqrt(n1+n02)-z1*sqrt(n1))/sqrt(n02)+Probit(&Targetpower))**2);

* avoid z1=0 or negative direction. The n2new is not a monotonic function of z1;

n2=min(&N2max, n2); *capped at N2max;

n2=max(n2, n02); * Do allow to reduce from initial sample size, also avoid n2=0;

End;

u02 = RAND('Normal')*sigma/sqrt(n2)+u0; * stage 2 Observed mean response in Control;

u12 = RAND('Normal')*sigma/sqrt(n2)+u1; * stage 2 Observed mean response in Test;

u0Cum = (u01*n1+u02*n2)/(n1+n2);

u1Cum = (u11*n1+u12*n2)/(n1+n2);

SE=sigma/sqrt((n1+n2)/2); * assume sigma known or large sample assumption;

z2=(u1Cum-u0Cum)/SE;

pv2=1-ProbNorm(z2);

If pv2<alpha2 Then Power=Power+1/&nSims;

AveN = AveN + n2/&nSims; * Average sample size per group;

End;

End;

Power=Power+ESP;

Output;

Run;

Proc print data=MPSSR; Run;

%Mend;

SAS Macro 4.6: One-Group Two-Stage Sample Size Reestimation with Promising-Zone Method for Binary Endpoint

%Macro Mehta_PocockSSROneGroupDesign(nSims=1000000, n1=100, n2=100, N2max=100, p0=0.1, p1=0.25, alpha=0.025, TargetPower=0.9, alpha1= 0.00153, alpha2=0.02454, beta1=0.8, PromisingL=0.0213, PromisingU=0.214);

* n1 and n2 = balanced design stagewise sample size per group at stages 1 and 2;

* N2max = maximum allowable sample size per group at stage 2 for SSR;

* Promising zone: 0.0213<p1<0.214 or 1.206<z1<2.027 or 0.526< Delta_obs/delta_ini<0.884 or 0.36<conditional power <0.9;

* Applicable small and larger sample size trials as long as the promising zone and/or adjusted approperiately to control FWER;

Data MPSSR;

keep n1 n02 N2max p0 p1 alpha1 alpha2 beta1 ESP FSP AveN Power;

n1=&n1; n2=&n2; N2max=&N2max; p0=&p0; p1=&p1; alpha1=&alpha1; alpha2=&alpha2; beta1=&beta1;

power = 0; AveN = 0; FSP = 0; ESP = 0; S0=sqrt(p0*(1-p0));

PromisingL=max(alpha1, &PromisingL); * Make sure Promising lower bound > efficacy stopping boundary on p-scale;

PromisingU=min(beta1, &promisingU); * make sure Promising upper bound < futiltiy boundary;

Do iSim = 1 To &nSims;

* Generate data for stage 1;

AveN = AveN + n1/&nSims; * Average sample size;

r11 = RAND('BINOMIAL',p1, n1)/n1;

```
* z1=(r11-p0)/S0*sqrt(n1);
z1=(r11-p0)/sqrt(r11*(1-r11))*sqrt(n1);
pv1=1-ProbNorm(z1);
If pv1<=alpha1 Then ESP=ESP+1/&nSims; * Efficacy stopping;
If pv1>beta1 Then FSP=FSP+1/&nSims; * Futility stopping;
If alpha1<pv1<=beta1 Then Do; * Start Stage 2;
n2=&n2; n02=&n2;
If PromisingL<pv1<PromisingU And n02 NE &N2max Then Do; * Sample size
estimation within promising zone;
If z1 NE 0 Then n2=Round((n1/z1**2)*((Probit(1-&alpha)*sqrt(n1+n02)-
z1*sqrt(n1))/sqrt(n02)+Probit(&Targetpower))**2,1);
n2=max(n2, n02); * Do allow to reduce from initial sample size, also avoid n2=0;
n2=min(&N2max, n2); * capped at N2max;
End;
* r12 = (r11*n1+RAND('BINOMIAL', p1, n2max))/(n1+n2max); * at promis-
ing zone, alway increase n2 to N2max;
r12 = (r11*n1+RAND('BINOMIAL', p1, n2))/(n1+n2); * at promising zone,
alway increase n2 to N2max;
z2=(r12-p0)/sqrt(r12*(1-r12))*sqrt(n1+n2);
pv2=1-ProbNorm(z2);
If pv2<alpha2 Then Power=Power+1/&nSims;
AveN = AveN + n2/&nSims; * Average sample size;
End;
End;
Power=Power+ESP;
Output;
Run;
Proc print data=MPSSR; Run;
%Mend;
```

SAS Macro 4.7: Two-Group Two-Stage Sample Size Reestimation with Promising-Zone Method for Binary Endpoint

```
%Macro Mehta_PocockSSRTwoGroupDesign(nSims=1000000, n1=100, n2=100,
N2max=100, p0=0.1, p1=0.25, alpha=0.025, TargetPower=0.9, alpha1= 0.00153,
alpha2=0.02454, beta1=0.8, PromisingL=0.0213, PromisingU=0.214);
* ni = balanced design stagewise sample size per group at stage i;
* N2max = maximum allowable sample size per group at stage 2 for SSR;
* Promising zone: 0.0213<p1<0.214 or 1.206<z1<2.027 or 0.526< Delta_obs/
delta_ini<0.884 or 0.36<conditional power <0.9;
* Applicable small and larger sample size trials as long as the promising zone
and/or adjusted approperiately to control FWER;
Data MPSSR;
n1=&n1; n2=&n2; p0=&p0; p1=&p1; alpha1=&alpha1; alpha2=&alpha2;
beta1=&beta1;
```

```
power = 0; AveN = 0; FSP = 0; ESP = 0;
PromisingL=max(alpha1, &PromisingL); * Make sure Promising lower bound
> efficacy stopping boundary on p-scale;
PromisingU=min(beta1, &promisingU); * make sure Promising upper bound <
futiltiy boundary;
Do iSim = 1 To &nSims;
* Generate data for stage 1;
AveN = AveN + n1/&nSims; * Average sample size per group;
r01 = RAND('BINOMIAL',p0, n1)/n1;
r11 = RAND('BINOMIAL',p1, n1)/n1;
SE=Sqrt(r01*(1-r01)/n1+r11*(1-r11)/n1);
z1=0;
If SE>0 Then z1=(r11-r01)/SE;
pv1=1-ProbNorm(z1);
If pv1<=alpha1 Then ESP=ESP+1/&nSims; * Efficacy stopping;
If pv1>beta1 Then FSP=FSP+1/&nSims; * Futility stopping;
If alpha1<pv1<=beta1 Then Do; * Start Stage 2;
n2=&n2; n02=&n2;
If PromisingL<pv1<PromisingU Then Do; * Sample size estimation within
promising zone;
If z1 NE 0 Then n2=round((n1/z1**2)*((Probit(1-&alpha)*sqrt(n1+n02)-
z1*sqrt(n1))/sqrt(n02)+Probit(&Targetpower))**2);
* avoid z1=0 or negative direction. The n2new is not a monotonic function of
z1;
n2=min(&N2max, n2); *capped at N2max;
n2=max(n2, n02); * Do allow to reduce from initial sample size, also avoid n2=0;
End;
r02 = (r01*n1+RAND('BINOMIAL', p0, n2))/(n1+n2);
r12 = (r11*n1+RAND('BINOMIAL', p1, n2))/(n1+n2);
SE=Sqrt(r02*(1-r02)/(n1+n2)+r12*(1-r12)/(n1+n2));
z2=0; If SE>0 Then z2=(r12-r02)/SE;
pv2=1-ProbNorm(z2);
If pv2<alpha2 Then Power=Power+1/&nSims;
AveN = AveN + n2/&nSims; * Average sample size per group;
End;
End;
Power=Power+ESP;
Output;
Run;
Proc print data=MPSSR; Run;
%Mend;
```

12.2.3   SAS Macros for Pick-Winner Design

SAS Macro 4.8: Pick-Winner Design for Normal Endpoint

```
/* The Classical ACTIVE K-arm dropping-Loser Design; */
   /* H0: all means are equal. Ha: at least one mean > mean0. */
   /* For Dunnett's test, nStage2=0. */
   %Macro WinnerDesignNormal(nSims=1000000,NumOfArms=5, mu0=0,
sigma=1, Z_alpha=2.407, nStage1=100, nStage2=100);
   data OptnArm;
   Set dInput;
   Array mu(&NumOfArms); Array xObs(&NumOfArms); Array WinProbs
(&NumOfArms);
   Keep NumOfArms mu0 mu1-mu&NumOfArms sigma WinProbs1-WinProbs&
NumOfArms Z_alpha N1 N2 TotalN Power;
   nSims=&nSims; NumOfArms=&NumOfArms; Z_alpha=&Z_alpha;
   N1=&nStage1; N2=&nStage2; N=N1+N2; mu0=&mu0; sigma=&sigma;
   Power=0;
   Do i=1 To NumOfArms; WinProbs{i}=0; End;
   Do iSim=1 To nSims;
   Do i=1 To NumOfArms;
   xObs(i) = RAND('NORMAL',mu(i), sigma/sqrt(N1));
   End;
   MaxRsp =xObs(1); Winner=1; * For equal response rates, lower arm is the
winner;
   Do i=1 To NumOfArms;
   If xObs(i)> MaxRsp Then Do; Winner=i; MaxRsp=xObs(i); End;
   End;
   WinProbs{Winner}=WinProbs{Winner}+ 1/nSims;
   x2 = RAND('NORMAL',mu(Winner), sigma/Max(1,sqrt(N2)));
   FinalxAve = (MaxRsp*N1+x2*N2)/N;
   x0Ave = RAND('NORMAL', mu0, sigma/sqrt(N1+N2));
   TestZ=(FinalxAve-x0Ave)*sqrt(N/2)/sigma;
   If TestZ >= Z_alpha Then Power=Power+1/nSims;
   End;
   TotalN=(NumOfArms+1)*N1+2*N2;
   output;
   Run;
   Proc Print data=OptnArm; Run;
   %Mend WinnerDesignNormal;
```

SAS Macro 4.9: Pick-Winner Design for Binary Endpoint

```
/* The Classical ACTIVE K-arm dropping-Loser Design; */
   /* H0: all proportions are equal. Ha: at least one proportion > p0. */
   %Macro WinnerDesignBinary(nSims=100000, NumOfArms=5, P0=0,
Z_alpha=2.407, nStage1=100, nStage2=100);
   data OptnArm;
```

```
Set dInput;
Array p(&NumOfArms); Array PObs(&NumOfArms); Array WinProbs
(&NumOfArms);
Keep NumOfArms P0 p1-p&NumOfArms WinProbs1-WinProbs&NumOfArms
Z_alpha N1 N2 TotalN Power;
nSims=&nSims; NumOfArms=&NumOfArms; Z_alpha=&Z_alpha;
N1=&nStage1; N2=&nStage2; N=N1+N2; P0=&P0;
Power=0;
Do i=1 To NumOfArms; WinProbs{i}=0; End;
Do iSim=1 To nSims;
Do i=1 To NumOfArms;
PObs(i) = RAND('BINOM', p{i}, N1)/N1;
End;
MaxRsp =pObs(1); Winner=1; * For equal response rates, lower arm is the
winner;
Do i=1 To NumOfArms;
If PObs{i}> MaxRsp Then Do; Winner=i; MaxRsp=PObs{i}; End;
End;
WinProbs{Winner}=WinProbs{Winner}+ 1/nSims;
PWin = RAND('BINOM',p{Winner}, N2)/N2;
FinalP = (MaxRsp*N1+PWin*N2)/N;
P0Obs = RAND('BINOM', P0, N)/N;
SE=Sqrt(FinalP*(1-FinalP)/N+P0Obs*(1-P0Obs)/N);
TestZ=(FinalP-P0Obs)/SE;
If TestZ >= Z_alpha Then Power=Power+1/nSims;
End;
TotalN=(NumOfArms+1)*N1+2*N2;
Output;
Run;
Proc Print data=OptnArm; Run;
%Mend WinnerDesignBinary;
```

12.3   Chapter 5

SAS Macro 5.2 was developed for simulating biomarker-adaptive trials with two parallel groups. The key SAS variables are defined as follows:

Alpha1 = early efficacy stopping boundary (one-sided),

 beta1 = early futility stopping boundary,

Alpha2 = final efficacy stopping boundary,

 u0p = response difference in biomarker-positive population,

u0n = response in biomarker-negative population,

sigma = asymptotic standard deviation for the response difference, assuming homogeneous variance among groups. For binary response, sigma $=\sqrt{r_1(1-r_1)+r_2(1-r_2)}$; For normal response, sigma $=\sqrt{2}\sigma$.

np1, np2 = sample sizes per group for the first and second stage for the biomarker-positive population.

nn1, nn2 = sample sizes per group for the first and second stage for the biomarker-negative population.

cntlType = strong, for the strong type-I error control and cntlType = weak, for the weak type-I error control,

AveN = average total sample-size (all arms combined),

pPower = the probability of significance for biomarker-positive population,

oPower = the probability of significance for overall population.

SAS Macro 5.1: Population-Adaptive Design

```
%Macro BMAD(nSims=1000000, nStages=2, u0p=0.2, u0n=0.1, sigma=1,
np1=50, np2=50, nn1=100, nn2=100, alpha1=0.01, beta1=0.15,alpha2=0.1871);
Data BMAD;
Keep alpha1 alpha2 FSP ESP Power AveN pPower oPower u0p u0 sigma;
alpha1=&alpha1; alpha2=&alpha2;
u0p=&u0p; u0n=&u0n; sigma=&sigma;
np1=&np1; np2=&np2; nn1=&nn1; nn2=&nn2;
n1=np1+nn1; n2=np2+nn2; Np=np1+np2; Nn=nn1+nn2; N=Np+Nn;
FSP=0; ESP=0;Power=0; AveN=0; pPower=0; oPower=0;
Do isim=1 to &nSims;
up1=Rannor(0)/Sqrt(np1/2)*sigma+u0p;
un1=Rannor(0)/Sqrt(nn1/2)*sigma+u0n;
uo1=(up1*np1+un1*nn1)/n1;
Tp1=up1*(np1/2)**0.5/sigma; To1=uo1*(n1/2)**0.5/sigma;
T1=Max(Tp1,To1); p1=1-ProbNorm(T1);
If p1>&beta1 Then FSP=FSP+1/&nSims;
If p1<=&alpha1 Then Do;
Power=Power+1/&nSims; ESP=ESP+1/&nSims;
If Tp1>To1 Then pPower=pPower+1/&nSims;
If Tp1<=To1 Then oPower=oPower+1/&nSims;
End;
AveN=AveN+2*(np1+nn1)/&nSims;
If &nStages=2 And p1>&alpha1 And p1<=&beta1 Then Do;
up2=Rannor(0)/Sqrt(np2/2)*sigma+u0p;
```

```
un2=Rannor(0)/Sqrt(nn2/2)*sigma+u0n;
uo2=(up2*np2+un2*nn2)/n2;
Tp2=up2*(np2/2)**0.5/sigma; To2=uo2*(n2/2)**0.5/sigma;
If Tp1>To1 Then Do;
T2=Tp2; AveN=AveN+2*np2/&nSims;
T=sqrt(np1/Np)*T1+sqrt(1-np1/Np)*T2;
p2=1-ProbNorm(T);
End;
If Tp1<=To1 Then Do;
T2=To2; AveN=AveN+2*(np2+nn2)/&nSims;
T=sqrt(n1/N)*T1+sqrt(1-n1/N)*T2;
p2=1-ProbNorm(T);
End;
If .<p2<=&alpha2 Then Do;
Power=Power+1/&nSims;
If Tp1>To1 Then pPower=pPower+1/&nSims;
If Tp1<=To1 Then oPower=oPower+1/&nSims;
End;
End;
End;
Run;
Proc Print Data=BMAD (obs=1); Run;
%Mend BMAD;
  %BMAD(nStages=2, u0p=0, u0n=0, sigma=1, np1=50, np2=50, nn1=100,
nn2=100, alpha1=0.004, beta1=1,alpha2=0.0128);
  %BMAD(nStages=2, u0p=-log(0.6), u0n=-log(0.9), sigma=1, np1=50, np2=50,
nn1=100, nn2=100, alpha1=0.004, beta1=1,alpha2=0.0128);
```

SAS Macro 5.2: Basket Design = Pick-K-Winners Design for Normal Endpoint

```
/* The Classical ACTIVE K-arm pick more than one winners design; */
/* H0: all means are equal. Ha: at least one mean is larger. */
%Macro BasketDesignNormal(nSims=10000, NumOfArms=5, nWinners=3,
Z_alpha=2.407);
data OptnArm;
Set dInput;
Array sigmas(&NumOfArms); Array u0s(&NumOfArms);
Array us(&NumOfArms);
Array N1s(&NumOfArms); Array N2s(&NumOfArms);
Array Powers(&nWinners); Array Z1(&NumOfArms); Array Z2(&nWinners);
Keep NumOfArms nWinners Powers1-Powers&nWinners Z_alpha AveN Power;
nSims=&nSims; NumOfArms=&NumOfArms; nWinners=&nWinners;
Z_alpha=&Z_alpha;
Power=0; AveN=0;
Do i=1 To nWinners; Powers(i)=0; End;
```

```
Do iSim=1 To nSims;
Do i=1 To NumOfArms;
u0 = RAND('Normal')*sigmas(i)/sqrt(N1s(i))+u0s(i); * Observed mean re-
sponse in Control;
u1 = RAND('Normal')*sigmas(i)/sqrt(N1s(i))+us(i); * Observed mean response
in Test;
SE=sigmas(i)/sqrt(N1s(i)/2); * assume sigma known or large sample assump-
tion;
z1(i)=(u1-u0)/SE; * Larger value is better;
AveN=AveN+N1s(i)/nSims;
End;
* Sort Z1(i) in descending order;
Do j=1 To NumOfArms; Do i=1 To NumOfArms-j;
If Z1(i+1)>Z1(i) Then Do
temp=Z1(i); Z1(i)=Z1(i+1); Z1(i+1)=Temp;
temp=N1s(i); N1s(i)=N1s(i+1); N1s(i+1)=Temp;
temp=N2s(i); N2s(i)=N2s(i+1); N2s(i+1)=Temp;
End;
End; End;
signif=0;
Do i=1 To nWinners;
u0 = RAND('Normal')*sigmas(i)/sqrt(N2s(i))+u0s(i); * Observed mean re-
sponse in Control;
u1 = RAND('Normal')*sigmas(i)/sqrt(N2s(i))+us(i); * Observed mean response
in Test;
SE=sigmas(i)/sqrt(N2s(i)/2); * assume sigma known or large sample assump-
tion;
Z2(i)=(u1-u0)/SE; * Larger value is better;
N=N1s(i)+N2s(i); AveN=AveN+N2s(i)/nSims;
Z=sqrt(N1s(i)/N)*Z1(i)+Sqrt(N2s(i)/N)*Z2(i);
If Z>Z_alpha Then Do;
Powers(i)=Powers(i)+1/nSims;
signif=1;
End;
End;
If signif=1 Then Power=Power+1/nSims;
End;
Output;
Run;
Proc Print data=OptnArm; Run;
%Mend BasketDesignNormal;
```

Example of invoking SAS Macro 5.2

```
data dInput;
Array Sigmas(5)(1, 1, 1, 1, 1);
Array u0s(5)(0.3, 0.3, 0.3, 0.3, 0.3);
```

```
Array us(5)(0.3, 0.3, 0.3, 0.3, 0.3);
Array N1s(5)(10, 10, 10, 10, 10);
Array N2s(5)(10, 10, 10, 10, 10);
%BasketDesignNormal(nSims=10000000, NumOfArms=5, nWinners=3,
Z_alpha=2.5690);
```

SAS Macro 5.3: Basket Design - Pick-K-Winners Design for Binary Endpoint

```
/* The Classical ACTIVE K-arm pick more than one winners design; */
/* H0: all proportions are equal, p0. Ha: at least one proportion > p0. */
%Macro BasketDesignBinary(nSims=10000, NumOfArms=5, nWinners=3,
Z_alpha=2.407);
data OptnArm;
Set dInput;
Array p0s(&NumOfArms); Array p1s(&NumOfArms);
Array N1s(&NumOfArms); Array N2s(&NumOfArms);
Array Powers(&nWinners); Array Z1(&NumOfArms); Array Z2(&nWinners);
Keep NumOfArms nWinners Powers1-Powers&nWinners Z_alpha AveN Power;
nSims=&nSims; NumOfArms=&NumOfArms; nWinners=&nWinners;
Z_alpha=&Z_alpha;
Power=0; AveN=0;
Do i=1 To nWinners; Powers(i)=0; End;
Do iSim=1 To nSims;
Do i=1 To NumOfArms;
p0 = RAND('BINOM', p0s{i}, N1s(i))/N1s(i); * Observed rate in Control;
p1 = RAND('BINOM', P1s{i}, N1s(i))/N1s(i); * Observed rate in Test;
SE=sqrt(p0*(1-p0)/N1s(i)+p1*(1-p1)/N1s(i));
z1(i)=(p1-p0)/SE; * Larger value is better;
AveN=AveN+N1s(i)/nSims;
End;
* Sort Z1(i) in descending order;
Do j=1 To NumOfArms; Do i=1 To NumOfArms-j;
If Z1(i+1)>Z1(i) Then Do
temp=Z1(i); Z1(i)=Z1(i+1); Z1(i+1)=Temp;
temp=N1s(i); N1s(i)=N1s(i+1); N1s(i+1)=Temp;
temp=N2s(i); N2s(i)=N2s(i+1); N2s(i+1)=Temp;
End;
End; End;
signif=0;
Do i=1 To nWinners;
p0 = RAND('BINOM', p0s{i}, N2s(i))/N2s(i); * Observed rate in Control;
p1 = RAND('BINOM', P1s{i}, N2s(i))/N2s(i); * Observed rate in Test;
SE=sqrt(p0*(1-p0)/N2s(i)+p1*(1-p1)/N2s(i));
Z2(i)=(p1-p0)/SE; * Larger value is better;
N=N1s(i)+N2s(i); AveN=AveN+N2s(i)/nSims;
Z=sqrt(N1s(i)/N)*Z1(i)+Sqrt(N2s(i)/N)*Z2(i);
```

```
If Z>Z_alpha Then Do;
Powers(i)=Powers(i)+1/nSims;
signif=1;
End;
End;
If signif=1 Then Power=Power+1/nSims;
End;
Output;
Run;
Proc Print data=OptnArm; Run;
%Mend BasketDesignBinary;
```

Example of invoking SAS Macro 5.3
Title "Simulation for one-sided alpha=0.025"; run;

```
data dInput;
Array p0s(3)(0.3, 0.3, 0.3);
Array p1s(3)(0.3, 0.3, 0.3);
Array N1s(3)(1000, 1000, 1000);
Array N2s(3)(1000, 1000, 1000);
%BasketDesignBinary(nSims=10000000, NumOfArms=3, nWinners=1,
Z_alpha=2.3485);
```

SAS Macro Biomarker-Informed Design

```
%Macro  BID(nSims=100000,  thetax=0.8,  thetay=0.8,  rho=0.6,  n1=250,
n2=250, alpha1=0.005, beta1=0.5, alpha2=0.024);
* for time-to-event endpoint, thetax=hazard ratio (TTP) and thetay=hazard
ratio for survival.;
   Data BID;
   Keep alpha1 alpha2 FSP ESP Power rho thetax thetay n1 n2;
   alpha1=&alpha1; alpha2=&alpha2; beta1=&beta1; thetax=&thetax;
thetay=&thetay;
   n1=&n1; n2=&n2; n=n1+n2; rho=&rho;
   vx1=-log(thetax)*sqrt(n1/4); vy1=-log(thetay)*sqrt(n1/4); vy2=-log(thetay)*
sqrt(n2/4);
   FSP=0; ESP=0; Power=0;
   Do isim=1 to &nSims;
   z1=Rannor(0);
   z1x=z1+vx1;
   z1y=rho*z1+sqrt(1-rho**2)*Rannor(8765)+vy1;
   p1x=1-ProbNorm(z1x);
   If p1x>beta1 Then FSP=FSP+1/&nSims;
   If p1x<=alpha1 Then Do;
   Power=Power+1/&nSims; ESP=ESP+1/&nSims;
   End;
```

```
If alpha1<p1x<=beta1 Then Do;
z2y=Rannor(0)+vy2;
z=sqrt(n1/n)*z1y+sqrt(1-n1/n)*z2y;
p=1-ProbNorm(z);
If p<=&alpha2 Then Power=Power+1/&nSims;
End;
* output;
End;
Run;
Proc Print Data=BID (obs=1); Run;
%Mend BID;
```

Examples of Invoking SAS Macro

%BID(nSims=100000, thetax=0.4, thetay=0.7, rho=0.2, n1=150, n2=150, alpha1=0.0, beta1=0.25, alpha2=0.025);

%BID(nSims=100000, thetax=0.4, thetay=0.7, rho=0.8, n1=150, n2=150, alpha1=0.0, beta1=0.25, alpha2=0.025);

%BID(nSims=100000, thetax=0.7, thetay=0.7, rho=0.2, n1=150, n2=150, alpha1=0.0, beta1=0.25, alpha2=0.025);

%BID(nSims=100000, thetax=0.7, thetay=0.7, rho=0.8, n1=150, n2=150, alpha1=0.0, beta1=0.25, alpha2=0.025);

%BID(nSims=100000, thetax=0.9, thetay=0.7, rho=0.2, n1=150, n2=150, alpha1=0.0, beta1=0.25, alpha2=0.025);

%BID(nSims=100000, thetax=0.9, thetay=0.7, rho=0.8, n1=150, n2=150, alpha1=0.0, beta1=0.25, alpha2=0.025);

%BID(nSims=100000, thetax=1.0, thetay=0.7, rho=0.2, n1=150, n2=150, alpha1=0.0, beta1=0.25, alpha2=0.025);

12.4 Chapter 6

Algorithm of Inverse CDF method:

Generate x from U(0,1); if $T = -\frac{1}{\lambda_1} \ln(1-x) \leq T_d$, then return T; otherwise, return $T = T_d - \frac{1}{\lambda_2} \ln\left(\frac{1-x}{e^{-\lambda_1 T_d}}\right)$.

SAS Macro 6.2: Random Sample from Two-Piecewise Exponential Distribution

```
%macro PWExp( nSims=100000, lambdaPRE=0.3, lambdaLAG=0.2, lag=12,
StudyDur=5);
* Generate observations, OS, from two-piecewise exponential distribution;
* lambdaPRE = hazard rate before the drug takes effect;
```

```
* lambdaLAG = hazard rate after the drug takes effect;
* lag = drug delayed effect time;
* StudyDur = Maximum time for each patient stage in the during (oncology has
different time for different patients);
Data PWEXP;
Keep OS;
Do iSim=1 To &nSims;
x = ranuni(347823);
T=-log(1-x)/&lambdaPRE;
OS=T;
If T>&lag Then OS=&lag-log((1-x)*exp(&lambdaPRE*&lag))
/&lambdaLAG;
* add censoring;
Censored=0;
If OS>&StudyDur Then Do; Censored=1; OS=&StudyDur; End;
Output;
End;
Run;
Proc univariate data=PWEXP;
histogram OS;
Run;
%Mend;
```

Example of invoking Macro 6.1

```
%PWExp(lambdaPRE=0.3, lambdaLAG=0.2, lag=12, StudyDur=5);
run;
```

SAS Macro 6.2: Delayed Drug Effect Using Piecewise Exponential Survival LogRank and Weighted LogRank Test

```
options nosource;
options nonotes;
%macro  PWExp(n1=100,  n2=100,  lambdaPRE1=0.3,  lambdaLAG1=0.2,
lag1=99999999, lambdaPRE2=0.3, lambdaLAG2=0.2, lag2=0.4, DeathsNeed=120,
estLag=1);
* Generate observations, OS, from two-piecewise exponential distribution;
* n = sample size for each group
* lambdaPRE = hazard rate before the drug takes effect;
* lambdaLAG = hazard rate after the drug takes effect;
* lag = true drug delayed effect time; estLag = estimated delayed effect time;
* StudyDur = Maximum time for each patient stage in the during (oncology has
different time for different patients);
* Trial stops when required number of deaths are reached;
* min(n1, n2) should > deathsNeed (total deaths);
```

```
* Generate Piecewise exponential survival data (OS);
Data PWEXP;
Keep Grp n1 n2 OS lag estLag;
* Simulated survival time for all patients;
Do Grp=1 To 2;
n1=&n1; n2=&n2; n=&n1; If Grp=2 Then n=&n2;
lambdaPRE=&lambdaPRE1; lambdaLAG=&lambdaLAG1; lag=&lag1; est-
Lag=&estLag;
If Grp=2 Then Do; lambdaPRE=&lambdaPRE2; lambdaLAG=&lambdaLAG2;
lag=&lag2; End;
Do i=1 To n;
x = ranuni(0); T=-log(1-x)/lambdaPRE;
OS=T; If T>lag Then OS=lag-log((1-x)*exp(lambdaPRE*lag))/lambdaLAG;
Output;
End;
End;
Run;
*Proc univariate data=PWEXP;
*histogram OS;
*Run;
Proc Sort Data=PWEXP;
by OS;
run;
* LogRank Test;
Data LogRank;
Set PWEXP(Obs=&DeathsNeed);
* D1 and D2 = deaths (not cumulative) at the time for the two groups;
* D=D1+D2, since assuming only one death a time, actual D=1 from simulated
data;
* R1 and R2 = number of patients at risk for the two groups;
Set PWEXP;
Keep OS estLag Lag CumD1 CumD2 SumDiff SumV SumDiffW1 SumVW1
SumDiffW2 SumVW2;
Retain CumD1 CumD2 SumDiff SumV SumDiffW1 SumVW1 SumDiffW2
SumVW2 0;
D1=0; D2=0;
If Grp=1 Then Do; D1=1; CumD1=CumD1+1; End;
If Grp=2 Then Do; D2=1; CumD2=CumD2+1; End;
R1=n1-CumD1; R2=n2-CumD2;
D=D1+D2; R=R1+R2;
E1=D/R*R1; * Expected deaths in group 1 if the death rates are the same for
the two groups;
V=D*R1/R*R2/R*(R-D)/(R-1);
Diff=D1-E1;
SumDiff=SumDiff+Diff;
```

```
    SumV=SumV+V;
    * For weighted logRank test;
    Rank=_N_;
    W1=Log(1+Rank); * Using Log(1+Rank) as weight. To be changed. Should not
use a random variable as weight since it will change the distribution of test statistic;
    W2=1; If OS > estLag then W2=2; * we can change the weight based on the
rank order.;
    DiffW1=W1*(D1-E1);
    SumDiffW1=SumDiffW1+DiffW1;
    SumVW1=SumVW1+W1*W1*V;
    DiffW2=W2*(D1-E1);
    SumDiffW2=SumDiffW2+DiffW2;
    SumVW2=SumVW2+W2*W2*V;
    run;
    * Calcualte test statistics and p-values;
    Data LogRank;
    Set LogRank;
    Z=SumDiff/sqrt(Sumv);
    pvLogRank=1-ProbNorm(z); * H0: Equal hazard rates vs Ha: Group 1 hazard
rate > Group Hazard rate;
    Zw1=SumDiffw1/sqrt(Sumvw1);
    pvLogRankw1=1-ProbNorm(Zw1); * p-value from weighted Logrank Test;
    Zw2=SumDiffw2/sqrt(Sumvw2);
    pvLogRankw2=1-ProbNorm(Zw2); * p-value from weighted Logrank Test;
    Run;
    Data LogRank;
    set LogRank end=eof;
    if eof then output;
    run;
    %Mend;
    Data CumData; run; * empty dataset;
    %macro Comb;
    %do i = 1 %to 1000; * 1000 simulations, cannot use nSims=1000;
    %PWExp(n1=200, n2=200, lambdaPRE1=0.3, lambdaLAG1=0.3, lag1=0.1,
lambdaPRE2=0.3, lambdaLAG2=0.2, lag2=0.1, DeathsNeed=198, estLag=0.2);
    * Cummulate data from all simulation runs;
    Data CumData;
    Set CumData LogRank;
    Run;
    %end;
    %mend;
    %Comb;
    run;
    Data CumData;
    Set CumData;
    retain powerLR powerLRW1 powerLRW2 0;
```

```
alpha=0.025;
LogRankSig=0; If .<pvLogRank<=alpha Then Do; LogRankSig=1; pow-
erLR=powerLR+1; End;
LogRankw1Sig=0; If .<pvLogRankw1<=alpha Then Do; LogRankw1Sig=1;
powerLRW1=powerLRW1+1; End;
LogRankw2Sig=0; If .<pvLogRankw2<=alpha Then Do; LogRankw2Sig=1;
powerLRW2=powerLRW2+1; End;
run;
Proc freq data=Cumdata;
Tables     LogRankSig     LogRankw1Sig     LogRankw2Sig     LogRankSig*
LogRankw1Sig*LogRankw2Sig/list;
run;
proc print data=CumData (obs=1000); run;
PROC UNIVARIATE data=Cumdata; * noprint;
var z;
histogram z;
run;

PROC UNIVARIATE data=Cumdata;
var zw1;
histogram zw1;
run;
PROC UNIVARIATE data=Cumdata;
var zw2;
histogram zw2;
run;
```

12.5 Chapter 7

SAS Macro 7.1: Determining Stopping Boundaries and Power with SPPM for Two Hypotheses

```
%Macro ChangDengBalserMethod2H(r=0.5, alpha=0.025, alpha1=0.001825, al-
phaRatio=1, nSims=10000, N=100, eSize1=0.3, eSize2=0.3);
/* SPPM Multiple testing method with two hypotheses */
/* For one-group design, z=eSize*sqrt(N), N = sample size ; */
/* If for two-group design, reduce N to N/2 because z=eSize*sqrt(N/2) */

Data Power; keep Power Power1 Power2;
Array a{4}; Array xNor{2}; Array x{2}; Array pv{2};
Array eSizes{2}; Array ss{4}; * Correlation matrix;
alpha=&alpha; alpha1=&alpha1; alpha2=alpha1/&alphaRatio;
```

```
sSize=4; nVars=2; r=&r; * constant correlation;
eSizes{1}=&eSize1; eSizes{2}=&eSize2;
Do i=1 To sSize; ss{i}=&r; end;
Do k=1 To nVars; ss(nVars*(k-1)+k)=1; End; * set 1 for the diagonal elements.
* Checovsky decomposition;
Do k=1 To nVars; Do L=1 To k;
Saa=0; Sa2=0;
Do j=1 to L-1;
Saa=Saa+a{nVars*(k-1)+j}*a{nVars*(L-1)+j};
Sa2=Sa2+a{nVars*(L-1)+j}*a{nVars*(L-1)+j};
End;
nkL=nVars*(k-1)+L;
a{nkL}=(ss{nkL}-Saa)/Sqrt(ss{nVars*(L-1)+L}-Sa2);
End; End;
Power1=0; Power2=0; Power=0;
Do iSim=1 to &nSims;
Do iVar=1 to nVars; xNOR{iVar}=Rannor(0); End;
Do iVar=1 to nVars;
x{iVar}=0;
Do i=1 To iVar; x{iVar}=x{iVar}+a{nVars*(iVar-1)+i}*xNor{i}; End;
End;

Do iVar=1 To nVars;
x{iVar}=x{iVar}+eSizes{iVar}*sqrt(&N);
pv{iVar}= 1 - probnorm(x{iVar});
End;
If pv1*pv2<=alpha1 And pv1<alpha Then Power1=Power1+1/&nSims;
If pv1*pv2<=alpha2 And pv2<alpha Then Power2=Power2+1/&nSims;
If (pv1*pv2<=alpha2 And pv2<alpha) Or (pv1*pv2<=alpha1 And pv1<alpha)
Then Power=Power+1/&nSims;
*Output;
End;
Run;
Proc Print data=Power(obs=10); Run;
%Mend ChangDengBalserMethod2H;
```

Examples of Invoking Macro 7.1

Title " Determine the critical value"; Run;
%ChangDengBalserMethod2H(r=0.85, alpha=0.025, alpha1=0.00264, alphaRatio=10, nSims=10000000, N=100, eSize1=0, eSize2=0);

Title " Simulate power"; Run;
%ChangDengBalserMethod2H(r=0.85, alpha=0.025, alpha1=0.00264, alphaRatio=10, nSims=10000000, N=100, eSize1=0.35, eSize2=0.3);

To determine the critical value, input the null hypothesis parameters and adjust the critical values until the simulated power equals α. To obtain power, use the determined critical values and parameters under alternative hypothesis to simulate the power.

SAS Macro 7.2: Determining Stopping Boundaries and Power with SPPM for Three Hypotheses

```
%Macro ChangDengBalserMethod3H(r=0, alpha=0.025, alpha1=0.004855, al-
pha4=0.0026778, nSims=10000, N=100, eSize1=0.3, eSize2=0.3, eSize3=0.3);
    /* SPPM Multiple testing method with two hypotheses */
    /* For one-group design, z=eSize*sqrt(N), N = sample size ; */
    /* If for two-group design, reduce N to N/2 because z=eSize*sqrt(N/2) */
    Data Power; keep power1 power2 power3 power;
    Array a{9}; Array xNor{3}; Array x{3}; Array pv{3}; Array signs{3};
    Array powers{3}; Array eSizes{3}; Array ss{9}; * Correlation matrix;
    alpha=&alpha; alpha1=&alpha1; alpha4=&alpha4;
    sSize=9; nVars=3; r=&r; * constant correlation;
    eSizes{1}=&eSize1; eSizes{2}=&eSize2; eSizes{3}=&eSize3;
    Do i=1 To sSize; ss{i}=&r; end;
    Do k=1 To nVars; ss(nVars*(k-1)+k)=1; End; * set 1 for the diagonal elements.
    * Checovsky decomposition;
    Do k=1 To nVars; Do L=1 To k;
    Saa=0; Sa2=0;
    Do j=1 to L-1;
    Saa=Saa+a{nVars*(k-1)+j}*a{nVars*(L-1)+j};
    Sa2=Sa2+a{nVars*(L-1)+j}*a{nVars*(L-1)+j};
    End;
    nkL=nVars*(k-1)+L;
    a{nkL}=(ss{nkL}-Saa)/Sqrt(ss{nVars*(L-1)+L}-Sa2);
    End; End;
    powers1=0; powers2=0; powers3=0; power=0;
    Do iSim=1 to &nSims;
    Do iVar=1 to nVars; xNOR{iVar}=Rannor(0); End;
    Do iVar=1 to nVars;
    x{iVar}=0;
    Do i=1 To iVar; x{iVar}=x{iVar}+a{nVars*(iVar-1)+i}*xNor{i}; End;
    End;
    Do iVar=1 To nVars;
    x{iVar}=x{iVar}+eSizes{iVar}*sqrt(&N);
    pv{iVar}= 1 - probnorm(x{iVar});
    End;
    signs1=0; signs2=0; signs3=0;
```

    If pv1*pv2*pv3<=alpha4 And pv1*pv2<alpha1 And pv1*pv3<alpha1 And
pv1<alpha Then signs1=1;
    If pv1*pv2*pv3<=alpha4 And pv1*pv2<alpha1 And pv2*pv3<alpha1 And
pv2<alpha Then signs2=1;
    If pv1*pv2*pv3<=alpha4 And pv1*pv3<alpha1 And pv2*pv3<alpha1 And
pv3<alpha Then signs3=1;
       do i=1 to nVars; if signs{i}=1 then powers{i}=powers{i}+1/&nSims; end;
       If max(signs1, signs2, signs3)=1 Then power=power+1/&nSims;
       *Output;
       End;
       Run;
       Proc Print data=Power(obs=1); Run;
       %Mend ChangDengBalserMethod3H;

Examples of Invoking Macro 7.2

    Title "Determine critical value with SPPM Method for 3 hypothese"; run;
       %ChangDengBalserMethod3H(r=0, alpha=0.025, alpha1=0.004855,
alpha4=0.0026778, nSims=10000000, N=100, eSize1=0, eSize2=0, eSize3=0);
    Title "Simulte the power using SPPM Method for 3 hypothese"; run;
       %ChangDengBalserMethod3H(r=0, alpha=0.025, alpha1=0.004855,
alpha4=0.0026778, nSims=1000000, N=100, eSize1=0.25, eSize2=0.2, eSize3=0.15);

    To determine the critical value, input the null hypothesis parameters and
adjust the critical values until the simulated power equals α. To obtain power,
use the determined critical values and parameters under alternative hypothesis
to simulate the power.

SAS Macro 7.3: Determining Critical Value and Power for Two Coprimary Endpoints with Chuang-Stein and Li-Huque Methods

    %Macro Coprimary2H(r=0.5, alpha=0.025, ChristyAlpha=0.0334, LHalphaMin=
0.023, LHAlphaMax=0.030, nSims=10000, N=100, eSize1=0.3, eSize2=0.3);
       /* determine the critical value and Power for two coprimary endpoints with */
       /* Christine-Stein methid and Li-Huque's method determine the critical value
*/
       /* and Power for two coprimary endpoints with Christine-Stein and Li-Huque's
methods */
       /* LHalphaMin, LHalphaMax, = critical value for LH method on p-scale. */
       /* ChristyAlpha = Christy method critical value on p-scale.*/
       /* For one-group design, z=eSize*sqrt(N), N = sample size ; */
       /* If for two-group design, reduce N to N/2 because z=eSize*sqrt(N/2) */
       Data Power; keep LHPower ClassicPower ChristyPower;
       Array a{4}; Array xNor{2}; Array x{2}; Array pv{2};

```
  Array eSizes{2}; Array ss{4}; * Correlation matrix;
  alpha=&alpha;  ChristyAlpha=&ChristyAlpha;  LHalphaMin=&LHalphaMin;
LHalphaMax=&LHalphaMax;
  sSize=4; nVars=2; r=&r; * constant correlation;
  eSizes{1}=&eSize1; eSizes{2}=&eSize2;
  Do i=1 To sSize; ss{i}=&r; end;
  Do k=1 To nVars; ss(nVars*(k-1)+k)=1; End; * set 1 for the diagonal elements.
  * Checovsky decomposition;
  Do k=1 To nVars; Do L=1 To k;
  Saa=0; Sa2=0;
  Do j=1 to L-1;
  Saa=Saa+a{nVars*(k-1)+j}*a{nVars*(L-1)+j};
  Sa2=Sa2+a{nVars*(L-1)+j}*a{nVars*(L-1)+j};
  End;
  nkL=nVars*(k-1)+L;
  a{nkL}=(ss{nkL}-Saa)/Sqrt(ss{nVars*(L-1)+L}-Sa2);
  End; End;
  LHPower=0; ClassicPower=0; ChristyPower=0;
  Do iSim=1 to &nSims;
  Do iVar=1 to nVars; xNOR{iVar}=Rannor(0); End;
  Do iVar=1 to nVars;
  x{iVar}=0;
  Do i=1 To iVar; x{iVar}=x{iVar}+a{nVars*(iVar-1)+i}*xNor{i}; End;
  End;
  Do iVar=1 To nVars;
  x{iVar}=x{iVar}+eSizes{iVar}*sqrt(&N);
  pv{iVar}= 1 - probnorm(x{iVar});
  End;
  pMin=min(pv1,pv2); pMax=max(pv1,pv2);
  If pMax<=&alpha Then ClassicPower=ClassicPower+1/&nSims; * conven-
tional method;
  If pMin<LHalphaMin And pMax<=LHalphaMax Then LHPower=LHPower+1/
&nSims; * Li-Huque method ;
  If pMax<=ChristyAlpha Then ChristyPower=ChristyPower+1/&nSims;  *
Christy-Stein method;
  *Output;
  End;
  Run;
  Proc Print data=Power(obs=1); Run;
%Mend Coprimary2H;
Title "Type-I errors under the global H0"; run;
  %Coprimary2H(r=0.5, alpha=0.025, ChristyAlpha=0.0334, LHalphaMin=0.023,
LHAlphaMax=0.030, nSims=10000000, N=100, eSize1=0, eSize2=0);
Title "Type-I errors under a local H0"; run;
```

%Coprimary2H(r=0.5, alpha=0.025, ChristyAlpha=0.0334, LHAlphaMin=0.023, LHAlphaMax=0.030, nSims=10000000, N=100, eSize1=0, eSize2=0.3);
    Title "Type-I errors under another local H0"; run;
    %Coprimary2H(r=0.5, alpha=0.025, ChristyAlpha=0.0334, LHAlphaMin=0.023, LHAlphaMax=0.030, nSims=10000000, N=100, eSize1=0, eSize2=0.3);
    Title "Powers"; run;
    %Coprimary2H(r=0.5, alpha=0.025, ChristyAlpha=0.0334, LHAlphaMin=0.023, LHAlphaMax=0.030, nSims=1000000, N=100, eSize1=0.3, eSize2=0.3);

To determine the critical values, input the null hypothesis parameters and adjust the critical values until the simulated power equals α. To obtain power, use the determined critical values and parameters under alternative hypothesis to simulate the power.

12.6   Chapter 8

SAS Macro 8.1: Multivariate Normal Variable Generation

```
%Macro MVNvars(group=1, nVars=3, nObs=200);
* Generate standard multtvariate normal data;
proc simnorm data=scov outsim=dSim
numreal = &nObs seed = 7435;
var y1-y&nVars ;
Run;
Data dSim; set dSim; Pid=_N_; run;
* Transform standard y to actual y using means and standard deviations;
Data MusSigmas; set MusSigmas;
Do pID=1 To &nObs; output; End;
Run;
Data ActualY; merge dSim MusSigmas; by pID;
Keep pID y1-y&nVars;
%Do i=1 %To &nVars;
y&i=mus&i+sigmas&i*y&i;
%End;
Run;
* Form a baseline, basey and calculate changes, chgy;
Data d1; set ActualY; keep basey pID; basey=y1; run;
%Do i=2 %To &nVars;
Data d&i; set ActualY; keep y pID chgy visit; y=y&i; chgy=y&i-y1; visit=&i;
Run;
%End;
* Merge baseline y and changes;
```

```
Data Trials&group; set d2-d&nVars; group=&group; run;
Proc sort data=Trials&group; by pID; run;
Data Trials&group; merge Trials&group d1; by pId; run;
%Mend;
```

Example of Invoking SAS Macro 8.1

```
Title "Correlation matrix for Proc Simnorm - group 1"; Run;
data scov(type=COV); * Cov{i,j}=Coef{i,j}*s{i}*s{j}, MEAN always =0 here;
input _TYPE_ $ 1-4 _NAME_ $ 5-10 y1 y2 y3 y4;
datalines ;
COV y1 1.0 0.4 0.3 0.2
COV y2 0.4 1.0 0.4 0.3
COV y3 0.3 0.4 1.0 0.4
COV y4 0.2 0.3 0.4 1.0
MEAN 0.0 0.0 0.0 0.0
run;
Data MusSigmas;
* if data in scov is covariance, then mu and sigma should be 0 and sigma=1;
Array mus{4}(0, 0.1, 0.1, 0.1);
Array sigmas{4}(1, 1, 1, 1);
Run;
%MVNvars(group=1, nVars=4, nObs=200);
* assume groups 1 and 2 have the same correlation coefficients;
Data MusSigmas;
Array mus{4}(0, 0.3, 0.3, 0.3);
Array sigmas{4}(1, 1, 1, 1);
Run;
%MVNvars(group=2, nVars=4, nObs=200);
* Create unique is, GrpPt for every subject;
Data Trial; set Trials1 Trials2;
GrpPT=STRIP(Put(Group, z2.))||"-"||STRIP(put(pID, z5.));
run;
```

12.7 Chapter 9

SAS Macro 9.1: Conditional Power for Normal Endpoint

```
%Macro ConPower(alpha2=0.024, ux=0.2, uy=0.4, sigma=1, p1=0.8, N1=100,
N2=100);
** cPower=Two stage conditional power. eSize=delta/sigma;
data cPower;
```

```
a2=&alpha2; sigma=&sigma;
u=(&ux+&uy)/2;
I1=sqrt(&N1/(&N1+&N2));
I2=sqrt(&N2/(&N1+&N2));
eSize=(&uy-&ux)/sigma;
BFun=(Probit(1-a2)- I1*Probit(1-&p1))/I2;
cPower=1-ProbNorm(BFun-eSize*sqrt(&N2/4));
Run;
Proc Print data=cPower; Run;
%Mend ConPower;
```

Example of Invoking Macro 9.1
%ConPower(alpha2=0.024, ux=0.2, uy=0.3, sigma=1, p1=0.3085, N1=100, N2=100);

SAS Macro 9.2: Time Projection of N Observed Deaths - Math-Simulation Mixed Approach

```
%Macro PredDeaths(Model="EXPONENTIAL", scale=0.2, shape=0.5,
nPts=400, obsdDeaths=120, DeathsNeed=300);
****************************************************
```
Given obsdDeaths observed deaths, simulate the additional time needed for have total DeathsNeed deaths

from the time of last death observed;

Algorithm:

(1) simulate survival time for all patients,

(2) merge with enrollment data to get calendar time of death: surval time + time of enrollment

(3) sort the merged dataset by the calendar time of death,

(4) get the calendar time for the last observed death and predicted death time the for DeathsNeed-th death

(5) the difference between the two death times is additional time needed to have the target number of deaths
```
****************************************************
```
Data SurTime;

scale=&scale; shape=&shape; nPts=&nPts; obsdDeaths=&obsdDeaths; DeathsNeed=&DeathsNeed;

do iPt = 1 to nPts;

If &Model="EXPONENTIAL" Then surTime = Rand('EXPOnential', 1/scale);

If &Model^="EXPONENTIAL" Then surTime = Rand(&Model, scale, shape);

Output;

end;

Run;

Data ProjTime; merge PtsEnroll SurTime; by iPt; CalSurTime=EnDay+surTime;
run; * Calendar time;

Proc sort data=ProjTime; by CalSurTime; Run;

Data T1; set ProjTime; lastObsdT=CalSurTime; if _N_=obsdDeaths; run;

Data T2; set ProjTime; ExpTime =CalSurTime; if _N_= DeathsNeed; run;

Data TimeNeed; merge T1 T2; TimeNeed= ExpTime- lastObsdT; run;

Data final; set final TimeNeed; if TimeNeed; run;

%Mend;

*proc print data=SurTime; run;

*Simulation nSims times to get mean and standard devation of additional time
needed for the traget number of events;

%macro PredTime(nSims=10, Model="EXPONENTIAL", scale=0.2, nPts=21,
obsdDeaths=3, DeathsNeed=18);

Data Final; TimeNeed=.; run;

Data Null;

Do i=1 to &nSims;

call execute ('%nrstr(%PredDeaths(Model="EXPONENTIAL", scale=&scale,
nPts=&nPts, obsdDeaths=&obsdDeaths, DeathsNeed=&DeathsNeed))');

End;

Run;

*Proc print data=final; run;

Proc means data=final; var TimeNeed; run;

%Mend;

Example of Invoking Macro 9.2

%PredTime(nSims=100, Model="EXPONENTIAL", scale=0.2, nPts=21, obs-
dDeaths=3, DeathsNeed=18);

Here is an example of invoking the macro with a dummy patient enrollment
data.

Data PtsEnroll;

Input Month NewPts @@;

* for more precise, one can use weekly enrollment instead of monthly;
datalines;

1 5 2 8 3 7 4 8 5 8 6 8 7 8 8 8 9 8 10 8 11 8 12 8 13 6
14 6 15 0 16 0 17 0 18 0 19 0 20 0 21 0 22 0 23 0 24 0

 ;

run;

Title "Exponential model"; run;

%PredDeaths(Model="EXPONENTIAL", a=0.8, b=0.5, TotDeaths=12, t=8);

Title "Lognormal model"; run;

%PredDeaths(Model="LOGNORMAL", a=0.8, b=0.5, TotDeaths=12, t=8);

Title "Gamma model"; run;

SAS Macro 9.3: Time Projection of N Observed Deaths - General Simulation Approach

%Macro PredDeaths(Model="EXPONENTIAL", scale=0.2, shape=0.5, nPts=400, obsdDeaths=120, DeathsNeed=300);

****

Given obsdDeaths observed deaths, simulate the additional time needed for have total DeathsNeed deaths

from the time of last death observed;

Model = "Exponential", "Lognormal", "Gamma", "and "Weibull"

Algorithm:

(1) simulate survival time for all patients,

(2) merge with enrollment data to get calendar time of death: surval time + time of enrollment

(3) sort the merged dataset by the calendar time of death,

(4) get the calendar time for the last observed death and predicted death time the for DeathsNeed-th death

(5) the difference between the two death times is additional time needed to have the target number of deaths

****

Data SurTime;

scale=&scale; shape=&shape; nPts=&nPts; obsdDeaths=&obsdDeaths; DeathsNeed=&DeathsNeed;

do iPt = 1 to nPts;

If &Model="EXPONENTIAL" Then surTime = Rand('EXPOnential', 1/scale);

If &Model^="EXPONENTIAL" Then surTime = Rand(&Model, scale, shape);

Output;

end;

Run;

Data ProjTime; merge PtsEnroll SurTime; by iPt; CalSurTime=EnDay+surTime; run; * Calendar time;

Proc sort data=ProjTime; by CalSurTime; Run;

Data T1; set ProjTime; lastObsdT=CalSurTime; if _N_=obsdDeaths; run;

Data T2; set ProjTime; ExpTime =CalSurTime; if _N_= DeathsNeed; run;

Data TimeNeed; merge T1 T2; TimeNeed= ExpTime- lastObsdT; run;

Data final; set final TimeNeed; if TimeNeed; run;

%Mend;

*proc print data=SurTime(obs=2); run;

*Simulation nSims times to get mean and standard devation of additional time needed for the traget number of events;

%macro PredTime(nSims=10, Model="EXPONENTIAL", scale=0.2, nPts=21, obsdDeaths=3, DeathsNeed=18);

Data Final; TimeNeed=.; run;

Data Null;

```
Do i=1 to &nSims;
call execute ('%nrstr(%PredDeaths(Model="EXPONENTIAL", scale=&scale,
nPts=&nPts, obsdDeaths=&obsdDeaths, DeathsNeed=&DeathsNeed))');
End;
Run;
*Proc print data=final; run;
Proc means data=final; var TimeNeed; run;
%Mend;
```

SAS Macro 9.4: Time Projection of N Observed Deaths - Conditional Distribution Approach

```
* To predict the time required for the target number of events;
%Macro PredDeaths(Model="EXPONENTIAL", scale=0.2, shape=0.5, lam-
daET=0.1, nPts=400, nPtsEnrolled=20, LastDayToEnroll=80, obsdDeaths=120,
LastObsDay=30, DeathsNeed=300);

***************************************************
Given obsdDeaths observed deaths, simulate the additional time needed for have
total DeathsNeed deaths
from the time of last death observed;
* Assume ETs will not be replaced; otherwise LamdaET=99999999;

***************************************************
Data SurTime;
Model=&Model; scale=&scale; shape=&shape; nPts=&nPts;
obsdDeaths=&obsdDeaths; LastObsDay=&LastObsDay;
DeathsNeed=&DeathsNeed; lamdaET=&lamdaET; nPtsEnrolled=
&nPtsEnrolled; LastDayToEnroll=&LastDayToEnroll;
do iPt = 1 to nPtsEnrolled-obsdDeaths; * simulate survival time for alive pa-
tients;
urv=Rand("UNIFORM"); * uniform rabdom variable; * surTime =
Rand('EXPOnential', 1/scale ); * 0 <= scale;
If &Model="EXPONENTIAL" Then surTime = Rand('EXPOnential',
1/scale); * memoryless of exp dist, conditional dist = exponetial, 0 <= scale;
If &Model^="EXPONENTIAL" Then Do;
SurP=1-cdf(&Model,LastObsDay, scale, shape);
x1=0; x2=36500; * x2=max poossible a person can live;
Do i=1 To 50; * 2^50>1.1E15;
xm=(x1+x2)/2;
fx1=(1-cdf(&Model,LastObsDay+x1,scale, shape))/SurP-urv;
fx2=(1-cdf(&Model,LastObsDay+x2,scale, shape))/SurP-urv;
fxm=(1-cdf(&Model,LastObsDay+xm,scale, shape))/SurP-urv;
If fx1*fxm<=0 Then x2=xm; If fx2*fxm<=0 Then x1=xm;
If abs(x1-x2)<0.01 Then leave; * allow max error 0.01 days;
End;
```

```
    surTime=(x1+x2)/2;
    End;
    ET=Rand('EXPOnential', 1/LamdaET); * it is better just to randomly remove
a centain number of ETs to avoid pts<ndeaths;
    censor=0; if ET<surTime then censor=1;
    surTime=min(surTime, ET)+LastObsDay; * truncated by ET;
    Output;
    end;
    Do iPt=nPtsEnrolled+1 to nPts; * simulate survival time for futire patients
using unconditional distribution, without censoring;
    If &Model="EXPONENTIAL" Then surTime0 = Rand('EXPOnential',
1/scale);
    If &Model^="EXPONENTIAL" Then surTime0 = Rand(&Model, scale, shape);
    ET=Rand('EXPOnential', 1/LamdaET);
    censor=0; if ET<surTime0 then censor=1;
    surTime=min(surTime0, ET); * truncated by ET;
    EnDay=LastObsDay+Rand("UNIFORM")*(LastDayToEnroll-LastObsDay);
    surTime=surTime0+EnDay; * Calculate calendar time;
    output;
    End;
    Run;
    Proc sort data=surTime; by censor surTime; Run; * censor=1 is not a event;
    Data TimeNeed;
    set surTime; TimeNeed=surtime;
    if _N_=DeathsNeed-obsdDeaths; * keep the time for the target number of events
only. If there are not enough events due to ET, censor=1. Otherwise censor=0;
    run; * need to deal with no observation due to too many TEs;
    Data final; set final TimeNeed; if TimeNeed; run; * append all simulated times;
    %Mend;
    *Simulation nSims times to get mean and standard devation of additional time
needed for the traget number of events;
    %macro PredTime(nSims=10, Model="EXPONENTIAL", scale=0.02, shape=1,
lamdaET=0.1, nPts=21, nPtsEnrolled=20, LastDayToEnroll=80, obsdDeaths=3,
DeathsNeed=18);
    Data Final; TimeNeed=.; run;
    Data Null;
    Do i=1 to &nSims;
    call execute ('%nrstr(%PredDeaths(Model=&Model, scale=&scale,
shape=&shape, lamdaET=&lamdaET, nPts=&nPts, nPtsEnrolled=&nPtsEnrolled,
LastDayToEnroll=&LastDayToEnroll, obsdDeaths=&obsdDeaths, DeathsNeed=&
DeathsNeed))');
    End;
    Run;
    Proc sort data=final; by censor; run;
    Proc means data=final; var TimeNeed; by censor; run;
    %Mend;
```

Example 1: Fifty Patients (7 deaths; 43 remaining patients stayed in study)

```
*proc print; run;
Title "Exponential"; Run;
%PredTime(nSims=100, Model="EXPONENTIAL", scale=0.02,
lamdaET=0.0001, nPts=50, nPtsEnrolled=20, LastDayToEnroll=80, obsdDeaths=7,
DeathsNeed=35);
Title "Lognormal"; Run;
%PredTime(nSims=100, Model="LOGNORMAL", scale=3.3, shape=0.78,
lamdaET=0.0001, nPts=50, nPtsEnrolled=20, LastDayToEnroll=80, obsdDeaths=7,
DeathsNeed=35);
Title "Weilbull"; Run;
%PredTime(nSims=100, Model="WEIBULL", scale=0.99, shape=50.4, lam-
daET=0.0001, nPts=50, nPtsEnrolled=20, LastDayToEnroll=80, obsdDeaths=7,
DeathsNeed=35);
Title "GAMMA"; Run;
%PredTime(nSims=100, Model="GAMMA", scale=1, shape=50.7,
lamdaET=0.0001, nPts=50, nPtsEnrolled=20, LastDayToEnroll=80, obsdDeaths=7,
DeathsNeed=35);
```

12.7.1 Drop-Loser Design with Efficacy and Toxicity - Dunnett Test and Gatekeeping Procedure

SAS Macro 9.5: Two-Stage Drop-Loser Adaptive Design

```
%Macro DrpLsrDTGKP(nSims=100000, nArms=5, alpha=0.0073, n1=320,
n2=192, Emin=0.15, MTTR=0.15, aUtility=3, Umin=0.01, method="DLDGKP");
/* %Macro DrpLsrDTGKP(nSims=100000, nArms=5, alpha=0.0060, n1=320,
n2=192, Emin=0.15, MTTR=0.15, aUtility=3, Umin=0.01, method="DLDDT");
*/
* nArms = number of arms in the trial where Arm 1 is the control;
* alpha = critical value on p-scale for pick-the-winner design;
* Emin = minimal clinically miningful and commercially viable effect size
(delta/sigma);
* MTTR = max tolerated toxicity rate;
* aUtiltiy = a constant for utility function;
* Umin = minimal utility required to be successul (drug approval);
* method="DLDDT" for DLD with Dunnett testing, method="DLDGKP" for
DLD with gatekepping procedure;
* power = probability of success: reject at least one comparison and
utility>Umin;
* PowWinner = power of the pick-the-winner design;
* powers{i} = probability of success of arm i;
* Dropped{i}=1 if Arm i is dropped, otherwise =0;
Data DrpLsrDTGKP; Set dInput;
Keep AveN power powers2-powers&nArms PowWinner;
```

```
Array us{&nArms}; Array u1s{&nArms}; Array u2s{&nArms};
Array ps{&nArms}; Array p1s{&nArms}; Array p2s{&nArms};
Array Tox{&nArms}; Array powers{&nArms}; Array Utility{&nArms}; Array
UtilityF{&nArms};
Array Dropped{&nArms}; Array pVals{&nArms}; Array pRanked{&nArms};
Array sigs{&nArms};
alpha=&alpha; nArms=&nArms; n1=&n1; n2=&n2; n=n1+n2;
Emin=&Emin; Umin=&Umin; MTTR=&MTTR;
AveN=0; Power=0; PowWinner=0;
Do i=1 To nArms; powers{i}=0; End;
Do isim=1 to &nSims;
Do i=1 To nArms; * Stage 1;
u1s{i}=Rannor(7383)/Sqrt(n1)+us{i}; * efficacy;
p1s{i}=Ranbin(2531,n1,ps{i})/n1; * Toxicity;
Utility(i)=1/(1+100*exp(-&aUtility/Emin*u1s{i}))-1/(1+100*exp(-&aUtility/
MTTR*p1s{i}));
* drop loser when the utility is less than 80% of Umin;
Dropped{i}=0; If Utility{i}-Utility(1)<0.8*Umin Then Dropped{i}=1;
AveN=AveN+n1/&nSims;
End;
Dropped{1}=0; * Always keep the control;
* Determine the winner and max utility;
Winner=1; Do i=2 To nArms; If u1s{i}>u1s{winner} Then winner=i; End;
Umax=Utility{1}; Do i=2 To nArms; If Utility{i}>Umax Then Umax=Utility{i};
End;
* Further drop losers with utility<50%;
Do i=2 To nArms; If Utility{i}<0.5*Umax Then Dropped{i}=1; End;
Do i=1 To nArms; * Stage 2;
u2s{i}=((Rannor(7383)/Sqrt(n2)+us{i})*n2+u1s{i}*n1)/n;
p2s{i}=(Ranbin(2531,n2,ps{i})+p1s{i}*n1)/n;
Z=(u2s{i}-u2s{1})*Sqrt(n/2);
pVals{i}=1-ProbNorm(z);
Tox{i}=0; If max(p1s{i}-p1s{1}, p2s{i}-p2s{1})>MTTR Then Tox{i}=1;
UtilityF{i}=1/(1+100*exp(-&aUtility/Emin*u2s{i}))-1/(1+100*exp(-&aUtility/
MTTR*p2s{i}));
If Dropped{i}=0 Then AveN=AveN+n2/&nSims;
End;
overallSig=0;
Do i=2 To nArms; * Donnutt testing;
DunnettK=pVals{i}<=alpha And UtilityF(i)-UtilityF(1)>Umin;
If &method="DLDDT" And Dropped{i}=0 And DunnettK Then Do;
powers{i}=powers{i}+1/&nSims;
OverallSig=1;
End;
* gatekeeping testing;
```

GKPsign=max(pVals{winner}, pVals{i})<=alpha And Dropped{winner}=0 And UtilityF{i}-UtilityF{1}>Umin;

DunnettK_1=pVals{i}<=alpha And Dropped{winner}=1 And UtilityF(i)-UtilityF(1)>Umin;

If &method="DLDGKP" And Dropped{i}=0 And (GKPsign Or DunnettK_1) Then Do;

powers{i}=powers{i}+1/&nSims;

OverallSig=1;

End;

End;

If pVals{winner}<=alpha Then PowWinner=PowWinner+1/&nSims;

power=power+overallSig/&nSims;

End;

Do i=2 To nArms; powers{i}=Round(powers{i},.001); End; Power= Round(Power,.001); AveN=Round(AveN);

Output;

Run;

Proc Print Data=DrpLsrDTGKP(obs=1); Run;

%Mend DrpLsrDTGKP;

Example of Invoking Macro 9.5

Title " Type-I Error Rate"; run;

Data dInput;

Array us{6}(0,0,0,0,0,0);

Array ps{6}(0.00001,0.00001,0.00001,0.00001,0.00001,0.00001);

%DrpLsrDTGKP(nSims=100000,nArms=6, MTTR=0.915);

Title "Power for linear efficacy & S-Shape toxicity"; run;

Data dInput;

Array us{6}(0,0.05,0.1,0.15,0.2,0.25);

Array ps{6}(0.000001,0.1,0.1,0.15,0.2,0.2);

%DrpLsrDTGKP(nSims=100000,nArms=6, MTTR=0.15);

12.7.2 Fisher's and Barnard's Tests

SAS Macro 9.6: Fisher's Test

%Macro Prob2by2Table(mRsps, nRsps, M, N, Prob);

* Calculate the Table Probability;

* mRsps out of M is one group and nRsps out of N in another group;

mRsps=&mRsps; nRsps=&nRsps; M=&M; N=&N;

Msum=0; Do i=mRsps+1 To M; Msum=Msum+Log(i); End;

Nsum=0; Do i=nRsps+1 To N; Nsum=Nsum+Log(i); End;

NRsum=0; Do i=2 To M+N-mRsps-nRsps; NRsum=NRsum+Log(i); End;

```
Num=NRsum+Msum+Nsum;
mNRsum=0; Do i=2 To M-mRsps; mNRsum=mNRsum+Log(i); End;
nNRsum=0; Do i=2 To N-nRsps; nNRsum=nNRsum+Log(i); End;
MNsum=0; Do i=mRsps+nRsps+1 To M+N; MNsum=MNsum+Log(i);
End;
Den=mNRsum+nNRsum+MNsum;
&Prob=Exp(Num-Den);
%Mend;
%Macro One_sidedFisherExactTest(m1Rsps, m2Rsps, N1, N2, pExact);
* Calculate the p-value for one-sided Fisher exact test;
* m1Rsps out of MN1 is one group and m2Rsps out of N2 in another group;
m1Rsps=&m1Rsps; m2Rsps=&m1Rsps; N1=&N1; N2=&N2;
P_value=0;
Do R1 = 0 To &m1Rsps;
R2=&m1Rsps+&m2Rsps-R1;
%Prob2by2Table(R1, R2,&N1, &N2, Prob);
P_value=P_value + Prob;
End;
&pExact=Max(0,Min(1,P_value));
%Mend;
```

SAS Macro 9.7: Barnard's Test

```
%Macro One_sidedBarbardExactPvalue(Rsp1, Rsp2, N1, N2, nDiv, p_Barnard);
* Rsp1<1 adn Rsp2>0;
Data BarnardTest;
keep P N1 N2 Rsp1 Rsp2 Tobs p_value P_value2 pBarnard;
* Calculate the p-value for one-sided Barnard exact test Ha: P2>P1;
N1=&N1; N2=&N2; N=N1+N2; Rsp1=&Rsp1; Rsp2=&Rsp2;
P1=Rsp1/N1; P2=Rsp2/N2;
Tobs=9999999998; * deal with StdErr=0 when P1=0 and P2=1 => T>=Tobs;
StdErr=sqrt(P1*(1-P1)/N1+P2*(1-P2)/N2);
If StdErr>0 Then Tobs=(P2-P1)/StdErr;
Do k=1 To &nDiv-1;
P=k/&nDiv;
P_value=0; P_value2=0;
Do R1 = 0 To N1-1;
P1=R1/N1;
Do R2 = Max(ceil(P1*N2), 1) To N2;
P2=R2/N2;
T=9999999999; * deal with StdErr=0 when R1=0 and R2=N2 => T>=Tobs;
StdErr=sqrt(P1*(1-P1)/N1+P2*(1-P2)/N2);
If StdErr>0 Then T=(P2-P1)/StdErr;
If T>=Tobs Then Do;
R=R1+R2;
```

```
Pobs=R/N;
* Formulate Coeficient C;
Msum=0; Do i=R1+1 To N1; Msum=Msum+Log(i); End;
Nsum=0; Do i=R2+1 To N2; Nsum=Nsum+Log(i); End;
Num=Msum+Nsum;
mNRsum=0; Do i=2 To N1-R1; mNRsum=mNRsum+Log(i); End;
nNRsum=0; Do i=2 To N2-R2; nNRsum=nNRsum+Log(i); End;
Den=mNRsum+nNRsum;
C=Exp(Num-Den);
P_value=P_value + C*P**R*(1-P)**(N-R);
P_value2=P_value2 + C*Pobs**R*(1-Pobs)**(N-R);
End;
End;
End;
Pmax=max(Pmax, p_value);
* Output; * to see how the Barnard probability changes as the true Ho proportion
```
changes, unblock the ouput;
```
End;
&p_Barnard=Pmax;
pBarnard=Pmax;
%Mend;
```

Example of Invoking SAS Macro 9.7

```
Title "Checking p-Value with One-sided Barnard Exact Test"; run;
%One_sidedBarbardExactPvalue(2, 6, 10, 10, 100, p_Barnard);
Run;
proc print data=BarnardTest; var Rsp1 Rsp2 N1 N2 Tobs pBarnard; run;
Title "One-sided Fisher exact test p-value"; Run;
Data FisherPv;
 Keep mRsps nRsps N1 N2 pExact;
%One_sidedFisherExactTest(2, 6, 10, 10, pExact);
Run;
Proc print data=FisherPv;
run;

DATA pCheck;
INPUT trt $ response $ count;
DATALINES;
T N 4
T Y 6
C N 8
C Y 2
;
Title " Check Fisher and Barnard p-values with Proc Freq"; Run;
```

```
PROC FREQ DATA=pCheck;
WEIGHT count / ZEROS;
TABLES trt*response;
EXACT Fisher BARNARD;
RUN;
Title "Checking p-Value with One-sided Barnard Exact Test"; run;
%One_sidedBarbardExactPvalue(1,8, 132, 148, 100, p_Barnard);
Run;
proc print data=BarnardTest; var Rsp1 Rsp2 N1 N2 Tobs pBarnard; run;
Title "One-sided Fisher exact test p-value"; Run;
Data FisherPv;
 Keep mRsps nRsps N1 N2 pExact;
%One_sidedFisherExactTest(1, 8, 132, 148, pExact);
Run;
Proc print data=FisherPv;
run;


DATA pCheck;
INPUT trt $ response $ count;
DATALINES;
T N 140
T Y 8
C N 131
C Y 1
;
 Title " Check Fisher and Barnard p-values with Proc Freq"; Run;
PROC FREQ DATA=pCheck;
WEIGHT count / ZEROS;
TABLES trt*response;
EXACT Fisher BARNARD;
RUN;
Proc univariate data=BarnardTest noprint;
 histogram p_value;
 run;
```

SAS Macro 9.8: Power Simulations with Barnard's Test

```
%Macro BarnardPower(Pt1, Pt2, N1, N2, alpha);
* Pt1, Pt2, N1, N2 = Proportions and sample size for the two groups;
* alpha = one-sided significance level;
Data BarnardPower;
 Keep N1 N2 N Pt1 Pt2 alpha BarnardPower ;
N1=&N1; N2=&N2; N=N1+N2; Pt1=&Pt1; Pt2=&Pt2; alpha=&alpha;
nDiv=100;
BarnardPower=0;
```

```
Do iR=0 to N1-1;
Do jR=Max(ceil(iR/N1*N2),1) to N2; * Test Ha: PT2>PT1;
ID=(iR-1)*N2+jR;
c1=PDF('BINOMIAL',iR,Pt1,N1); c2=PDF('BINOMIAL',jR,Pt2,N2);
* Start Barnard test;
Pmax=0;
P1=iR/N1; P2=jR/N2;
Tobs=88888888; * deal with StdErr=0 when iR=0 and jR=N2 => T>=Tobs;
StdErr=sqrt(P1*(1-P1)/N1+P2*(1-P2)/N2);
If StdErr>0 Then Tobs=(P2-P1)/StdErr;
Do k=1 To nDiv-1;
P=k/nDiv;
P_value=0; P_value2=0;
Do R1 = 0 To N1-1;
P1=R1/N1;
Do R2 = Max(ceil(P1*N2),1) To N2; * Test Ha: PT2>PT1;
 P2=R2/N2;
T=99999999; * deal with StdErr=0 when R1=0 and R2=N2 => T>=Tobs;
StdErr=sqrt(P1*(1-P1)/N1+P2*(1-P2)/N2);
If StdErr>0Then T=(P2-P1)/StdErr;
If T>=Tobs Then Do;
R=R1+R2;
Pobs=R/N;
* Formulate Coeficient C;
Msum=0; Do i=R1+1 To N1; Msum=Msum+Log(i); End;
Nsum=0; Do i=R2+1 To N2; Nsum=Nsum+Log(i); End;
Num=Msum+Nsum;
mNRsum=0; Do i=2 To N1-R1; mNRsum=mNRsum+Log(i); End;
nNRsum=0; Do i=2 To N2-R2; nNRsum=nNRsum+Log(i); End;
Den=mNRsum+nNRsum;
C=Exp(Num-Den);
P_value=P_value + C*P**R*(1-P)**(N-R);
End;
End;
End;
Pmax=max(Pmax, p_value);
End;
pBarnard=Pmax;
* End of Barnard p-value calculation;
If pBarnard<=alpha Then BarnardPower=BarnardPower+c1*c2;
End; *End of jR;
End; * End of iR;
output;
Run;
%Mend;
```

```
Run;
%BarnardPower(0.2, 0.7, 10, 10, 0.1);
run;
proc print data=BarnardPower; run;
```

SAS Macro 9.9: Power Simulations with Fisher's Test

```
%Macro FisherPower(Pt1, Pt2, N1, N2, alpha);
* Proportions and sample size for the two groups;
* alpha = one-sided significance level;
Data FisherPower;
 Keep N1 N2 N Pt1 Pt2 alpha FisherPower;
N1=&N1; N2=&N2; N=N1+N2; Pt1=&Pt1; Pt2=&Pt2; alpha=&alpha;
FisherPower=0;
Do iR=0 to N1-1;
Do jR=Round(iR/N1*N2+0.5) to N2; * Test Ha: PT2>PT1;
ID=(iR-1)*N2+jR;
c1=PDF('BINOMIAL',iR,Pt1,N1); c2=PDF('BINOMIAL',jR,Pt2,N2);
* Start Fisher test;
P_value=0;
Do R1 = 0 To iR;
R2=iR+jR-R1;
* %Prob2by2Table(R1, R2,N1, N2, Prob);
* Form cpefficient;
Msum=0; Do i=R1+1 To N1; Msum=Msum+Log(i); End;
Nsum=0; Do i=R2+1 To N2; Nsum=Nsum+Log(i); End;
NRsum=0; Do i=2 To N1+N2-R1-R2; NRsum=NRsum+Log(i); End;
Num=NRsum+Msum+Nsum;
mNRsum=0; Do i=2 To N1-R1; mNRsum=mNRsum+Log(i); End;
nNRsum=0; Do i=2 To N2-R2; nNRsum=nNRsum+Log(i); End;
MNsum=0; Do i=R1+R2+1 To N1+N2; MNsum=MNsum+Log(i); End;
Den=mNRsum+nNRsum+MNsum;
Prob=Exp(Num-Den);
P_value=P_value + Prob;
End;
pFisher=Max(0,Min(1,P_value));
If pFisher<=alpha Then FisherPower=FisherPower+c1*c2;
End; *End of jR;
End; * End of iR;
output;
Run;
%Mend;
```

Example of Invoking Macro 9.9

```
%FisherPower(0.2, 0.7, 10, 10, 0.1);
Proc print data=FisherPower; run;
```

Generating Power Curves

```
Data PowerCurves; run;
%BarnardPower(0.1, 0.1, 15, 15, 0.025);
%FisherPower(0.1, 0.1, 15, 15, 0.025);
Data Powers; merge BarnardPower FisherPower; run;
Data PowerCurves;
set PowerCurves Powers; run;
%BarnardPower(0.1, 0.4, 15, 15, 0.025);
%FisherPower(0.1, 0.4, 15, 15, 0.025);
run;
```

SAS Macro 9.10: Power One-Arm Trial with Survival Endpoint

```
%macro  PowerOneSurv(n=100, lambda1=0.077, lambda2=0.0462, tStudy
=36, tEnroll=18, alpha=0.025, nSims=10000);
* Sun et al Method and Jiarong Wu method
* Uniform enrollment during tEnroll;
* n = sample size
* lambda1 = hazard rate for the Ho;
* lambda2 = hazard rate for Ha;
Data PowerOneSurvival;
keep n tEnroll tStudy lambda1 lambda2 alpha Power Powero aveD z;
n=&n; tEnroll=&tEnroll; tStudy=&tStudy; lambda1=&lambda1; lambda2=
&lambda2; alpha=&alpha; nSims=&nSims;
Power=0; Powero=0;
aveD=0;
Do iSim=1 To nSims;
D=0; * number of deaths in the trial;
ExpDeaths=0;
Do i=1 To n;
EntryTime=ranuni(0)*tEnroll;
T= -log(1-ranuni(0))/lambda2;
tFollowUp=tStudy-EntryTime;
If T<=tFollowUp Then D=D+1; *observed deaths;
* X=min(T,tFollowUp);
ExpDeaths=ExpDeaths+(1-exp(-lambda1*tFollowUp));
End;
aveD+D/nSims;
z=(D-ExpDeaths)/sqrt(ExpDeaths); * use Expected deaths as variance;
pvLogRank=ProbNorm(z);
zo=(D-ExpDeaths)/sqrt(D); * use observed deaths as variance;
pvLogRanko=ProbNorm(zo);
If pvLogRank<alpha Then Power=Power+1/nSims;
If pvLogRanko<alpha Then Powero=Powero+1/nSims;
```

* Output; *output Individual trial results;
End;
Output;
Run;
proc print data=PowerOneSurvival (obs=5); run;
%Mend;

Type-I Error Control Checking and Power Simulation

%PowerOneSurv(n=45, lambda1=0.077, lambda2=0.077, tStudy=36, tEn-roll=18, alpha=0.2222, nSims=1000000);

%PowerOneSurv(n=45, lambda1=0.077, lambda2=0.077, tStudy=36, tEn-roll=18, alpha=0.2067, nSims=1000000);

%PowerOneSurv(n=45, lambda1=0.077, lambda2=0.0462, tStudy=36, tEn-roll=18, alpha=0.2222, nSims=100000);

%PowerOneSurv(n=45, lambda1=0.077, lambda2=0.0462, tStudy=36, tEn-roll=18, alpha=0.2067, nSims=100000);

12.8   Chapter 11

SAS Macro 11.1: Blinded Treatment Effect Estimation

%Macro BlindedEstofTrtEffect(nSims=1000, N1=200, N2=100, u1=3, u2=0);
/* MeanDiffBlind2 = Blinded treatment estimation Using variance and Skew-ness*/
/* This method can tell the treatment difference, including the sign; */
Data MixedNormal;
Keep N1 N2 u1 u2 aveMeanDiffBySkewness MeanDiffBySkewness u1BySkew u2BySkew bias skewness Bias3 delta3;
Array x1{400000}; Array x2{400000};
nSims=&nSims; N1=&N1; N2=&N2; N=N1+N2; u1=&u1; u2=&u2; w1=N1/N;
w2=N2/N;
aveMeanDiffBySkewness=0;
Do isim=1 To nSims;
sumu1=0; sumu2=0; Sigma2=0; Skewness=0;
Do i=1 To N1; x1{i} = Rannor(0)+u1; sumu1=sumu1+x1{i}; End;
Do i=1 To N2; x2{i} = Rannor(3472)+u2; sumu2=sumu2+x2{i}; End;
uxhat=(sumu1+sumu2)/(N1+N2);
Do i=1 To N1;
Sigma2=Sigma2+(x1(i)-uxhat)**2/N;
Skewness=Skewness+(x1(i)-uxhat)**3/N;

```
End;
Do i=1 To N2;
Sigma2=Sigma2+(x2(i)-uxhat)**2/N;
Skewness=Skewness+(x2(i)-uxhat)**3/N;
End;

MeanDiffBySkewness=0;
If Skewness NE 0 & N1 NE N2 Then MeanDiffBySkewness=sign(Skewness*(w2-
w1))*(abs(Skewness/(w1*w2*(w2-w1))))**(1/3);

u1BySkew=uxhat+w2*MeanDiffBySkewness;
u2BySkew=uxhat-w1*MeanDiffBySkewness;
aveMeanDiffBySkewness=aveMeanDiffBySkewness+MeanDiffBySkewness/nSims;
Bias =(u1BySkew-u2BySkew)-(u1-u2);
delta3=skewness/(w1*w2*(w2-w1));
Bias3=delta3- (u1-u2)**3;
output;
end;

Output;
Run;
Proc print data=MixedNormal(obs=1); Run;
%Mend;
```

Example of Invoking Macro 11.1

```
%BlindedEstofTrtEffect(nSims=10000, N1=1500, N2=500, u1=2.5, u2=3);
Title 'MixedNormal Histogram';
ods graphics off;
proc univariate data=MixedNormal noprint;
histogram bias/ normal(percents=20 40 60 80 midpercents);
run;
proc univariate data=MixedNormal noprint;
histogram Bias3/ normal(percents=20 40 60 80 midpercents);
run;
proc univariate data=MixedNormal noprint;
histogram skewness/ normal(percents=20 40 60 80 midpercents);
run;
proc univariate data=MixedNormal noprint;
histogram MeanDiffBySkewness/ normal(percents=20 40 60 80 midpercents);
run;
proc univariate data=MixedNormal noprint;
histogram delta3/ normal(percents=20 40 60 80 midpercents);
run;
Proc means data=MixedNormal; var delta3; run;
```

SAS Macro 11.2   Dynamic Treatment Simulation

```
%Macro CausalityModel(nPts=1000000);
Data CM;
Do ptIDsim=1 To &nPts;
x = RAND('EXPONENTIAL');
Cycle1=0; If ranuni(0)>0.5 Then Cycle1=1;
Cycle2=0; If x>1 then Cycle2=1;
Output;
End;
%Mend CausalityModel;
```

Example of Invoking Macro 11.2

```
%CausalityModel(nPts=1000);
Title "A Model with Cycle1 and Cycle2 only with 1000 patients"; run;
proc reg; model x = Cycle1 Cycle2; run;
```

Index

Printed in the United States
by Baker & Taylor Publisher Services